Pediatric Rheumatology in Clinical Practice

Pediatric Rheumatology in Clinical Practice

Edited by Leslie Schwartz

AMERICAN
MEDICAL PUBLISHERS
www.americanmedicalpublishers.com

American Medical Publishers,
41 Flatbush Avenue,
1st Floor, New York,
NY 11217, USA

Visit us on the World Wide Web at:
www.americanmedicalpublishers.com

ISBN: 978-1-63927-429-1

Cataloging-in-Publication Data

Pediatric rheumatology in clinical practice / edited by Leslie Schwartz.
p. cm.
Includes bibliographical references and index.
ISBN 978-1-63927-429-1
1. Pediatric rheumatology. 2. Rheumatoid arthritis in children--Treatment.
3. Rheumatism in children. 4. Rheumatology. I. Schwartz, Leslie.
RJ482.R48 P43 2022
618.927 23--dc23

Table of Contents

Preface

Pediatrics is the branch of medicine that focuses on the physical, mental and emotional well-being of infants, children and adolescents. Various sub-fields such as adolescent medicine, pediatric allergy and immunology, pediatric cardiology and pediatric critical care fall under its domain. Rheumatology is a branch of medicine that focuses on the treatment of rheumatic diseases. Rheumatology primarily deals with disorders and diseases related to the musculoskeletal system, soft tissues, autoimmune diseases, vasculitides and heritable connective tissue disorders. Pediatrics rheumatology is a branch of medicine that deals with the medical care of infants, children and adolescents suffering from rheumatic diseases such as rheumatoid arthritis, ankylosing spondylitis, reactive arthritis, psoriatic arthropathy relapsing polychondritis, etc. Most rheumatic diseases are treated with steroids, disease-modifying anti-rheumatic drugs, analgesic, NSAIDs (non-steroid anti-inflammatory drugs), and monoclonal antibodies. In extremely severe cases, rheumatology surgery can also be carried out. This book contains some path-breaking studies in the field of pediatrics rheumatology. It includes some of the vital pieces of work being conducted across the world, on various topics related to this domain. This book is appropriate for students seeking detailed information in this area as well as for experts.

After months of intensive research and writing, this book is the end result of all who devoted their time and efforts in the initiation and progress of this book. It will surely be a source of reference in enhancing the required knowledge of the new developments in the area. During the course of developing this book, certain measures such as accuracy, authenticity and research focused analytical studies were given preference in order to produce a comprehensive book in the area of study.

This book would not have been possible without the efforts of the authors and the publisher. I extend my sincere thanks to them. Secondly, I express my gratitude to my family and well-wishers. And most importantly, I thank my students for constantly expressing their willingness and curiosity in enhancing their knowledge in the field, which encourages me to take up further research projects for the advancement of the area.

Editor

1

Macrophage Activation Syndrome: different mechanisms leading to a one clinical syndrome

Claudia Bracaglia*, Giusi Prencipe and Fabrizio De Benedetti

Abstract

Background: Macrophage activation syndrome (MAS) is a severe complication of rheumatic disease in childhood, particularly in systemic Juvenile Idiopathic Arthritis (sJIA). It is characterize by an uncontrolled activation and proliferation of T lymphocytes and macrophages.

Main content: MAS is currently classified among the secondary or acquired forms of haemophagocytic lymphohistiocytosis (sHLH). The reason is that MAS shares clinical and laboratory features with primary genetic HLH (pHLH). In this context is conceivable that some of the pathogenic mechanisms of pHLH may be involved in other forms of HLH. Heterozygosity for mutations of genes involved in pHLH may lead to a cytotoxic defect and to a development of clinical overt disease. But other different contributors might be involved to the development of MAS such as infections or underlying inflammation. In MAS, the inflammatory status of the patient is a major contributor of the disease. Indeed, the majority of the MAS episodes occurs during active disease phases or at disease onset. In addition, recent evidence in animals and humans suggest that genetics may also play a major role in contributing to hyperinflammation and particularly to macrophages hyper-responses.

Conclusions: We hypothesize that HLH may be one unique clinical syndrome, to whose generation different mechanisms may contribute, and maintained by one final effector mechanism.

Keywords: Macrophage activation syndrome, Haemophagocytic lymphohistiocytosis, IL-6, IL-18, IFNγ, Inflammasome, Natural killer

Background

The term Macrophage Activation Syndrome (MAS) identifies a potentially fatal complication of rheumatic diseases. It occurs usually in the context of systemic Juvenile Idiopathic Arthritis (sJIA), but it may occur also, albeit more rarely, in systemic Lupus Erythematosus and Kawasaki disease.

MAS is typically characterized by high fever, lymphoadenopathy, hepatosplenomegaly variably associated with hemorrhages, signs of liver, central nervous system and kidney involvement, and may lead to multiple organ failure. Laboratory abnormalities include decrease in white blood cells, platelet and hemoglobin, hypertransaminasemia, marked increase in ferritin, and evidence for intravascular coagulation activation.

* Correspondence: claudia.bracaglia@opbg.net
Division of Rheumatology, Ospedale Pediatrico Bambino Gesù IRCCS, Piazza S. Onofrio 4, 00165 Rome, Italy

MAS clinical and laboratory features

Minoia et al. collected in a multinational multicentre study 362 cases of patients with diagnosis of MAS, in the context of sJIA, established by the treating physicians. All patients had fever, a relevant percentage of them (58%) had splenomegaly and lymphadenopathy (51%). Surprisingly, 35% of them had symptoms suggestive of CNS involvement, 16% had pericarditis, which is consistent with systemic JIA, and 20% had clinical evidence of consumption coagulopathy. See Appendix 1: Case 1 for laboratory abnormalities in sJIA and MAS. In the large multinational study, the great majority of the patients had high ferritin. All the patients had liver involvement and, in the great majority of them, transaminases (94%) and LDH (94%) were abnormal. Anaemia

(92%) was very frequent; however, thrombocytopenia (70.3%) and neutropenia (54.5%) were not as frequent as in primary HLH (pHLH). Triglycerides (93%) were elevated in the majority of patients; evidence of intravascular coagulation, as demonstrated by elevated d-dimer, was present in the great majority of the patients (97%). Fibrinogen was not below the normal limit in a significant portion of patients (48.6%), as expected in highly inflammatory disease where fibrinogen behaves as a positive acute phase protein [1].

Classification

In general, MAS is classified among the secondary forms of haemophagocytic lymphohistiocytosis (sHLH), as a sHLH occurring in the context of a rheumatic disease (Table 1), the reason being that HLH and MAS share a number of clinical and laboratory features. The most significant differences are due to the inflammatory background of MAS: particularly platelet counts, as well as fibrinogen levels, are usually higher in MAS compared to pHLH. Primary HLH is caused by mutation in genes that code for proteins that are involved in "perforin-mediated" cytolytic function. They are either proteins such as perforin, directly involved in cytotoxicity, or proteins involved in vesicle transport and fusion with the plasma membrane.

Table 1 Classification of primary (genetic) and secondary (reactive) HLH [46–48]

	GENE	FUNCTION
Genetic HLH		
Primary or Familial HLH (pHL)		
pHL-1	Unknown	
pHL-2	PRF1	Pore-forming protein
pHL-3	UNC13D	Vesicle priming (impair granule exocytosis)
pHL-4	STX11	Vesicle transport and fusion
pHL-5	STXBP2	Vesicle transport and fusion
Sporadic associated with Immunodeficiencies		
CHS	LYST	Vesicle transport
GS-2	RAB27A	Vesicle docking
XLP-1/XLP-2	SH2DIA/ BIRC4	Signal transduction and activation of lymphocytes
Secondary HLH or Acquired HLH or Reactive HLH		
Infections (EBV, Leishmania, H1N1...)		
Rheumatic diseases (sJIA...) →MAS or rheuma-HLH		
Malignancies (lymphoma...)		

There are several conditions associated with secondary or acquired or reactive HLH. Although definitive epidemiologic data are lacking, sHLH appear to be much more frequent than pHLH. Among infection associated HLH, Epstein Barr Virus is certainly the most common trigger [2]. Additional typical triggers include other Herpes viruses, Leishmania and H1N1 influenz [3–5]. There are a number of cases associated with lymphoma and leukaemia, most frequently T cell receptor gamma-delta bearing T cell lymphomas. These appear to be rare in children, but this occurrence is rather frequent in adults [6]. HLH can also be associated to an underlying rheumatic disease with sJIA being by far the most frequent one. This form of sHLH is what paediatric rheumatologist call MAS or rheuma-HLH. There is a significant number of cases in which an apparent underlying disease or an apparent underlying infection cannot be found [7].

Genetics of MAS: contribution to defective cytotoxicity

As mentioned above, in pHLH, all causative genes code for proteins involved in the cytotoxic pathway, in which cytolytic granules are transported to and fused with the cell membrane, and eventually pore-forming proteins, such as perforin, are secreted in these immunological synapses [8, 9]. If HLH is considered one clinical syndrome is conceivable that some of the pathogenic mechanisms of pHLH may be involved in other forms of HLH. See Appendix 2: Case 2 for potential impact of heterozygosity for mutations of pHLH genes on development of clinical overt disease and of a defective cytotoxicity [10].

One may also expect that a significant role for genetics may impact on the recurrence of the disease. Indeed, recurrent MAS in patients with sJIA is a well-known phenomenon. However, information on the frequency of recurrences is lacking from the large series reported in recent papers [1, 11–14].

Kaufman et al. performed whole exome sequencing in 14 MAS cases on sJIA and found that 5 out of 14 patients (36%) were heterozygous for at least one mutation of the known genes related to pHLH. In addition, they found that 22 rare variants occurred in at least two patients. Most of these variants code for proteins involved in microtubule organization and vesicle transport [11]. This suggested that cellular assembly and cytoskeletal organization may be involved in the potential defect in cellular cytotoxicity of these patients. A number of other studies have previously looked at the frequency of variants in the genes causing pHLH and overall they all found a number of patients carrying either hypomorphic variants or pathogenic mutations in heterozygosity in both *UNC13d* [15] and *PRF1* [13]. In the context of the Italian National Registry of familial HLH we performed mutation analysis of genes involved in pHLH in 31 patients with sJIA and MAS. The analysis included *PRF1, UNC13d, STX11, STXBP2*and *RAB27a*, and identified monoallelic mutations in 11 of the 31 patients (35.5%). Three out of 31 patients (9.7%) carried a mutation in 2 genes. Interestingly, it has been recently reported that mice carrying heterozygous mutation in more than one gene involved in pHLH carry a significant higher risk to develop HLH following viral infection [16]. Overall, clinical and laboratory feature of MAS in patients carrying the mutations were not different from those of patients who do not carry the mutation. However, recurrences of MAS seem to be more frequent in patients who carry the mutations (mutated 27% versus non-mutated 10%). In our series of patients one patient died because of MAS and she was heterozygous for a known pathogenic *PRF1* mutation (N252S) [17]. Altogether these observations, far from being conclusive, point to the presence of a genetic contribution to MAS similar to that of pHLH. All together these observations suggest that events related to the pathogenesis of pHLH are relevant in sHLH in general, and in MAS in particular: a) accumulation of partial genetic defect in one, or more than one, of the known pHLH related gene b) the possible dominant negative effects of some heterozygous variants [10, 18]. Defective cytotoxicity may impair clearance of infected cells, and/or prolong lymphocyte-APC interactions, both events leading to increased pro-inflammatory cytokine production (e.g. IFNγ) by T lymphocytes [10, 19].

Different contributors to the development of a unique clinical syndrome

In pHLH the contribution of genetics is so strong that, even in the absence of any demonstrable trigger, genetically caused immune abnormalities are sufficient to drive the individual in full blown clinical HLH. In HLH secondary to infection, in some instances, the strength of the infectious agent is sufficient to cause HLH. Most of the patients who died of H1N1 or H5N1 died with HLH [20]. There are other agents that cause HLH rather often, as mentioned above. In these instances, there must be a contribution from the infectious agent, or more precisely from the response elicited by a given infectious agent. In this respect, it is interesting to note that gene expression profiles of peripheral blood mononuclear cells from patients with symptomatic mononucleosis show evident similarities with gene expression profiles of patients with HLH or MAS [21]. However, there must be also a contribution from the genetic background. Schulert et al. found rare variants in pHLH related genes in 5 out 14 cases of fatal H1N1 influenza infection, all of whom had evidence of hemophagocytosis. Five patients were heterozygous for *LYST* mutation, two of them carried also a *PRF1* mutation [22].

In MAS, the HLH clinical syndrome develops on the background of a highly inflammatory disease such as sJIA. Also in sJIA an infectious trigger appears to play a role. Several MAS appears to be triggered by acute infections in patients with active sJIA. In a recent large multinational survey, this occurrence was documented in approximately 1/3 of the cases [1]. In MAS, it is obvious that an additional contribution must be provided by the inflammatory status of the patient; indeed, the majority of the MAS episodes occurs during active disease phases or at disease onset.

Contribution of active inflammation to the development of MAS

We generated a model of MAS using the interleukin-6 (IL-6) transgenic mouse (IL-6TG). In these mice, administration of Toll-like receptor (TLR) ligands, including lipopolysaccharides (LPS) and poly(I:C), induces the development of MAS by mimicking an acute infection on a background of high levels of IL-6 [23]. This experimental approach recapitulates what occurs in patients with systemic JIA: an infection triggers MAS on a background of active disease, which is indeed characterized by high levels of IL-6.

Compared to wild type mice, LPS-challenged IL-6 transgenic mice display an increased fatality rate and show hematologic and biochemical features typically present in MAS patients, including lower neutrophils and platelet count, higher levels of ferritin and LDH, as well as a cytokine storm.

When we looked at the stimulatory effect of IL-6, we showed that, in vitro, prolonged exposure of human macrophages to IL-6 leads to increased production of cytokines and chemokines, including Tumor Necrosis Factor-α (TNF-α) and (C-X-C Motif) Ligand 8 (CXCL-8), both at a basal level and upon stimulation with TLR ligands, suggesting a role for IL-6 in amplifying the inflammatory response [24]. In addition, we demonstrated that IL-6 amplifies TLR-induced inflammatory response also in cells originating from inflammatory site, such as synovial fluid mononuclear cells and fibroblast-like synoviocytes isolated from arthritides patients. Indeed, treatments of these cells with IL-6 increased basal production of CXCL8, C-C motif chemokine ligand 2 (CCL2) and Interleukin-1β (IL-1β) following poly(I:C) and muramyl dipeptide stimulation [24].

The other major feature of MAS in the context of sJIA is the transitory defect in cellular cytotoxic function. Grom et al. demonstrated that most of the sJIA patients have profoundly decreased Natural Killer (NK) cell activity [25]. The reduced NK cytotoxic activity observed was associated, in some patients, to a decreased perforin expression on NK cells and, in other patients, to a decreased perforin expression on T-cells. However, overall, the great majority of patients display a NK cytotoxic activity defect.

Consistently, we found that NK activity was impaired also in the murine model of MAS, the IL-6TG. Indeed, IL-6TG mice challenged with poly(I:C), a substitute for viral dsRNA, display a significant decrease in NK cell cytotoxicity, associated to lower expression levels of perforin and granzyme B, in the absence of altered granule exocytosis [26]. An example of IL-6 leading to decreased cytolytic activity of lymphocytes on top of an underlying genetic defect has been shown [10]. Similarly, in vitro experiments revealed that exposure of human PBMCs to high levels of IL-6, such as those typically present in sJIA, inhibits NK cell cytotoxicity by down-regulating the expression of perforin and granzyme B. Altogether, this evidence suggests that high circulating levels of IL-6 in JIA patients, besides their role in increasing macrophage activation and TLR response, play a major role in inducing a transitory defect in cytotoxicity on top of a subclinical genetic defect.

In addition to IL-6, other inflammatory cytokines may play a role in predisposition to MAS. Indeed, even in patients treated with tocilizumab, in which IL-6 was fully neutralized, MAS may occur [27]. One of the potential candidates is IL-1β. There is a number of observations pointing to the efficacy of high dose of anakinra in at least some patients with MAS [28, 29]. On the other hand, there is a number of studies describing patients who developed clinically overt MAS while being treated with both IL-1 blockers anakinra and canakinumab [30–32]. In apparent contrast, in criopyrinopathies, which are the purely IL-1β mediated, cases of MAS are not described. Overall, these data would suggest that neither IL-6 nor IL-1β alone may be the major contributors to the predisposition to MAS.

Increasing number of evidence suggests that interleukin-18 (IL-18) might be another relevant mediator in sJIA. In a study performed in Japan, the subset of sJIA patients characterized by high levels of IL-18 (and conversely low levels of IL-6) had a higher frequency of MAS episodes [12]. These data need to be confirmed in a Western population. Albeit in a small number of patients, data from Put et al. are consistent with this observation: in sJIA patients high IL-18 levels do not markedly increase during active MAS, pointing to IL-18 being a predisposing cytokine [33]. The mechanisms behind the predisposing effect of IL-18 are not clear yet. It is well know that IL-18 affects NK cell activity, but preliminary evidence suggests that it may also regulate macrophage responses [34].

Contribution of genetics to hyperinflammation

In addition to the known role of genetics of cytotoxicity genes in HLH, recent evidence in animals and humans suggest that genetics may also play a major role in contributing to hyperinflammation and particularly to macrophages hyper-responses. Indeed, data in the animals clearly support this hypothesis. The most studied model of genetically driven HLH are perforin knock-out mice which, upon LCMV infection, develop full blown HLH and die [35]. When *UNC13d* deficient mice are crossed with mice deficient for MYD88, which is a central element in TLR intracellular signalling, the animals are protected from disease development, demonstrating that, at least in animals, TLR signalling and macrophage responses are crucial [36]. Indirect evidence in humans has been provided by a study suggesting that a polymorphism in IRF5, a transducer of intracellular TLR, is associated with the risk of MAS in patients with sJIA [37]. In addition and much more importantly, direct evidence in humans is provided by the recent observation that gain of function mutations of NLRC4, an inflammasome sensor, cause a disease characterized by recurrent or dramatic HLH. This observation demonstrates in humans that genetically induced abnormalities in autoinflammation cause HLH. The disease, still described in very few patients appear to be characterized by early onset of fever, skin rash, severe gastro-intestinal involvement, splenomegaly and recurrent, severe MAS/HLH [38, 39]. Immunological studies revealed that the most striking abnormality is represented by surprisingly high levels of IL-18 pointing to the fact that the NLRC4 protein is particularly important in regulating IL-18 production and further supporting the role of IL-18 as a predisposing factor to HLH/MAS [38].

Different contributors and one pathogenic mediator?

It is reasonable to hypothesize that several factors, acting at different steps, contribute to the development of MAS and sHLH. A multilayer model of pathogenic events leading to the development of MAS has been proposed, including genetics, inflammatory activity and infection, contributing to reaching a threshold of activation that results in overt MAS [40]. In perforin knock-out mice infected with LCMV, the most used mouse model of primary HLH, neutralization of a number of cytokines does not produce any relevant clinical effect. However, neutralization of IFNγ leads to protection from disease and to survival of the animals [35]. Based on a number of experiments both in mice and on human cells, it has been hypothesized that mutations of genes impacting on cytotoxic activity generate an inability of cytotoxic T cells to lyse the target cells. This defect leads to prolonged hyperactivation of T cells with hyperproduction of IFNγ [10, 19]. High levels of IFNγ leads to activation of macrophages, as a compensatory mechanism aimed at phagocytosis of the infected cells. Indeed, these patients do not succumb from overwhelming infections. These activated macrophages produce very large amounts of inflammatory cytokines and generate a cytokine storm, which is the driver of the clinical and laboratory features of HLH and eventually leads the host to death, if left untreated.

Translating from pHLH to MAS and based on the similarities in clinical and laboratory features as well as in genetic contribution, we have recently investigated whether IFNγ could potentially be involved also in MAS. IFNγ levels were found to be higher in patients with active MAS at sampling compared to patients with active sJIA without MAS at sampling [41]. Using the above mentioned mouse model of MAS in IL-6 transgenic mice we have also found that neutralization of IFNγ improved survival and reverted biochemical abnormalities (Prencipe G. 2016 submitted). Interestingly, in patients with MAS a marked increase in CXCL9 levels was also found. CXCL9 is known to be specifically induced by IFNγ [42]. Indeed in patients with active MAS levels of IFNγ and CXCL9 were strictly related to laboratory features of MAS, including ferritin levels, white blood cell and platelet counts, and LDH [41]. These correlations were not present in patients with active sJIA without MAS. These data suggest that during MAS, but not during active sJIA, there is a specific activation of IFNγ and of the IFNγ pathway. Noteworthy in the NLRC4 patient, reported by Canna et al., one of the cytokines that increases significantly during active HLH episodes is indeed CXCL9 [38]. We also found high levels of CXCL9 in a patient with NLRC4 induced disease (unpublished). Observations in MAS and in NLRC4-induced disease show that hyperinflammation induced by dysregulated inflammatory responses may directly cause overproduction of IFNγ.

Conclusion

All together these observations are consistent with the hypothesis that HLH may be one clinical syndrome maintained by one effector mechanism, which involves increased macrophage activation and increased T-cells activation. In this loop, IFNγ seems to play a major role. In classical pHLH, genetic mutations and the consequent defect in cytotoxic pathways are sufficient to drive a patient above the threshold eliciting this vicious loop. NLRC4-induced disease provides proof of concept that genetic predisposition to inflammasome hyper-response alone can drive patients directly into the same vicious loop. In patients with MAS an additive/synergist role is played by several contributors, including infectious triggers, genetics, of both cytotoxicity and inflammatory response, and inflammatory activity of the underlying rheumatic disease. Recently generated evidence points to IFNγ as the major mediator also of HLH secondary to infections [43, 44], as well as of MAS. These findings may have significant translational value. A monoclonal antibody to IFNγ is in clinical trial in primary HLH with initial satisfactory response [45] and a trial in MAS is being planned.

Appendix 1: Case 1

Case 1

An 8 years old Caucasian boy with sJIA onset one year before, suddenly developed persistent fever, generalised seizures, hypotension, purpura and splenomegaly. Laboratory picture was completely different if compared to his laboratory at sJIA onset. Blood count showed leukopenia with neutrophenia and anemia. Erithrocyte sedimentation rate (ESR) was relatively low, however CRP was high as it was. Fibrinogen was low because of intravascular activation of the coagulation, d-dimers were high. He presented also liver involvement with some degree of liver insufficiency. The most striking feature was hyperferritinimia, which was markedly higher compared to sJIA presentation (Table 2). This case represents a typical picture of MAS complicating sJIA. Changes in laboratory features are the hallmark and these have been recently mathematically characterized in multination effort [1]. However, MAS may represents a significant challenge when occurring at sJIA onset.

Table 2 Patient's laboratory features

Laboratory Features	sJIA presentation	MAS presentation
White blood cells, x10^9/L	15.04	3.02
Neutrophils %	86%	19%
Haemoglobin, g/dL	9.08	7.09
Platelet, x109/L	640	125
Ferritin, ng/mL	880	11345
ESR, mm/h	98	32
CRP, mg/dL	13.08	19.07
Fibrinogen, mg/dL	560	88
D-dimers, ng/mL	<10	>40
Sodium, mEq/L	136	129
ALT, U/L	23	180
AST, U/L	18	145
LDH, U/L	380	1910
Bilirubin, mg/dL	0.06	2.06

ESR, erythrocyte sedimentation rate; CRP, C-reactive protein; ALT, alanine aminotransferase; AST, aspartate aminotransferase; LDH, lactate dehydrogenase

Appendix 2: Case 2

Case 2

A 15 years-old, Caucasian male presented with persistent fever since 4 weeks, diarrhoea vomiting, skin rash, hepatosplenomegaly, and elbows arthritis. Blood tests showed high ferritin (5896 ng/ml), liver inflammation (AST 224 IU/l, ALT 635 IU/l, LDH 676 IU/l), and intravascular activation of coagulation with high d-dimers (2.26 μg/ml), and a bone marrow biopsy showed hemophagocytosis. He was treated with glucocorticoids, cyclosporine A and cyclophosphamide with good response. Three years later, he presented again with persistent fever, skin rash, diffuse arthralgia, and myalgia. He referred to the malaise and arthralgia as being the "same disease" as the one 3 years before. As soon as ferritin started to rise significantly (5481 ng/ml), dexamethasone and cyclosporine A were started with a prompt response. He was found to carry a single copy heterozygous missense mutation in *RAB27a*. This same mutation was found in his father, who was apparently healthy, but who had a baseline moderately high serum ferritin level (800 ng/ml). Functional tests showed a marginal defect in CD107a degranulation in the patient and his healthy father [10]. Indeed experiments with this very mutation have shown an impact on cytotoxic function as well as on the duration of the immune synapses [10]. This patient appears to have had two episodes of HLH, which cannot be strictly defined as primary or genetic HLH; it is however, tempting to speculate that carriage of this mutation plays an important role in the two recurrences of secondary HLH.

Abbreviations

CCL2: C-C motif chemokine ligand 2; CXCL8: (C-X-C Motif) Ligand 8; CXCL9: (C-X-C Motif) Ligand 9; HLH: Haemophagocytic lymphohistiocytosis; IL-18: Interleukin-18; IL-1β: Interleukin-1β; IL-6: Interleukin-6; IL-6TG: IL-6 transgenic mouse; IRF5: Interferon regulatory factor 5; LCMV: Lymphocytic choriomeningitis virus; LPS: Lipopolysaccharides; MAS: Macrophage activation syndrome; MYD88: Myeloid differentiation primary response 88; NK: Natural killer; PBMC: Peripheral blood mononuclear cell; pHLH: Primary or familial haemophagocytic; lymphohistiocytosis; sHLH: Secondary or acquired haemophagocytic lymphohistiocytosis; sJIA: Systemic juvenile idiopathic arthritis; TLR: Toll-like receptor; TNF-α: Tumor necrosis factor-α

Acknowledgements

Not applicable.

Funding

Giusi Prencipe was supported in her research by the Italian Ministry of Health (Rome, Italy) Young Investigator Grants "GR-2011-02347874".

Authors' contributions

CB conducted the literature review and wrote the manuscript; GP wrote the section on mouse model; FDB reviewed the manuscript. All authors read and approved the final manuscript.

Competing interests

Claudia Bracaglia and Giusi Prencipe declare that they have no competing interests. Fabrizio De Benedetti declares competing interests with Novartis, Novimmune, Hoffmann-La Roche, SOBI, AbbVie.

Consent for publication

A consent for publication was collected from the patients and their parents described in Appendix 1: Case 1 and Appendix 2: Case 2.

References

1. Minoia F, Davi S, Horne A, Demirkaya E, Bovis F, Li C, et al. Clinical features, treatment, and outcome of macrophage activation syndrome complicating systemic juvenile idiopathic arthritis: a multinational, multicenter study of 362 patients. Arthritis Rheumatol. 2014;66(11):3160–9.
2. Hashemi-Sadraei N, Vejpongsa P, Baljevic M, Chen L, Idowu M. Epstein-Barr virus-related hemophagocytic lymphohistiocytosis: hematologic emergency in the critical care setting. Case Rep Hematol. 2015;2015:491567. Pubmed Central PMCID: 4338404.
3. Kilani B, Ammari L, Kanoun F, Ben Chaabane T, Abdellatif S, Chaker E. Hemophagocytic syndrome associated with visceral leishmaniasis. Int J Infect Dis. 2006;10(1):85–6.
4. Ozdemir H, Ciftci E, Ince EU, Ertem M, Ince E, Dogru U. Hemophagocytic lymphohistiocytosis associated with 2009 pandemic influenza A (H1N1) virus infection. J Pediatr Hematol Oncol. 2011;33(2):135–7.
5. Singh G, Shabani-Rad MT, Vanderkooi OG, Vayalumkal JV, Kuhn SM, Guilcher GM, et al. Leishmania in HLH: a rare finding with significant treatment implications. J Pediatr Hematol Oncol. 2013;35(3):e127–9.
6. Lehmberg K, Sprekels B, Nichols KE, Woessmann W, Muller I, Suttorp M, et al. Malignancy-associated haemophagocytic lymphohistiocytosis in children and adolescents. Br J Haematol. 2015;170(4):539–49.
7. Xu XJ, Tang YM, Song H, Yang SL, Xu WQ, Zhao N, et al. Diagnostic accuracy of a specific cytokine pattern in hemophagocytic lymphohistiocytosis in children. J Pediatr. 2012;160(6):984–90 e1.
8. Chandrakasan S, Filipovich AH. Hemophagocytic lymphohistiocytosis: advances in pathophysiology, diagnosis, and treatment. J Pediatr. 2013; 163(5):1253–9.
9. Stepp SE, Dufourcq-Lagelouse R, Le Deist F, Bhawan S, Certain S, Mathew PA, et al. Perforin gene defects in familial hemophagocytic lymphohistiocytosis. Science. 1999;286(5446):1957–9.
10. Zhang M, Bracaglia C, Prencipe G, Bemrich-Stolz CJ, Beukelman T, Dimmitt RA, et al. A heterozygous RAB27A mutation associated with delayed cytolytic granule polarization and hemophagocytic lymphohistiocytosis. J Immunol. 2016;196(6):2492–503. Pubmed Central PMCID: PMC4779709.
11. Kaufman KM, Linghu B, Szustakowski JD, Husami A, Yang F, Zhang K, et al. Whole-exome sequencing reveals overlap between macrophage activation syndrome in systemic juvenile idiopathic arthritis and familial hemophagocytic lymphohistiocytosis. Arthritis Rheumatol. 2014;66(12): 3486–95. Pubmed Central PMCID: 4321811.
12. Shimizu M, Nakagishi Y, Inoue N, Mizuta M, Ko G, Saikawa Y, et al. Interleukin-18 for predicting the development of macrophage activation syndrome in systemic juvenile idiopathic arthritis. Clin Immunol. 2015; 160(2):277–81.
13. Vastert SJ, van Wijk R, D'Urbano LE, de Vooght KM, de Jager W, Ravelli A, et al. Mutations in the perforin gene can be linked to macrophage activation syndrome in patients with systemic onset juvenile idiopathic arthritis. Rheumatology (Oxford). 2010;49(3):441–9.
14. Zhang K, Biroschak J, Glass DN, Thompson SD, Finkel T, Passo MH, et al. Macrophage activation syndrome in patients with systemic juvenile idiopathic arthritis is associated with MUNC13-4 polymorphisms. Arthritis Rheum. 2008;58(9):2892–6. Pubmed Central PMCID: 2779064.
15. Hazen MM, Woodward AL, Hofmann I, Degar BA, Grom A, Filipovich AH, et al. Mutations of the hemophagocytic lymphohistiocytosis-associated gene UNC13D in a patient with systemic juvenile idiopathic arthritis. Arthritis Rheum. 2008;58(2):567–70.
16. Sepulveda FE, Garrigue A, Maschalidi S, Garfa-Traore M, Menasche G, Fischer A, et al. Polygenic mutations in the cytotoxicity pathway

increase susceptibility to develop HLH immunopathology in mice. Blood. 2016;127(17):2113–21.

17. Bracaglia C, Sieni E, Da Ros M, De Fusco C, Micalizzi C, Cetica V, Ciambotti B, Coniglio ML, Insalaco A, De Benedetti F, Aricò M. Mutations of familial hemophagocytic lymphohistiocytosis (FHL) related genes and abnormalities of cytotoxicity function tests in patients with macrophage activation syndrome (MAS) occurring in systemic juvenile idiopathic arthritis (sJIA). Pediatr Rheumatol Online J. 2014;12 Suppl 1:53. Pubmed Central PMCID: PMC4184267. Epub Published online 2014 Sep 17.
18. Spessott WA, Sanmillan ML, McCormick ME, Patel N, Villanueva J, Zhang K, et al. Hemophagocytic lymphohistiocytosis caused by dominant-negative mutations in STXBP2 that inhibit SNARE-mediated membrane fusion. Blood. 2015;125(10):1566–77. Pubmed Central PMCID: 4351505.
19. Jenkins MR, Rudd-Schmidt JA, Lopez JA, Ramsbottom KM, Mannering SI, Andrews DM, et al. Failed CTL/NK cell killing and cytokine hypersecretion are directly linked through prolonged synapse time. J Exp Med. 2015;212(3): 307–17. Pubmed Central PMCID: 4354371.
20. Shrestha B, Omran A, Rong P, Wang W. Report of a fatal pediatric case of hemophagocytic lymphohistiocytosis associated with pandemic influenza a (H1N1) infection in 2009. Pediatr Neonatol. 2015;56(3):189–92.
21. Dunmire SK, Odumade OA, Porter JL, Reyes-Genere J, Schmeling DO, Bilgic H, et al. Primary EBV infection induces an expression profile distinct from other viruses but similar to hemophagocytic syndromes. PLoS One. 2014;9(1):e85422. Pubmed Central PMCID: 3894977.
22. Schulert GS, Zhang M, Fall N, Husami A, Kissell D, Hanosh A, et al. Whole-exome sequencing reveals mutations in genes linked to hemophagocytic lymphohistiocytosis and macrophage activation syndrome in fatal cases of H1N1 influenza. J Infect Dis. 2016;213(7):1180–8.
23. Strippoli R, Carvello F, Scianaro R, De Pasquale L, Vivarelli M, Petrini S, et al. Amplification of the response to toll-like receptor ligands by prolonged exposure to interleukin-6 in mice: implication for the pathogenesis of macrophage activation syndrome. Arthritis Rheum. 2012;64(5):1680–8.
24. Caiello I, Minnone G, Holzinger D, Vogl T, Prencipe G, Manzo A, et al. IL-6 amplifies TLR mediated cytokine and chemokine production: implications for the pathogenesis of rheumatic inflammatory diseases. PLoS One. 2014; 9(10):e107886. Pubmed Central PMCID: PMC4182736.
25. Grom AA, Villanueva J, Lee S, Goldmuntz EA, Passo MH, Filipovich A. Natural killer cell dysfunction in patients with systemic-onset juvenile rheumatoid arthritis and macrophage activation syndrome. J Pediatr. 2003;142(3):292–6.
26. Cifaldi L, Prencipe G, Caiello I, Bracaglia C, Strippoli R, De Benedetti F. Inhibition of natural killer (nk) cell cytotoxicity by interleukin-6: implications for the pathogenesis of macrophage activation syndrome. Pediatr Rheumatol. 2014;12 Suppl 1:56.
27. Yokota S, Itoh Y, Morio T, Sumitomo N, Daimaru K, Minota S. Macrophage activation syndrome in patients with systemic juvenile idiopathic arthritis under treatment with tocilizumab. J Rheumatol. 2015;42(4):712–22.
28. Ravelli A, Grom AA, Behrens EM, Cron RQ. Macrophage activation syndrome as part of systemic juvenile idiopathic arthritis: diagnosis, genetics, pathophysiology and treatment. Genes Immun. 2012;13(4):289–98.
29. Boom V, Anton J, Lahdenne P, Quartier P, Ravelli A, Wulffraat NM, et al. Evidence-based diagnosis and treatment of macrophage activation syndrome in systemic juvenile idiopathic arthritis. Pediatr Rheumatol Online J. 2015;13:55. Pubmed Central PMCID: PMC4669611.
30. Zeft A, Hollister R, LaFleur B, Sampath P, Soep J, McNally B, et al. Anakinra for systemic juvenile arthritis: the rocky mountain experience. J Clin Rheumatol. 2009;15(4):161–4.
31. Nigrovic PA, Mannion M, Prince FH, Zeft A, Rabinovich CE, van Rossum MA, et al. Anakinra as first-line disease-modifying therapy in systemic juvenile idiopathic arthritis: report of forty-six patients from an international multicenter series. Arthritis Rheum. 2011;63(2):545–55.
32. Grom AA, Ilowite NT, Pascual V, Brunner HI, Martini A, Lovell D, et al. Rate and clinical presentation of macrophage activation syndrome in patients with systemic juvenile idiopathic arthritis treated with canakinumab. Arthritis Rheumatol. 2016;68(1):218–28.
33. Put K, Avau A, Brisse E, Mitera T, Put S, Proost P, et al. Cytokines in systemic juvenile idiopathic arthritis and haemophagocytic lymphohistiocytosis: tipping the balance between interleukin-18 and interferon-gamma. Rheumatology. 2015;54(8):1507–17.
34. Novick D, Kim S, Kaplanski G, Dinarello CA. Interleukin-18, more than a Th1 cytokine. Semin Immunol. 2013;25(6):439–48.
35. Jordan MB, Hildeman D, Kappler J, Marrack P. An animal model of hemophagocytic lymphohistiocytosis (HLH): CD8+ T cells and interferon gamma are essential for the disorder. Blood. 2004;104(3):735–43.
36. Krebs P, Crozat K, Popkin D, Oldstone MB, Beutler B. Disruption of MyD88 signaling suppresses hemophagocytic lymphohistiocytosis in mice. Blood. 2011;117(24):6582–8. Pubmed Central PMCID: PMC3123024.
37. Yanagimachi M, Naruto T, Miyamae T, Hara T, Kikuchi M, Hara R, et al. Association of IRF5 polymorphisms with susceptibility to macrophage activation syndrome in patients with juvenile idiopathic arthritis. J Rheumatol. 2011;38(4):769–74.
38. Canna SW, de Jesus AA, Gouni S, Brooks SR, Marrero B, Liu Y, et al. An activating NLRC4 inflammasome mutation causes autoinflammation with recurrent macrophage activation syndrome. Nat Genet. 2014;46(10):1140–6. Pubmed Central PMCID: 4177369.
39. Romberg N, Al Moussawi K, Nelson-Williams C, Stiegler AL, Loring E, Choi M, et al. Mutation of NLRC4 causes a syndrome of enterocolitis and autoinflammation. Nat Genet. 2014;46(10):1135–9. Pubmed Central PMCID: PMC4177367.
40. Strippoli R, Caiello I, De Benedetti F. Reaching the threshold: a multilayer pathogenesis of macrophage activation syndrome. J Rheumatol. 2013; 40(6):761–7.
41. Bracaglia C, de Graaf K, Pires Marafon D, Guilhot F, Ferlin W, Prencipe G, et al. Elevated circulating levels of interferon-γ and interferon-γ induced chemokines characterize patients with macrophage activation syndrome complicating systemic juvenile idiopathic arthritis. Ann Rheum Dis. 2017; 76(1):166–72.
42. Groom JR, Luster AD. CXCR3 ligands: redundant, collaborative and antagonistic functions. Immunol Cell Biol. 2011;89(2):207–15. Pubmed Central PMCID: 3863330.
43. Behrens EM, Canna SW, Slade K, Rao S, Kreiger PA, Paessler M, et al. Repeated TLR9 stimulation results in macrophage activation syndrome-like disease in mice. J Clin Invest. 2011;121(6):2264–77. Pubmed Central PMCID: 3104738.
44. Buatois V, Chatel L, Cons L, Lory S, Richard F, Guilhot F, et al. Use of a mouse model to identify a blood biomarker for IFNgamma activity in pediatric secondary hemophagocytic lymphohistiocytosis. Transl Res. 2016; S1931-5244(16):30157-8.
45. Jordan ML F, Allen C, De Benedetti F, Grom AA, Ballabio M, Ferlin WG, De Min C. A novel targeted approach to the treatment of hemophagocytic lymphohistiocytosis (HLH) with an anti-interferon gamma (IFNγ) monoclonal antibody (mAb), NI-0501: first results from a pilot phase 2 study in children with primary HLH. In: American society of hematology - 57th annual meeting & exposition - LBA-3. 2015.
46. Gupta S, Weitzman S. Primary and secondary hemophagocytic lymphohistiocytosis: clinical features, pathogenesis and therapy. Expert Rev Clin Immunol. 2010;6(1):137–54.
47. Janka GE. Familial and acquired hemophagocytic lymphohistiocytosis. Annu Rev Med. 2012;63:233–46.
48. Xu XJ, Tang YM. Advances in studies on hemophagocytic lymphohistiocytosis: diagnosis and treatment. Zhonghua er ke za zhi Chinese J Pediatr. 2011;49(9):712–6.

2

Spectrum of paediatric rheumatic diseases in Nigeria

Babatunde Hakeem Olaosebikan[1], Olufemi Oladipo Adelowo[1], Barakat Adeola Animashaun[2] and Richard Oluyinka Akintayo[3*]

Abstract

Background: Paediatric rheumatology service in Sub-Sahara African is virtually not available as there is a shortage of paediatric rheumatologists and other rheumatology health professionals. We aim to describe the clinical spectrum and the frequencies of paediatric rheumatic diseases (PRDs) in Lagos State University Teaching Hospital (LASUTH), Lagos, Nigeria.

Methods: This is a retrospective review of patients with PRDs seen over a five year period (March 2010 to February 2016) at the rheumatology clinic and children ward of LASUTH. We reviewed the folders of 57 patients from our records. The demographics, baseline laboratory features, clinical diagnosis, treatment patterns and patient outcomes were extracted and analyzed. Clinical and laboratory characteristics between patients with Juvenile idiopathic arthritis (JIA) and patients with juvenile connective tissue diseases (JCTD) were compared using Fisher's exact test.

Results: Fifty seven patients were studied with a female to male ratio of 3 to 1 (Female: 43; M: 14). The mean age at presentation in years was 14 ± 4.4 years (range: 1.5–22 years). The mean duration of symptoms before diagnosis was 18.4 ± .9 months (range: 2–60 months). The diagnostic types of PRDs included 28(49.1%) cases of JIA. These were made up of 14 cases of polyarticular JIA, nine cases of oligoarticular JIA and 5 cases of systemic onset JIA. Others were 18 (24.6%) cases of juvenile systemic lupus erythematosus (JSLE), 3 (5.3%) cases of joint hypermobility syndrome, 2 (3.5%) cases of juvenile systemic sclerosis, 2 (3.5%) cases of fibromyalgia, 2 (3.5%) cases of plantar fasciitis, 1 (1.6%) case of juvenile dermatomyositis (JDM), 1 (1.6%) case of juvenile polymyositis-systemic lupus erythematosus (PM-SLE) overlap, 1 (1.6%) case of secondary bilateral knee osteoarthritis from Blount disease, 1 (1.6%) case of secondary osteoporosis from childhood leukemia and 1 (1.6%) case of Osgood-Schlatter's disease. Constitutional symptoms and extra-articular diseases were significantly more frequent among JCTD cases than among the JIA cases (Constitutional symptoms: 100% vs 83.3%, $p = 0.003$; extra-articular disease: 100% vs 10.7%, $p = 0.001$). The percentage mortality in this study was 10.5% while 20 (35.1%) of the patients were lost to clinic follow up.

Conclusion: The pattern of PRDs observed in this study is similar to that described in South African and North American series but it differs from patterns reported in Asian series. Although hitherto largely unrecognized, PRDs may constitute a substantial cause of morbidity and mortality in black Africans.

Keywords: Paediatric rheumatic disease, Nigeria, Juvenile idiopathic arthritis, Juvenile systemic lupus erythematosus

* Correspondence: richocounlimited@gmail.com
[3]Department of Medicine, University of Ilorin Teaching Hospital, Ilorin, Kwara State, Nigeria
Full list of author information is available at the end of the article

Background

The burdens and impacts of malnutrition, poverty-related and infectious diseases are well known in Sub-Sahara Africa. There is however, little or no attention to non-communicable diseases including paediatric rheumatic diseases (PRDs). The shortage of paediatric rheumatologists and other rheumatology health professionals as well as a general lack of awareness of this subject often contribute to missing these diagnoses and a consequent perception of rarity of PRDs in Africa [1]. In developing countries, prevalence estimates of PRDs are usually difficult to determine. This is especially so in Africa where access to pediatric rheumatology service is rare [2]. In Singapore, the prevalence of true PRDs among all cases referred to childhood rheumatology clinic is 57.8%, while in four Canada provinces, the prevalence estimates over 9 to 14 year period for systemic autoimmune rheumatic diseases (SARD) is 2 SARD cases per 10,000 residents aged 18 or less [3, 4]. However, this estimate did not include frequency of individual SARD. The frequencies and spectrums of PRDs vary in different studies from the western hemisphere and Asia. Whilst some studies from North America and Europe have reported JIA as the most frequent PRD, a study from Asia found systemic vasculitis as the most common [3, 5–8]. In Africa, there are few reports on PRD conditions such as JIA, juvenile systemic lupus erythematosus (JSLE), and juvenile dermatomyositis (JDM) [9–11]. However, there is a dearth of reports on the frequencies and spectrums of PRDs in various Sub-Saharan African settings [1]. A hospital-based report of the spectrum of PRDs in two tertiary institutions in South Africa has documented a relative frequency of 33.3% for JIA and 10.2% for juvenile connective tissue diseases (JCTD) [12]. Also, inflammatory arthritides were the most frequent musculoskeletal conditions among Kenyan children in outpatient clinics and wards [13, 14]. Patients with JCTD were, however, not included in the Kenyan studies. In a new rheumatology clinic in Zambia, Chipeta et al. registered 230 pediatric rheumatic cases over 2 years but the pattern of the PRDs was not stated in their report [15].

Epidemiological reports of PRDs in Africa are hampered by the lack of trained professionals in the field of rheumatology. Therefore, the burden of these diseases is unknown. Moreover, cases are often misdiagnosed or underdiagnosed and this is helped by a number of factors. One is the widespread belief that arthritis does not occur in children. Also, the much higher rate of infectious conditions often poses a lot of confusion and tends to lead to a delay in definitive diagnosis. Clinicians might believe they are dealing with an occult infection over a sustained period in a true case of rheumatic disease.

To the best of our knowledge, there have been no published reports of the spectrums of PRDs among West Africans. This is a retrospective study of the types and frequencies of PRDs in Nigerians attending a tertiary teaching hospital.

Methods

This is a retrospective review of PRD cases managed between the first week of March 2010 and the last week of February 2016 at the adult rheumatology unit of LASUTH. LASUTH is a tertiary teaching hospital in the cosmopolitan city of Lagos. The hospital has one of the two adult rheumatology clinics in the city. There is no paediatric rheumatology clinic in Nigeria and as such pediatric rheumatic patients are managed by adult rheumatologists in conjunction with paediatricians. The paediatric patients with either musculoskeletal complaints or systemic symptoms suspicious of a rheumatic disease were referred for rheumatology review from the paediatric clinic, peripheral hospitals or paediatric wards. The diagnosis of PRDs was based on validated criteria such as the American College of Rheumatology (ACR) classification criteria, International League of Association of Rheumatology criteria, and other validated criteria for rheumatic diseases. The entry criterion for case selection was the diagnosis of a PRD in the patient's record either as paediatric-onset disease in adult or a paediatric-age patient. Paediatric was defined as disease onset before the 16th birthday in all cases except JSLE where disease onset before the 18th birthday was adopted. The hospital records were retrieved for each patient and details of biodata, baseline clinical parameters, baseline laboratory indices, clinical diagnoses, drug treatments and patient outcomes were extracted. The duration of symptoms was taken as the onset from the first symptoms to clinical diagnosis at our facility. The full blood count, haematocrit, and erythrocyte sedimentation rate were documented in 50 cases (87.7%). Furthermore, C-reactive protein and serum ferritin were recorded for 37 cases (64.9%). Antinuclear antibody (ANA) was recorded in 48 cases(84.2%) while anti-extractable nuclear antigen (ENA) was documented in 16 patients(28.1%). Rheumatoid factor (RF) was recorded in seven patients (12.3%). ANA and ENA were analyzed by Enzyme-linked immunosorbent assay (ELISA) methods and RF was assayed by nephelometry.

Statistical methods

Fisher's exact test was applied to compare the clinical and laboratory characteristics between patients with JIA and patients with JCTD. All statistical analyses were done using the SPSS version 21(IBM USA, Armonk, NY 10504). A p value <0.05 was considered to be significant. Ethical approval was granted by the research and ethics committee of Lagos State University Teaching Hospital (LASUTH)

Results

A total of 57 patients with PRDs, which included 11 cases diagnosed in pediatric ward, 30 referred cases from general paediatric clinic, and 16 patients referred from peripheral hospitals were managed at the adult rheumatology unit. These accounted for 2.4% of the 2330 rheumatic cases diagnosed and managed in our institution over the study period. As shown in Table 1, three quarters of our PRD cases were female and the mean age at presentation was 14 years. The mean duration of symptoms before the diagnosis was made was 18 months and musculoskeletal pain was documented in 52 (92%) PRD cases.

PRDs in 57 Nigerian children

As shown in Table 2, JIA was the most frequent PRD seen in 28 (49%) of all cases. Polyarticular JIA(50%) was the most frequent of the three types of JIA observed. A total of 18 JCTD cases were seen. These accounted for 31.6% of all PRDs. They include 14 cases of JSLE, two cases of juvenile systemic sclerosis, and a case each of juvenile dermatomyositis and PM-SLE overlap.

Laboratory features

As shown in Table 3, 23 patients had positive ANA while 13 patients had positive ENA antibody. Anaemia was recorded in 37 PRD patients (74%) while rheumatoid factor was positive in two patients with polyarticular JIA. The mean haematocrit was 27.7% while the mean ESR was 72.9 mm/h.

The JCTD cases seen include JSLE, juvenile systemic sclerosis, juvenile dermatomyositis, and PM-SLE overlap. In addition to JIA, these five diagnoses constituted the chronic inflammatory rheumatic disorders managed. Constitutional symptoms such as progressive weight loss, recurrent fever and fatigue were present in all patients with JCTD while constitutional symptoms were found in 15 (53.6%) patients with JIA ($p < 0.001$). Elevated ESR was found in 15 (83.3%) of JCTD patients and 25 (89.3%) of JIA patients. However, the difference in these proportions was not statistically significant ($p = 0.666$). Extra-articular manifestations included organ based features such as nephritis, pneumonitis and uveitis which excluded the musculoskeletal and constitutional symptoms; and they were found in all 18 (100%) patients with JCTD and 3 (10.7%) patients with JIA ($p < 0.001$).

Table 1 Baseline demographic and clinical characteristics of 57 Nigerian children with PRDs

	n (%)	Range	Mean(±SD)
Female	43(75.4)		
Male	14(24.6)		
Age at presentation (years)		1.5–22	14(±4.4)
Duration of symptoms (months)		2–60	18.4(±1.9)
Musculoskeletal pain	52(91.2)		
Arthritis	40(70.2)		
Constitutional symptoms	33(57.9)		
Extra-articular disease	21(36.8)		

Table 2 Spectrum of PRDs in 57 Nigerian children

Pediatric rheumatic diseases	Frequency (%)
Chronic inflammatory rheumatic diseases	
Juvenile idiopathic arthritis	28(49.1)
Systemic onset JIA	5(17.8)
Polyarticular JIA	14(50)
Oligoarticular JIA	9(31.2)
Juvenile connective tissue diseases (JCTD)	
JSLE	14(24.6)
Juvenile systemic sclerosis	2(3.5)
Juvenile dermatomyositis	1(1.6)
PM-SLE overlap	1(1.6)
Other rheumatic diseases	
Joint hypermobility syndrome	3(5.3)
Isolated plantar fasciitis	2(3.5)
Fibromyalgia	2(3.5)
Juvenile autoimmune uveitis	1(1.6)
Secondary osteoarthritis	1(1.6)
Secondary osteoporosis	1(1.6)
Osgood-Schlatter's disease	1(1.6)

JSLE juvenile systemic lupus erythematosus, *PM-SLE overlap* polymyositis-systemic lupus erythematosus overlap

Table 3 Laboratory characteristics of Nigerian children with PRDs

Laboratory abnormalities	Total number of PRD cases tested	n (%)
Anaemia(haematocrit < 33%)	50	37(74)
Elevated ESR(ESR > 20 mm/h)	50	42(84)
Elevated CRP(CRP > 8 mg/l)	37	32(86.4)
Elevatedferritin (Ferritin > 150 μg/l)	37	27(72.9)
Elevated RF(Rh-factor > 30iu/ml)	7	2(28.6)
Positive Anti-nuclear antibody	48	23(47.9)
Positive Anti-ENA antibody	16	13(81.2)
Laboratory parameters in SARDs	Mean(±SD)	Range
Haematocrit (%)	27.7(±7.5)	14–42
ESR (mm/h)	72.9(±37.4)	4–142
WBC (/μL)	11,081(±8,742)	1,350–45,600
Platelet count (/μL)	336,166(±191,938)	81,200–820,000
CRP (mg/L)	8.1(±4.9)	3–21
Ferritin(mg/dl)	548.5(±273.4)	62–2,140

PRD paediatric rheumatic disease, *ESR* erythrocyte sedimentation rate, *CRP* C - reactive protein, *ENA* Extractable nuclear antigen, *WBC* white blood cell. Normal reference range from our laboratory: Haematocrit-33-45%, ESR-0-20 mm/h, WBC-4500-13500/μL, Platelet count-150,000-450,000/μL,CRP-0-8 mg/l, ferritin-10-150 μg/l

Treatment and outcome patterns in Nigerians with PRDs

Non-steroidal anti-inflammatory drugs (NSAIDs) were used for treatment in 40 (70.1%) cases while oral prednisolone was used in 32 (56.1%) cases. Twenty-five (43.8%) patients with JIA had methotrexate while all cases with JSLE had hydroxychloroquine. Five patients had biologic agents (rituximab in four and etanercept in one) out of 18 biologic-eligible patients. Rituximab was used in four JSLE patients with refractory lupus nephritis unresponsive to prednisolone, hydroxychloroquine, and azathioprine or mycophenolate mofetil while etanercept was administered in one refractory rheumatoid factor-positive polyarticular JIA patient. This latter patient happened to be the only survivor among all patients that had biologics. There were six mortalities accounting for 10.5% of the PRD cases while 20 (35.1%) patients were lost to follow up. Four mortalities were in patients with JSLE while two were in patients with systemic onset JIA. Progressive renal failure from lupus nephritis was the cause of mortality in the deceased JSLE patients. While one patient with systemic onset JIA died from overwhelming sepsis, the other died from suspected macrophage activating syndrome.

Discussion

This is a report of patients with PRDs seen over a 5-year period by an adult rheumatology team. PRDs accounted for 2.8% of all inpatient and outpatient rheumatic cases managed over the period. This contrasts with the prevalence of 57.8% documented in childhood rheumatic clinic in Singapore [3]. This difference may be attributed to the primary adult focus of our unit. We noted that the mean age of presentation in our series is higher than the mean age reported among US patients with PRD (14 ± 4.4 years vs 7 ± 5.76 years) [16]. Besides, Nigerian patients with PRDs have high mean duration of symptoms before diagnosis (18.2 months). Late presentation and delayed diagnosis may be due to poverty, ignorance, and inadequate healthcare infrastructures and personnel. The inclusion of patients older than 18 years with retrospective diagnoses of childhood-onset diseases may also explain the high mean age of presentation observed in this series. There are no paediatric rheumatology clinics or paediatric rheumatologists in Nigeria. However, delay in diagnosis was also documented in the USA, a country with about 300 certified pediatric rheumatologists [17]. The report stated that 60% of children referred for suspected rheumatic conditions did not have confirmed rheumatic diagnosis and further rheumatologic follow up was requested in 40% of cases. The complex tendencies of many JCTD may inherently present diagnostic difficulties and sometimes prolong the period of evaluation before a diagnosis is made. Moreover, the near similar manifestations of JCTD with common childhood infections and malignancies may lead to initial diagnostic confusions in lower hospitals contributing to the delay in presenting for rheumatologist care.

We observed that PRDs are more frequent among female patients than in the male patients. This observation may be due to the substantial proportion of JCTD and JIA cases in our study as these conditions are generally more common in the female than in the male [4]. The most frequent clinical feature among our patients was musculoskeletal pain occurring in 91.2% while constitutional symptoms were recorded in 57.9% of PRD cases. Similarly, it was observed in Canada that musculoskeletal pain was the most common presenting complaint in a children rheumatology clinic [17]. In addition, they found that joint swelling and fever were most predictive of the need for further rheumatology follow up in their clinic.

JIA is the most frequent PRD condition identified in this study accounting for 49.1% of PRD cases. This is followed by JSLE in 24.6% of the study subjects and JCTD, on the whole, constituted 36.1% of PRD subjects. This result is in consonance with various studies from Europe, South Africa and USA that documented JIA as the most frequent PRD while either juvenile lupus or all CTDs was the next in their reports [12, 16, 18]. Previous reports from Africa suggest that JIA, JSLE, and JDM may not be uncommon in Sub-Saharan Africa [9, 10, 19]. Systemic vasculitis was the commonest PRD observed in Singapore by Tan et al. and it was found in a low proportion (4.3%) in a South African series but we did not document any systemic vasculitis in our series [3, 12]. Geographical variations in the frequencies of vasculitides are likely to be the reason for this finding. We found a low proportion of non-inflammatory rheumatic conditions such as joint hypermobility syndrome, isolated plantar fasciitis, fibromyalgia, and secondary osteoarthritis in our series. Orthopedic surgeons in our hospital often manage children with mechanical and non-inflammatory PRDs. This may explain the low frequency of this category of cases in this study.

Patients with a high clinical likelihood of a particular PRD had laboratory investigations tailored to that condition. This policy was adopted in our center to reduce the cost and burden of investigations on our patients as most of these patients pay directly for their laboratory investigations. The proportion of PRD cases with anaemia and elevated ESR in this study is high. This is due to a high proportion of subjects with SARDs in this study. Although, the proportions of nutritional anaemia and occult parasitaemia were not estimated in our patients, they may contribute to the high percentage of subjects with anaemia in our study.

We face enormous challenges in Africa with regards to anti-rheumatic medications. In Nigeria, numerous NSAIDs and oral prednisolone are readily available over the counter and patients often self-medicate with them before seeking a physician's review. Moreover, some synthetic disease-modifying anti-rheumatic drugs (DMARDs) are not readily available and when they are available, they may be unaffordable for many patients. Doctors and patients sometimes source for DMARDs from other countries often at prohibitive costs. Standard therapy with NSAIDs, DMARDs and glucocorticoids were administered to the majority of our patients with chronic inflammatory rheumatic diseases. Access to biologic DMARDs is limited in most African countries and this often limits the quality of specialist care a patient could get [20]. The highly limited access to biologics is a problem in the developing world where patients often fail to get access to specialist care until late in their disease. Rituximab and Etanercept, the only biologic DMARDs available in Nigeria, are largely unaffordable for our patients who have to pay for their treatment.

JSLE contributed four out of the six deaths and all these four patients had lupus nephritis unresponsive to standard therapy. Also, they had rituximab infusions in addition to other supportive care. However; they died from progressive renal failure after haemodialysis was instituted. The other two patients had systemic JIA and the causes of death in them were overwhelming sepsis and suspected macrophage activating syndrome. Systemic lupus erythematosus has been shown to run a more severe and more aggressive course in blacks and, even worse, in children [21]. Long delays before the diagnoses were made and inadequate treatments due to financial difficulties may have contributed to the high short-term mortality. In addition, some studies have suggested that socio-demographic disparities may influence the outcomes of these younger subjects [21, 22]. The proportion of PRD cases lost to follow up in this study was 35.1%. This high rate of discontinuation of care plan reflects the common pattern of unsustained treatment adherence among our patients. Poverty, illiteracy and various health related cultural beliefs may contribute to this phenomenon. Our study is also limited by a small sample size and the retrospective nature of the design. The burden of PRDs may have been underappreciated due to the adult focus of our practice as there is no paediatric rheumatologist in our country. Furthermore, high default rate among our patients makes the actual treatment outcome difficult to determine. Prospective cohort studies on this subject will help to determine the course of PRDs and their outcomes among Nigerians.

Conclusions

The spectrum of PRDs observed in this Nigerian series shares some similarities with patterns described in earlier studies from South Africa, North America and Europe. In all of these studies JIA accounts for the largest number of PRDs. Our patients with JIA tend to be younger than the patients presenting with JCTDs. However, systemic vasculitides, the most frequent PRDs in Singapore, were not observed in our series. The Nigerian patients with PRDs are more likely to be female, are more likely to present to the hospital later than children from the West and are more likely to present with musculoskeletal complaints than other symptoms.

Abbreviations

ACR: American College of Rheumatology; ANA: Antinuclear antibody; DMARD: Disease-modifying anti-rheumatic drug; ELISA: Enzyme-linked immunosorbent assay; ENA: Extractable nuclear antigen; JCTD: Juvenile connective tissue diseases; JDM: Juvenile dermatomyositis; JIA: Juvenile idiopathic arthritis; JSLE: Juvenile systemic lupus erythematosus; JSLE: Juvenile systemic lupus erythematosus; LASUTH: Lagos State University Teaching Hospital; NSAID: Non-steroidal anti-inflammatory drug; PM-SLE overlap: Polymyositis-systemic lupus erythematosus overlap; PRDs: Pediatric rheumatic diseases; RF: Rheumatoid factor; SARD: Systemic autoimmune rheumatic diseases

Acknowledgements

Not applicable.

Funding

None.

Authors' contributions

OBH and AOO designed the study. OBH, ABA and ARO gathered the data and did the analysis. OBH and ARO wrote the first draft while AOO and ABA revised it. All authors read and approved the final manuscript.

Competing interests

The authors declare that they have no competing interests.

Consent for publication

Not applicable.

Author details

[1]Department of Medicine, Lagos State University Teaching Hospital, Ikeja, Lagos State, Nigeria. [2]Department of Paediatrics, Lagos State University Teaching Hospital, Ikeja, Lagos State, Nigeria. [3]Department of Medicine, University of Ilorin Teaching Hospital, Ilorin, Kwara State, Nigeria.

References

1. Scott C, Webb K. Paediatric rheumatology in sub-saharan africa. Rheumatology (Oxford). 2014;53:1357–8.
2. Lawrence RC, Helmick CG, Arnett FC, Deyo RA, Felson DT, Giannini EH, et al. Estimates of the prevalence of arthritis and selected musculoskeletal disorders in the united states. Arthritis Rheum. 1998;41:778–99.
3. Tan JHT, Fun HS, Arkachaisri T. Paediatrics rheumatology clinic population in singapore: The kkh experience. Proc Singap Healthc. 2012;21:265–71.
4. Shiff NJ, Lix LM, Joseph L, Duffy C, Tucker LB, Svenson LW, et al. The prevalence of systemic autoimmune rheumatic diseases in canadian pediatric populations: Administrative database estimates. Rheumatol Int. 2015;35:569–73.
5. Rosenberg AM. Longitudinal analysis of a pediatric rheumatology clinic population. J Rheumatol. 2005;32:1992–2001.
6. Sawhney S, Magalhães CS. Paediatric rheumatology—a global perspective. Best Pract Res Clin Rheumatol. 2006;20:201–21.
7. Malleson P, Fung M, Rosenberg A. The incidence of pediatric rheumatic diseases: Results from the canadian pediatric rheumatology association disease registry. J Rheumatol. 1996;23:1981–7.
8. Bowyer S, Roettcher P. Pediatric rheumatology clinic populations in the united states: Results of a 3 year survey. Pediatric rheumatology database research group. J Rheumatol. 1996;23:1968–74.
9. Adelowo OO, Umar A. Juvenile idiopathic arthritis among nigerians: A case study. Clin Rheumatol. 2010;29:757–61.

10. el-Garf A, Salah S. Juvenile systemic lupus erythematosus among egyptian children. J Rheumatol. 1990;17:1168–70.
11. Adelowo O, Nwankwo M, Olaosebikan H. Juvenile dermatomyositis in a nigerian girl. BMJ Case Rep. 2014. doi:10.1136/bcr-2013-202132.
12. Okong'o LO, Scott C. The spectrum of paediatric rheumatic diseases in two tertiary centres in cape town, south africa. Pediatr Rheumatol. 2014;12:1.
13. Broten L, Migowa A, Scuccimarri R, Ng'ang'a E, Wachira J, Ngwiri T, et al. Spectrum of outpatient musculoskeletal visits at the largest pediatric center in east africa in 2011. Arthritis Rheum. 2013;65:S930–S1.
14. Migowa A, Colmegna I, Wachira J, Ngwiri T, Hitchon C, Bernatsky S, et al. Spectrum of musculoskeletal inpatient diagnoses at the largest pediatric center in east africa in 2011. J Rheumatol. 2015;42:1271.
15. Chipeta J, Njobvu P, McGill PE, Bucala R. Progress made towards enhancement of rheumatology education and practice in zambia: Review of an ilar-supported project. Clin Rheumatol. 2014;33:1367–72.
16. Mahajan M, Shah M, Toth M, Mcninch N, El-Hallak M. Inpatient pediatric rheumatic diseases: Characteristics, cost and trends. Arthritis Rheum. 2014;66:S992.
17. Rodriguez M, Ranieri D, Onel K. Paediatric rheumatology referral patterns: presenting complaints of new patients at large, urban academic centre. Paediatr Rheumatol. 2016;14(supply):30.
18. Huemer C, Huemer M, Dorner T, Falger J, Schacherl H, Bernecker M, et al. Incidence of pediatric rheumatic diseases in a regional population in austria. J Rheumatol. 2001;28:2116–9.
19. Faller G, Mistry BJ, Tikly M. Juvenile dermatomyositis in south african children is characterised by frequent dystropic calcification: A cross sectional study. Pediatr Rheumatol. 2014;12:1.
20. Maini M, Adelowo F, Saleh J, Weshahi Y, Burmester G-R, Cutolo M, et al. The global challenges and opportunities in the practice of rheumatology: White paper by the world forum on rheumatic and musculoskeletal diseases. Clin Rheumatol. 2015;34:819–29.
21. Son MBF, Johnson VM, Hersh AO, Lo MS, Costenbader KH. Outcomes in hospitalized pediatric patients with systemic lupus erythematosus. Pediatrics. 2014;133:e106–13.
22. Levy DM, Peschken CA, Tucker LB, Chédeville G, Huber AM, Pope JE, et al. Influence of ethnicity on childhood-onset systemic lupus erythematosus: Results from a multiethnic multicenter canadian cohort. Arthritis Care Res. 2013;65:152–60.

3

Psoriasis and associated variables in classification and outcome of juvenile idiopathic arthritis

Maria Ekelund[1,2], Kristiina Aalto[3], Anders Fasth[4], Troels Herlin[5], Susan Nielsen[6], Ellen Nordal[7,8], Suvi Peltoniemi[3], Marite Rygg[9,10], Marek Zak[6], Lillemor Berntson[2*] and on behalf of the Nordic Study Group of Pediatric Rheumatology (NoSPeR)

Abstract

Background: To study the impact of psoriasis and features associated with psoriasis on classification and outcome in a population-based follow-up cohort of children with juvenile idiopathic arthritis (JIA).

Methods: In all, 440 children with JIA were followed for a median of 8 years in a prospective Nordic population-based cohort study. Data for remission was available for 427 of these children. The presence of psoriasis, psoriasis-like rash, dactylitis, nail pitting, enthesitis, tenosynovitis and heredity was assessed in relation to ILAR classification and remission.

Results: Clinical findings associated with psoriasis developed consecutively during the 8-year period. Six of 14 children with psoriasis were not classified as juvenile psoriatic arthritis according to the ILAR criteria at 8 year follow-up. Dactylitis was more common in children with early onset of JIA. After 8 years we found a cumulative median number of eleven arthritic joints in children with psoriasis or psoriasis-like rash compared with six in the rest of the cohort ($p = 0.02$). Also, the chance for not being in remission after 8 years increased significantly in patients with psoriasis, psoriasis-like rash or at least two of: 1) first-degree heredity for psoriasis or psoriatic arthritis, 2) dactylitis or 3) nail pitting, compared with the rest of the group (OR 3.32, $p = 0.010$).

Conclusions: Our results indicate a more severe disease over time in psoriasis-associated JIA, as features of psoriasis develop during the disease course. This group is a major challenge to encompass in a future JIA classification in order to facilitate early tailored treatment.

Keywords: Arthritis, Juvenile Rheumatoid, Psoriasis, Child

Background

Classification of children with JIA and features of psoriasis has challenged the research community for decades. The disease comprises a variety of features often developing over the years, with large heterogeneity. Since classification criteria have varied over time there have also been dissimilarities in the cohorts studied. The question has been raised whether juvenile psoriatic arthritis (JPsA) is an entity of its own [1] or whether psoriasis and juvenile arthritis develop only as separate entities [2–4]. Adult psoriatic arthritis (PsA) is considered a unique disease entity, clearly distinct from rheumatoid arthritis. Immunology research has revealed that molecules of the interleukin-23 and interleukin-17 pathways promote skin and joint inflammation in psoriasis [5]. These discoveries have led to efforts to target interleukin-23, interleukin-17 and related molecules to treat psoriasis and psoriatic arthritis [6].

Classification of JPsA has been a challenge. In 1989, the Vancouver criteria for JPsA were presented comprising

* Correspondence: lillemor.berntson@telia.com
[2]Department of Women's and Children's Health, Uppsala University, Uppsala, Sweden
Full list of author information is available at the end of the article

two categories of JPsA, one definite and one probable [7]. In three studies utilizing the Vancouver classification criteria, joint patterns differed at onset between oligoarticular JIA and oligoarticular JPsA, with greater involvement of small joints in the hands and wrists being more typical in the latter category [1, 8, 9]. Age at onset was significantly higher in oligoarticular JPsA compared with oligoarticular JIA. A child with an oligoarticular pattern with wrists or small joints in hands or feet affected, more often had nail pitting, psoriasis or heredity for psoriasis.

In the current ILAR classification, JPsA may be diagnosed in children with arthritis and (1) psoriasis or (2) if two features suggestive of a psoriatic diathesis are present, including dactylitis, nail changes, or psoriasis in a first-degree relative, in the absence of specific exclusions [10].

During later years two distinct phenotypic subgroups of JPsA have been discussed. One occurs in children (predominantly girls) younger than 5 years of age at onset, with small joint involvement, a higher risk of progression to polyarticular disease, high frequency of ANA positivity and dactylitis. In contrast, children above 5 years of age at onset had no obvious gender difference, were more likely to be ANA negative and to exhibit enthesitis and axial joint involvement [7, 11, 12].

So far, the prognosis for JPsA has been considered approximately the same as for patients with other categories of JIA based on two follow-up studies, one using both the Vancouver and the ILAR criteria with a follow-up time of 1 month, up to 16.8 years [2] and the second using the Vancouver criteria with a median follow-up time of 2 years [13]. Children with a polyarticular course had the worst prognosis. Positive ANA in children with JPsA has been discussed as a negative prognostic factor without any conclusive results [7, 9, 14]. Occurrence of HLA-B27 has been shown as a risk factor for sacroiliitis in JPsA [2].

In light of this knowledge, we wanted to challenge earlier findings by studying a well-defined cohort of children with JIA, followed prospectively over a long time, especially since previous studies were referral-based. Our aim was to study the occurrence of variables indicating psoriatic diathesis during the first 8 years of disease in a population-based cohort of children with JIA and to address aspects of classification and outcome.

Methods

Patients were recruited from a Nordic JIA cohort. All new patients with JIA from defined geographical areas of Denmark, Finland, Norway, and Sweden were collected prospectively during 1997–2000 [15]. The study design was population-based. All physicians within each catchment area eligible to meet children with arthritis received a letter informing about the study. Pediatric rheumatologists from 12 participating centers included patients. The database consisted of clinical and laboratory data from 500 patients, including 440 followed for at least 7 years, median 98 months. The 60 patients lost to follow-up did not differ from the 440 with follow-up data as regards number of active joints during the first 6 months after onset, Childhood Health Assessment Questionnaire (CHAQ), Juvenile Arthritis Disease Activity Score (JADAS27), or proportion with oligoarticular disease at baseline. Also, occurrence of psoriasis, psoriatic-like rash, dactylitis, enthesitis, first degree heredity for psoriasis or psoriatic arthritis did not differ between the 60 lost to follow-up compared to the 440 in the study cohort. JIA categories had been determined based on the ILAR criteria [10]. For 427 of 440 children, outcome data was available for analysis of remission. The presence of psoriasis and psoriasis-like rash during the 8-year follow-up period was assessed in relation to clinical characteristics, ILAR classification and remission. Remission status according to the preliminary criteria of Wallace et al was used [16]. Clinical variables were collected cumulatively during this period; they were not necessarily present at the time of the 8-year follow-up. A patient was considered to have psoriasis if a dermatologist had made that diagnosis. Rashes noted by the examining rheumatologist, well skilled in pediatric rheumatology, and thought likely (but not definitely) to represent psoriasis were considered psoriasis-like.

Results

In the cohort of 440 children followed for at least 7 years after disease onset (median 98 months, range 84–147 months), 14 children developed psoriasis and 13 psoriasis-like rash (Table 1). Only 8 of the 14 children with psoriasis and JIA were classified as juvenile psoriatic arthritis (JPsA) according to the ILAR criteria. The other six were classified as undifferentiated. Four of those were mutually excluded from JPsA as well as enthesitis related arthritis (ERA), thus they did not fit any category. One boy was excluded because he was older than six at onset and HLA-B27 positive, and another child was excluded because of positive rheumatoid factor (RF). Children with dactylitis and/or nail pitting were found among many ILAR categories. First-degree heredity for psoriasis or psoriatic arthritis occurred in 9 of 14 children with JPsA and in 51 of 57 of children classified as undifferentiated arthritis. In a comparison between the eight children with psoriasis, classified as JPsA (ILAR criteria) at 98 months of disease, and the six children with psoriasis classified as undifferentiated, there was no significant difference in age at onset ($p = 0.34$), first degree heredity for psoriasis/psoriatic arthritis ($p = 0.53$), dactylitis ($p = 1.0$), nail pitting ($p = 0.30$) or cumulative number of joints ($p = 0.59$), but the cohorts were too

Table 1 Clinical characteristics in a Nordic cohort of children with juvenile idiopathic arthritis, classified according to the ILAR classification criteria[b] and followed for at least seven years

Clinical characteristics	Number of patients n	Age at onset median (IQR)	Psoriasis n	Psoriasis- like rash n	Dactylitis n	Nail pitting n	Patients assessed for heredity n	First-degree heredity for psoriasis or psoriatic arthritis n (%)
Systemic arthritis	18	4.5 (2.2-6.7)	-	-	-	-	18	-
Oligoarticular persistent	133	5.1 (2.6-8.5)	-	1	6	3	123	-
Oligoarticular extended	78	4.1 (1.8-8.4)	-	2	1	3	74	-
Polyarticular RF negative	80	4.9 (2.2-9.1)	-	2	7	-	79	-
Polyarticular RF positive	3	10.2, 13.2, 13.3	-	-	-	-	3	-
Psoriatic arthritis	14	5.8 (4.3-7.9)	8	3	3	7	14	9 (64.3)
Enthesitis-related arthritis	49	10.0 (6.8-12.3)	-	3	1	2	47	-
Undifferentiated arthritis	65	7.8 (3.2-11.8)	6[a]	2	6	3	57	51 (78.5)

[a]None of the six patients with psoriasis at the 8-year follow-up fit any category, four because of mutual exclusion from JPsA and ERA because of enthesitis, one because he was a HLA-B27-positive boy older than 6 years at onset, one because of positive RF

[b]International League of Associations for Rheumatology classification criteria [10] assessed at last study visit (median 98, range 84–147 months)

small for meaningful statistical analyses. Children with psoriasis ($n = 14$) compared to those with psoriatic-like rash ($n = 13$) did not differ regarding gender ($p = 0.71$), outcome ($p = 0.16$) or median cumulative number of joints ($p = 0.26$).

Table 2 presents the development of clinical features associated with psoriasis during the first 8 years of disease. Twenty-four children developed dactylitis during disease course, 15 of them had dactylitis at onset. Median age at time of onset of JIA in the group with dactylitis was 2.4 (IQR 1.7–5.4) years compared with 5.8 (IQR 2.7–9.9) years in the rest of the cohort ($p = 0.007$).

Five of 24 children with dactylitis developed psoriasis or psoriasis-like rash during the first 8 years of their arthritis, Table 3. Table 3 also presents the significantly higher cumulative number of active joints in children with psoriasis or psoriasis-like rash as well as the increased frequency of dactylitis, nail pitting, enthesitis, and first-degree heredity for psoriasis compared with children without psoriasis or psoriasis-like rash.

Features of sacroiliitis (SI) developed in several children with psoriasis or psoriasis- like rash (Table 4). SI or enthesitis coexisting with psoriasis or psoriasis-like rash lead to mutual exclusion from both JPsA and ERA categories.

Seven of 27 children with psoriasis or psoriasis-like rash were HLA-B27 positive (missing value in another three) and this group had a high age of onset (median 10.8, IQR 5.9–11.8 years), and a high cumulative number of joints (median 15, IQR 9–18 joints), data not shown. Several of the ERA or SI-like features were clustered together. Six of the 27 children with psoriasis or psoriasis-like rash had inflammatory back pain or buttock pain at any time during the first 98 months of disease (Table 4), three of those were HLA-B27 positive, and in two sacroiliitis was confirmed by x-ray.

In children with psoriasis or psoriasis-like rash or at least two of either dactylitis, nail pitting, or first-degree heredity of psoriasis, the remission rate was significantly lower compared with children without these clinical features, $p = 0.010$ (Table 5).

First-degree heredity for psoriasis in children with oligoarticular onset did not increase the risk for oligoarticular extended disease during those first 8 years of disease (data not shown).

Table 2 Development of clinical features associated with psoriasis in 440 children with JIA followed for at least seven years after onset (median 98, range 84–147 months)

Clinical features	Patients at onset n	Cumulative number of patients at eight years n
Dactylitis	15	24
Nail pitting	10	18
Psoriasis	11	14
Psoriasis-like rash	6	13
Enthesitis	37	41

Statistical analysis

Statistical analyses were performed using the Statistical Package for Social Sciences, version 23 (SPSS Inc., Chicago, IL, USA). Demographics and disease characteristics were described using median and interquartile range (IQR), or total number and percent of study cohort. Statistical analyses of differences between children with and without psoriasis/psoriasis-like rash during the first year of disease were performed using the chi-square test (Fisher's exact test, 2-sided) for comparison of dichotomous variables. The Mann-Whitney U-test was used for comparison of non-parametric data and independent samples was used for comparison of median values between the two groups.

Table 3 Clinical features describing the first eight years of disease in 440 children with JIA according to occurrence of psoriasis or psoriasis-like rash

Clinical feature	Number of patients assessed	Total cohort	Psoriasis or psoriasis-like rash $n = 27$	No psoriasis or psoriasis-like rash $n = 413$	p-value*
Gender, n (% females)	440 (66.1)	440 (66.1)	27 (48.1)	413 (67.3)	0.06[a]
Age at time of onset median (IQR)	440	5.5 (2.5-9.7)	7.2 (3.8-11.0)	5.3 (2.3-9.4)	0.08[b]
Cumulative joints median (IQR)	440	6 (2-12)	11 (5-16)	6 (2-12)	0.02[c]
Dactylitis (%)	440	24	5 (18.5)	19 (4.6)	0.01[a]
Nail pitting (%)	440	18	7 (25.9)	11 (2.7)	<0.001[a]
First-degree heredity for psoriasis or psoriatic arthritis (%)	420	51	7 (25.9)	44 (10.6)	0.03[a]
Enthesitis (%)	438	41	6 (22.2)	35 (8.5)	0.03[a]
Tenosynovitis (%)	436	88	6 (22.2)	82 (19.8)	0.81[a]

*Patients with psoriasis or psoriasis-like rash compared with those without, [a]Fisher's exact test, [b]Independent samples Mann-Whitney U test, [c]Independent samples median test

Binary logistic regression analyses were performed in order to identify the association between occurrence of psoriasis or psoriasis-like rash and failure of remission 8 years after disease onset. The dichotomized variable remission (remission without medication) versus remission with medication or not in remission was used as the dependent variable in the regression model. Results of the regression analyses are shown as odds ratios (OR), 95% confidence intervals (CI) and p-values. The level of significance was set at 5% ($p < 0.05$).

Discussion

In this population-based study of 440 patients followed for a median of 98 months, we found that as many as six of 14 children with definite psoriasis were classified as undifferentiated JIA based on exclusion criteria in the ILAR classification. In children with psoriasis or psoriasis-like rash we found a strong association with first-degree heredity for psoriasis or psoriatic arthritis, dactylitis and nail pitting, but also with enthesitis. Psoriasis or psoriasis-like rash was also associated with higher cumulative number of active joints and possibly with less favorable outcome, as features of psoriasis are additive.

Table 4 Development of clinical variables during a follow-up time of at least seven years after onset (median 98, range 84–147 months) in groups of patients included in a cohort of 440 Nordic patients with JIA

	Psoriasis or psoriasis-like rash		Dactylitis	
	$n = 27$	n[a]	$n = 24$	n[a]
Radiological SI[b]				
At onset		0		
Cumulative at median 98 months		2		0
Inflammatory back pain/buttock pain				
At onset		3		0
Cumulative at median 98 months		6		0
Enthesitis				
At onset		5		3
Cumulative at median 98 months		6		4

[a]Number of patients with the feature developing during the first median 98 months
[b]*SI* sacroiliitis

A strength of our study was the prospective population-based design and also that the whole cohort was followed for at least 7 years. A weakness was that the group of children with psoriasis or psoriasis-like rash was small and no dermatologist verified the psoriasis-like rash. The pediatric rheumatologists involved in the study all had several years' experience and a psoriasis-like rash was only defined if there was a high suspicion of psoriasis.

Another clinical sign, dactylitis, has proven a strong predictor of JPsA [13]. In preparative studies for classification of psoriatic arthritis in adults (CASPAR criteria), the specificity of dactylitis was shown to be 95%, nail dystrophy 98% and tender enthesitis and diffuse enthesitis pain 77–93% [17]. The strong association between psoriatic arthritis, dactylitis, nail changes and enthesitis is in accordance with our results. In our study cohort occurrence of dactylitis was spread among ILAR categories, but had a strong association with psoriasis or psoriasis-like rash. Also, enthesitis showed a strong association with psoriasis or psoriasis-like rash in our study cohort. Although enthesitis is a well-recognized feature of PsA in adults, it is an exclusion criterion for JPsA in the ILAR classification, and a common reason for exclusion from the JPsA category [15]. Another important feature in psoriatic diathesis in adults is heredity for psoriasis [17] and our results pointed in the same direction.

In our cohort, first-degree heredity for psoriasis was common in the undifferentiated JIA category, which has

Table 5 Analyses of binary logistic regression for not being in remission related to psoriasis and psoriasis-related variables in 427 children with JIA, followed for at least seven years of disease

		Number of patients	Not in remission[c] after 8 years n (%)	*p*-value	OR	95% confidence interval
Psoriasis or psoriasis-like rash[a]	Yes	25	19 (76.0)	0.062	2.44	0.96-6.2
	No	402	227 (56.5)			
Psoriasis or psoriasis-like rash OR at least two of three[b]	Yes	31	25 (80.6)	0.010	3.32	1.33-8.27
	No	379	211 (55.7)			
Dactylitis	Yes	24	16 (66.7)	0.36	1.5	0.63-3.6
	No	403	230 (57.1)			
Nail pitting	Yes	18	13 (72.2)	0.21	1.96	0.69-5.6
	No	409	233 (57.0)			
Enthesitis	Yes	40	29 (72.5)	0.046	2.08	1.01-4.29
	No	385	215 (55.8)			
First-degree heredity for psoriasis or psoriatic arthritis	Yes	48	28 (58.3)	0.86	1.1	0.42-2.82
	No	361	208 (57.6)			
Total		427	181 (42.4)			

[a]Data in 13 patients with psoriasis and 12 with psoriasis-like rash
[b]1) dactylitis, 2) nail pitting, 3) first-degree heredity for psoriasis or psoriatic arthritis
[c]Remission was defined as inactive disease off medication for at least twelve months in accordance with the preliminary definition of Wallace [16]

also been discussed by others and illustrates the classification difficulties [18]. Stoll et al studied classification of juvenile psoriatic arthritis and found that the ILAR criteria excluded almost 60% of those included with the Vancouver criteria [19], which is in line with our results regarding ILAR classification.

Another challenge in classification is the progression of the disease over time. In an earlier publication we showed that patients classified as JPsA according to the ILAR criteria increased from 6 to 14 during the follow-up period. In about half of the children with JPsA, the classic rash presented after the onset of arthritis, with a time lag that could be 10 years or more [20]. Manifestations of psoriasis in the young child are often atypical or unspecific, such as erythema and scaling behind the ears, features taken into consideration by the Vancouver set of JPsA criteria, but excluded under the JIA nomenclature in the ILAR classification [7]. Our data presents the heterogeneity of JPsA and the development over time of clinical variables supporting a psoriatic diathesis, as well as the overlap between JPsA and enthesitis-related arthritis in a group of patients.

The earlier findings of two phenotypic subgroups of JPsA: a younger group, predominantly girls, with a polyarticular onset, high frequency of ANA positivity and dactylitis [13], in contrast to an older age group more likely to exhibit enthesitis and axial joint involvement [7, 13], can only partly be confirmed by our results since our cohort was too small for further analysis. We found a significantly lower age at time of onset in children who developed dactylitis during the 8 years, compared with those who did not. None of the 15 children with dactylitis at disease onset developed inflammatory back pain during the disease course and in the extended group of 24 children with dactylitis after 8 years, none developed any sign of sacroiliitis. This result is consistent with a previous observation that patients with dactylitis and sacroiliitis tend to be distinctive phenotypic groups of juvenile psoriatic arthritis [21]. Our finding of an older age at onset in the group of HLA-B27 positive children with psoriasis or psoriasis-like rash also supports earlier data, but we were surprised by the very high cumulative number of joints with arthritis in this group.

The polyarticular disease progression in children with psoriasis and arthritis in our study is in line with earlier studies [7, 9, 12]. Our result indicates a somewhat less favorable outcome in the cohort of children with psoriasis, psoriasis-like rash or at least two well-known features characterizing the JPsA group, but our numbers are too low to analyze each of the clinical features as a single trait, and larger studies are needed to confirm our results. The prognosis in JPsA defined according to the Vancouver classification criteria was not worse compared with other JIA categories in earlier studies [2, 13], but the time of follow-up varied: 1 month in one study up to 17 years, and a median of 23 months in the other. By comparison, our cohort was followed for at least 7 years, with a median of 98 months, and in a population-based setting.

Since classification of JPsA has changed over time, it is difficult to compare one study with another and to properly present outcomes in this group of patients. In our study clinical findings associated with psoriasis as well as first-degree heredity for psoriasis were strongly associated with children developing psoriasis or psoriasis-like rash during the first 8 years of disease. Our cohort also reveals the difficulty of using the ILAR classification to assign those children. The consequence is that we do not study children with a psoriatic diathesis specifically, which would be important in relation to new therapies under development for JPsA and bringing these children new treatment possibilities.

Conclusions

We suggest stronger emphasis on the variables of psoriatic diathesis, and not using strict exclusion criteria in future follow-up studies of JIA, and to consider this also in future JIA classifications. We need to better understand how to predict this category of disease and to be able to tailor proper treatment for this group of children.

Abbreviations

CHAQ: Childhood health assessment questionnaire; CI: Confidence interval; ERA: Enthesitis related arthritis; ILAR: The international league of associations for rheumatology; IQR: Interquartile range; JADAS27: Juvenile arthritis disease activity score; JIA: Juvenile idiopathic arthritis; JPsA: Juvenile psoriatic arthritis; PsA: Psoriatic arthritis; RF: Rheumatoid factor

Acknowledgements

We thank the children and parents participating in the study. We also thank the participating nurses as well as the other members of the Nordic Study Group of Pediatric Rheumatology (NoSPeR), Gudmund Marhaug (Trondheim), Freddy Karup Pedersen (Copenhagen), Pirkko Pelkonen (Helsinki), and Boel Anderson-Gäre (Jönköping), for their inspiring cooperation. Finally, we thank the following participating physicians who contributed by collecting data: Nils Thomas Songstad (Tromsø), Kjell Berntzen and Nina Moe (Trondheim), Mikael Damgaard, Maria Ekelund, and Nils Olof Jonsson (Jönköping), Anders Berner and Hans Ekström (Karlstad), Eric Ronge (Skövde), Agne Lind and Lars Hammarén (Borås), Johan Robinsson (Trollhättan), and Anna-Lena Nilsson (Östersund).

Funding

This work was supported by grants from the Department of Women's and Children's Health, Uppsala University Hospital, Uppsala, the Gillbergska foundation, Uppsala, the Futurum - academy of health and care, Region Jönköping county and the Swedish Rheumatism association.

Authors' contributions

All authors were involved in planning and performance of the study, inclusion of patients and data collection. ME and LB conceptualized and drafted the manuscript. All authors have reviewed and edited the manuscript, as well as read and approved the final version.

Competing interests

The authors declare that they have no competing interests.

Author details

[1]Department of Pediatrics, Ryhov County Hospital, Jönköping, Sweden. [2]Department of Women's and Children's Health, Uppsala University, Uppsala, Sweden. [3]Department of Pediatrics, Children's Hospital, Helsinki University Hospital, Helsinki, Finland. [4]Department of Pediatrics, Institute of Clinical Sciences, Sahlgrenska Academy, University of Gothenburg, Gothenburg, Sweden. [5]Department of Pediatrics, Århus University Hospital, Århus, Denmark. [6]Pediatric Rheumatology Department, Pediatric Clinic II, Copenhagen University Hospital, Rigshospitalet, Copenhagen, Denmark. [7]Department of Pediatrics, University Hospital of North Norway, Tromsø, Norway. [8]Department of Clinical Medicine, UIT The Arctic University of Norway, Tromsø, Norway. [9]Department of Laboratory Medicine, Children's and Women's Health, Norwegian University of Science and Technology, Trondheim, Norway. [10]Department of Pediatrics, St. Olav's Hospital, Trondheim, Norway.

References

1. Stoll ML, Nigrovic PA, Gotte AC, Punaro M. Clinical comparison of early-onset psoriatic and non-psoriatic oligoarticular juvenile idiopathic arthritis. Clin Exp Rheumatol. 2011;29:582–8.
2. Butbul Aviel Y, Tyrrell P, Schneider R, Dhillon S, Feldman BM, Laxer R, et al. Juvenile Psoriatic Arthritis (JPsA): juvenile arthritis with psoriasis? Pediatr Rheumatol Online J. 2013;11:11.
3. Petty RE. Juvenile psoriatic arthritis, or juvenile arthritis with psoriasis? Clin Exp Rheumatol. 1994;12 Suppl 10:S55–8.
4. Ravelli A, Consolaro A, Schiappapietra B, Martini A. The conundrum of juvenile psoriatic arthritis. Clin Exp Rheumatol. 2015;33:S40–3.
5. Gaffen SL, Jain R, Garg AV, Cua DJ. The IL-23-IL-17 immune axis: from mechanisms to therapeutic testing. Nat Rev Immunol. 2014;14:585–600.
6. Ritchlin CT, Krueger JG. New therapies for psoriasis and psoriatic arthritis. Curr Opin Rheumatol. 2016;28:204–10.
7. Southwood TR, Petty RE, Malleson PN, Delgado EA, Hunt DW, Wood B, et al. Psoriatic arthritis in children. Arthritis Rheum. 1989;32:1007–13.
8. Huemer C, Malleson PN, Cabral DA, Huemer M, Falger J, Zidek T, et al. Patterns of joint involvement at onset differentiate oligoarticular juvenile psoriatic arthritis from pauciarticular juvenile rheumatoid arthritis. J Rheumatol. 2002;29:1531–5.
9. Roberton DM, Cabral DA, Malleson PN, Petty RE. Juvenile psoriatic arthritis: followup and evaluation of diagnostic criteria. J Rheumatol. 1996;23:166–70.
10. Petty RE, Southwood TR, Manners P, Baum J, Glass DN, Goldenberg J, et al. International League of Associations for Rheumatology classification of juvenile idiopathic arthritis: second revision, Edmonton, 2001. J Rheumatol. 2004;31:390–2.
11. Stoll ML, Punaro M. Psoriatic juvenile idiopathic arthritis: a tale of two subgroups. Curr Opin Rheumatol. 2011;23:437–43.
12. Lambert J. Psoriatic arthritis in Childhood. Clin Rheum Dis. 1976;2:339–52.
13. Stoll ML, Zurakowski D, Nigrovic LE, Nichols DP, Sundel RP, Nigrovic PA. Patients with juvenile psoriatic arthritis comprise two distinct populations. Arthritis Rheum. 2006;54:3564–72.
14. Shore A, Ansell BM. Juvenile psoriatic arthritis–an analysis of 60 cases. J Pediatr. 1982;100:529–35.
15. Nordal E, Zak M, Aalto K, Berntson L, Fasth A, Herlin T, et al. Ongoing disease activity and changing categories in a long-term nordic cohort study of juvenile idiopathic arthritis. Arthritis Rheum. 2011;63:2809–18.
16. Wallace CA, Ruperto N, Giannini E. Preliminary criteria for clinical remission for select categories of juvenile idiopathic arthritis. J Rheumatol. 2004;31: 2290–4.
17. Taylor W, Gladman D, Helliwell P, Marchesoni A, Mease P, Mielants H, et al. Classification criteria for psoriatic arthritis: development of new criteria from a large international study. Arthritis Rheum. 2006;54:2665–73.
18. Chan MO, Petty RE, Guzman J, ReACCh-Out Investigators. A Family History of Psoriasis in a First-degree Relative in Children with JIA: to Include or Exclude? J Rheumatol. 2016;43(5):944–7.

4

Methods for analyzing observational longitudinal prognosis studies for rheumatic diseases: a review & worked example using a clinic-based cohort of juvenile dermatomyositis patients

Lily Siok Hoon Lim[1,2,3*], Eleanor Pullenayegum[4], Rahim Moineddin[5], Dafna D Gladman[6,7], Earl D Silverman[8,9,10] and Brian M Feldman[3,4,8,10,11]

Abstract

Most outcome studies of rheumatic diseases report outcomes ascertained on a single occasion. While single assessments are sufficient for terminal or irreversible outcomes, they may not be sufficiently informative if outcomes change or fluctuate over time. Consequently, longitudinal studies that measure non-terminal outcomes repeatedly afford a better understanding of disease evolution.

Longitudinal studies require special analytic methods. Newer longitudinal analytic methods have evolved tremendously to deal with common challenges in longitudinal observational studies. In recent years, an increasing number of studies have used longitudinal design. This review aims to help readers understand and apply the findings from longitudinal studies. Using a cohort of children with juvenile dermatomyositis (JDM), we illustrate how to study evolution of disease activity in JDM using longitudinal methods.

Keywords: Epidemiology, Longitudinal study, Childhood-onset dermatomyositis, Biostatistics

Background

Outcome studies in rheumatic diseases have generally focused on single-occasion outcome assessments, e.g., 5-year outcome. When the outcome of interest is not a terminal event (e.g., death), but a dynamic one (e.g., disease activity, functional status), a cross-sectional view is usually not the best way to look at the data. Two patients may have similar outcomes at a point in time but *how* they arrived at their outcomes may have been very different. To understand the disease course, information about how outcomes change over time is necessary. By measuring patients' outcomes repeatedly (by definition, on ≥ 3 occasions), a longitudinal study provides information about the shape of outcome trajectory, e.g., whether the disease goes into remission, waxes and wanes or remains persistently active [1].

Longitudinal studies require special longitudinal statistical analysis. Although some of these methods have been available for many years, they are not commonly used in the literature. These complex methods are harder to understand and use. This paper aims to: 1) Provide a review of common methods used to analyze longitudinal trajectory data; and 2) Demonstrate how to interpret results from longitudinal trajectory analysis [2–4]. We will focus on application of these methods to a real-life clinic-based rheumatic disease cohort.

Questions that can be addressed by a longitudinal study

A longitudinal study can answer questions about the sources of variability in observed outcomes. In studies where outcomes are assessed once, the differences in outcomes are usually attributed to differences between individuals [1]. The effects of within-individual differences

* Correspondence: llim@chrim.ca
[1]Children's Hospital Research Institute of Manitoba, University of Manitoba, Winnipeg, Canada
[2]Department of Pediatrics, University of Manitoba, Winnipeg, Canada
Full list of author information is available at the end of the article

cannot be differentiated from that of between-individual differences in cross-sectional studies. In contrast, by measuring the outcomes repeatedly over time– for each individual– the longitudinal design captures important prognostic information about within-individual differences and allows these effects to be distinguished from between-individual differences.

Prognostic factors that fluctuate or emerge later during the course of the disease can only be understood using the longitudinal design. Examples of prognostic factors that often vary over time may include a biomarker of disease activity, or alterations in treatment. Using a longitudinal study design, we can repeatedly and simultaneously measure both the time-varying prognostic factors and the outcome(s) of interest, allowing direct relationships to be established.

Special considerations in analyzing the longitudinal study

Methods to analyze longitudinal data have been available since the 1960s. Traditional longitudinal analyses include repeated measures analysis of variances (RANOVA) [5] and multivariate analysis of variance (MANOVA) [6]. Newer methods of longitudinal analysis include the generalized estimating equation (GEE) [7], mixed effects regression model (MRM) [8, 9], latent class trajectory analyses (LCTA) [10, 11], joint modeling [12–14] and multi-state modeling [15]. For illustrating longitudinal disease trajectory in this review, we will focus on the first four of these newer models. In this section, we will also compare the traditional with the modern methods of longitudinal analysis.

In a longitudinal study, each individual contributes at least three observations (by definition). As observations originating from the same individual are less variable than those originating from different individuals, longitudinal analysis needs to account for this relationship [16]. If analyzed without consideration for within-individual correlations, the conclusion will be inaccurate. However, traditional methods like RANOVA have highly restrictive assumptions [5], such as the assumption that the correlation between two measurements is constant, i.e., the correlation between measurements is similar, whether the measurements have been two days or two years apart. In contrast, newer methods attempt to account for the fact that within-individual correlations likely vary over time [17] (Additional file 1: Appendix).

In a longitudinal study, patients may be followed for differing lengths of time, resulting in a different number of visits for each patient and different visit schedules among patients. While traditional methods require an equal number of visits and/or the same schedule of visits, newer methods can accommodate an unequal number of visits and irregular measurement schedules [17].

Missing data is inevitable in observational longitudinal studies. As patients are followed over long periods, there will be times when patients may leave a cohort and then return, or be lost to follow-up. Traditional longitudinal methods have a requirement of no missing data, which is impractical in longitudinal observational studies [18]. In contrast, newer methods are able to handle missing data with varying degrees of flexibility [7, 8, 19] (Additional file 1: Appendix).

We will now apply four of the longitudinal methods– GEE, MRM, LCTA and Joint Modelling– to illustrate the use of these methods in an observational cohort. We have chosen these four models, as they all provide a view of the shape of the longitudinal outcome trajectory and form the basic models from which more complex models can be developed.

Juvenile dermatomyositis as a disease model for longitudinal analysis

We will use Juvenile Dermatomyositis (JDM) as a convenient disease model to show how longitudinal design and analysis can be used in rheumatic diseases. Multiple cross-sectional studies have determined that, when assessed 2-3 years after diagnosis, there are three disease course patterns in JDM: monocyclic, polycyclic or chronic [20–23]. Although previous studies have shown that a substantial proportion of patients have active disease many years after the diagnosis [24, 25], these studies could not differentiate patients with active disease throughout their entire disease course from those with a polycyclic course. A longitudinal study can help to clarify this question.

The study population was 95 JDM patients followed at The Hospital for Sick Children, Toronto, Canada. Information about this cohort has been previously reported [26, 27]. We used clinical data from the first four years of follow-up to demonstrate the application of longitudinal analytic methods. The frequency of patients' visits was based on the severity of their disease, i.e., the visit schedule was irregular across the population. See Additional file 1: Appendix for the baseline characteristics of this cohort.

The primary outcome was the modified Disease Activity Score (DASm) [27, 28]. The skin component of modified DAS (SDAS) scores up to 4 points and the musculoskeletal component (MDAS) up to 7 points.

We used: 1) The DASm at diagnosis (bDAS) as an example of a time-invariant (unchanging) prognostic factor; and 2) The steroid dose (in mg/kg) or methotrexate use (yes or no) from visits before each DASm measurement as examples of time-varying (changing) prognostic factors. As we used bDAS as a predictor, we excluded the first visit DASm (bDAS) in this dataset. We tested 3 different lag times (of 3, 6 and 12 months) when the time-varying predictor (treatment) was measured (e.g., methotrexate use 3 months before, 6 months before or 12 months before DASm measurement).

Questions and answers

Question 1: What is the disease activity course for a population of JDM patients?

The GEE, which determines the mean population disease activity trajectory, is frequently used to answer this kind of question [7]. The GEE calculates the average DASm of the whole population at each visit. These population averages are then joined to make a "trajectory" of DASm for the whole population over time. The GEE assumes that the measurement schedule is unrelated to the outcome, i.e., both sick and well patients are presumed to have the same visit schedule on average. As sicker patients were likely seen more frequently than those who were well, this assumption was probably not supported in our clinic-based cohort. However, there have been extensions of the GEE (the weighted GEE) that allow GEE to be used even when the measurement schedule is related to the outcome [29].

The GEE is the most popular method used for longitudinal analysis for several reasons [30]. With the GEE, the mean population response at each occasion is modelled as the result of only the prognostic factors of interest and not of previous responses or random effects (individual heterogeneity) [9]. If the researcher's interest is in the average population prognosis, then the GEE provides a simple interpretation [31].

We will briefly discuss the results when we used the GEE to analyze our study cohort. From the smoothed local regression plot of Fig. 1 [32], we can see that the average population DASm decreases rapidly and then plateaued to a lower degree of disease activity. This is clinically sensible as there are effective treatments for lowering disease activity in JDM, yet many patients remain chronically active.

In summary, the GEE is a good choice for analyzing studies where the overall population prognosis is the primary interest, e.g., when addressing questions about population trends or healthcare utilization.

Question 2a: How do we determine the disease activity course of an individual with JDM?

The best way to address this question is to use the MRM, a so-called subject-specific model, that allows for potential inference at the level of the individual [1, 33]. For a continuous outcome like DASm, the MRM also provides us with the average population trajectory. The smoothed plot (Fig. 2) shows the DASm trajectories of both the individual patients (gray lines) and the mean population trajectory (bold black line) [32]. As the outcome is continuous, fitting the MRM resulted in a similar longitudinal trajectory to that derived from the GEE. However, if the outcome is not continuous, calculating the mean population trajectory from the MRM is very complex.

In the MRM, each individual's trajectory is different from the mean population trajectory because of "random effects." Random effects are a combination of *unmeasured* prognostic factors, confounders, environmental factors and genetic factors, which account for heterogeneity within the population [31]. Any difference between an individual's trajectory and the average population trajectory is the result of that individual's random effects; this forms the basis for individual level inference from the MRM. Random effects may be applied at intercepts, which represent between-individual differences. When random effects are applied to slopes, this allows individuals' time trend to deviate from the average population trajectory. Although the random effects are taken into account in modeling,

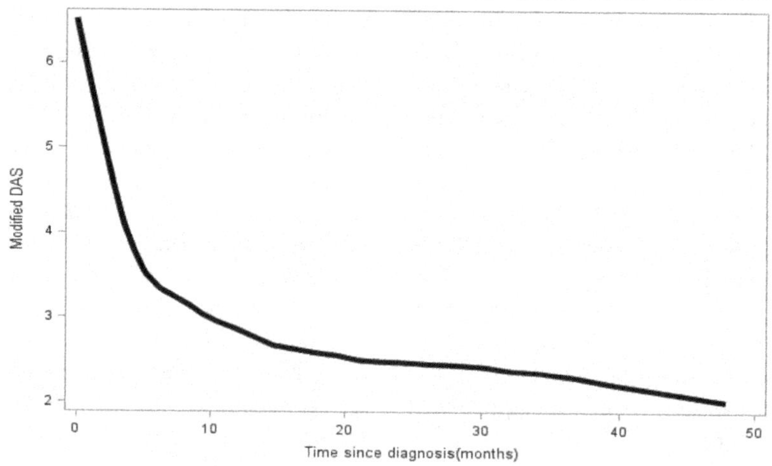

Fig. 1 Population-averaged modified DAS trajectory in JDM patients (representation of GEE). Disease activity score, DAS. Total population = 95

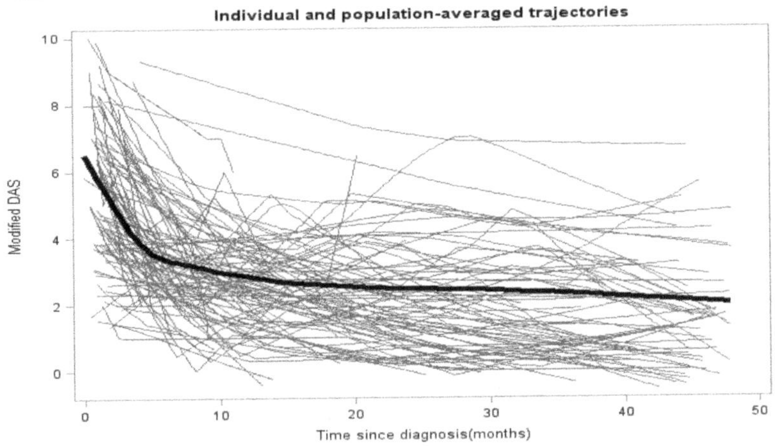

Fig. 2 Plot of all JDM patients' individual and the population-averaged modified DAS trajectories (representation of MRM). Disease activity score, DAS. Total population = 95

the results reported are that of the mean population trajectory in this case.

Although the results of the MRM may appear much like the GEE in continuous outcomes models, the interpretations are very different. The MRM models the average of individuals' trajectories (subject specific) but the GEE models the trajectory from DASm averages at each time point (population average). Practically, in the context of the continuous outcomes models, the forms and the results from the 2 models are very similar. The differences between MRM and GEE are obvious when the outcomes are non-continuous, e.g., binary or ordinal [9, 34–36]. Taking the example of a random intercepts (logistic) MRM, where the outcome could be disease remission (yes/no), and a time-invariant covariate could be calcinosis at baseline (yes/ no), the odds of remission would correspond to the effect of calcinosis plus an individual's random effects. The effect of calcinosis therefore changes with different individuals. The odds ratios estimated by the logistic MRM are subject specific as these additionally adjust for heterogeneity between individuals. In the binary outcome GEE, the odds ratio corresponds to odds of an event among those with baseline calcinosis divided by the odds of an event in those without. As these are ratios of subpopulation risks, the GEE estimates are termed population average. From this, it should also be obvious that the results of non-continuous MRM will always be greater that than of non-continuous GEE due to inclusion of the random effects. The choice of model depends on the purposes of the study. If the mean prevalence of disease remission in a population over time predicted by baseline calcinosis is of interest, the GEE is suitable. If the investigators want to *study individuals' risk factors for personal predictions*, then the MRM is the model of choice. As the estimates of the MRM are adjusted for random effects (unobserved individual characteristics), the results reflect the effect of baseline calcinosis status of an individual with a specific random effect (or individuals with the same random effect).

Question 2b: How do we predict the disease activity course of an individual with JDM?

i) Time-invariant prognostic factor
   The MRM can be used to determine the individual level predictive effect of a time-invariant prognostic factor, such as the baseline DASm (bDAS), on the trajectory of disease activity. From Fig. 3, we can see that the average trajectory for individuals with a higher bDAS had a faster initial improvement

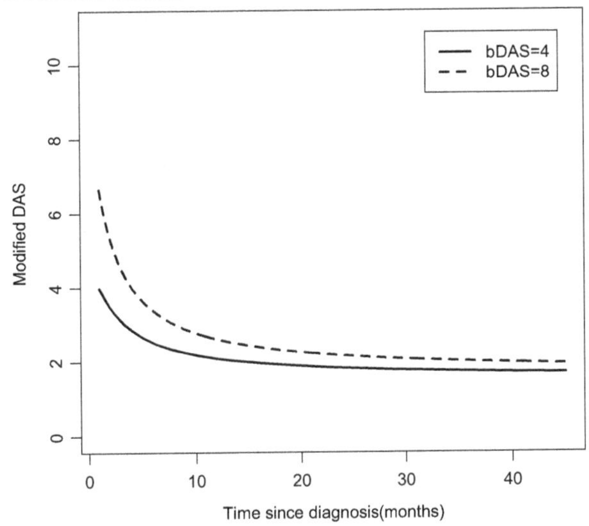

Fig. 3 Effect of baseline (time-invariant) modified DAS on the modified DAS trajectory in JDM patients (MRM). Activity Score, DAS; Baseline modified DAS (bDAS)

(up to month 10) followed by persistently higher activity, compared to the average trajectory of individuals with a lower bDAS ($p < 0.0001$). Baseline state therefore predicted the rate of change of the slope of the trajectory. We can therefore tell patients that their disease activity will likely improve within 1 year (with treatment). Those who are more active initially (higher bDAS) will likely see a relatively faster improvement in their symptoms compared to those who are less weak.

ii) Time-varying prognostic factor
Using the MRM, we tested the individual level effects of time-varying prognostic factors, including corticosteroid and methotrexate exposures from 3, 6 and 12 months before each visit. In this case, the time-varying predictors tested did not influence the DASm trajectory. Had these time-varying predictors been significant, their effects would have been to shift the trajectory up or down, corresponding to slower or faster resolution of disease activity.
In summary, if the primary interest of a study is to understand how covariates impact disease course, based on the *individual* patient's prognosis trajectory, the MRM is the best choice. The MRM is also more suitable when there is significant heterogeneity in individuals' disease courses in the population.

Question 3a: Are there different patterns (or subgroups) of disease activity course among individuals with JDM?

The models used in the preceding sections assumed that the shape of patient trajectories were homogenous, i.e., all patients follow the same disease course. If the investigator suspects that his study population contains heterogeneous patient trajectories, then latent class trajectory analysis (LCTA) (Additional file 1: Appendix) can be used to identify distinct subgroups with different disease trajectories (those with a clinically distinct prognosis) [10, 37].

When we applied LCTA to our cohort, we found three distinct subclasses. Each of these three subclasses has a class-specific average population disease activity trajectory, derived using individuals' trajectories (with the MRM as in question 2a). From Fig. 4, we can see that Class 2 patients have high disease activity at diagnosis, and then rapidly improve. Class 1 patients have moderate disease activity at diagnosis that improves gradually to low disease activity over time. Class 3 patients have high disease activity at diagnosis that improves very gradually. For this kind of model, we determine a probability of belonging in each of the three classes but for each individual, but the probability of any individual of belonging to each class varies. When classified according to the highest probability of class

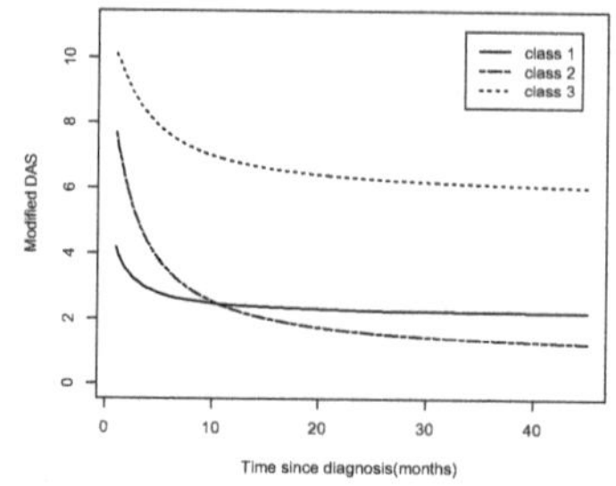

Fig. 4 Latent classes of JDM disease activity trajectories (LCTA). Disease Activity Score, DAS. Class 1, $n = 49$; Class 2, $n = 43$; Class 3, $n = 3$

membership for each individual, 42% are in class 1, 55% in class 2 and 3% in class 3. None of the patients was classified into 2 classes with similar probabilities, i.e., was ambiguous in the class membership probability (see Additional file 1: Appendix).

The LCTA is very flexible (Additional file 1: Appendix): 1) More than one and more than one kind of outcome trajectory can be modelled at a time (see next section); and 2) Trajectories of different subclasses can take on different shapes (reflecting different patterns of outcome evolutions) [37–39].

Question 3b: What factors predict an individual's membership in the different subgroups of disease activity?

The LCTA allows us to study the effects of time-invariant baseline factors, such as bDAS, in predicting membership in distinct subgroups. We use the bDAS to predict membership in the three subclasses. The higher the bDAS, the less likely is a patient to belong in class 1 (OR 0.11, 95% CI 0.02-0.63) or 2 (OR 0.27, 95% CI 0.05-1.41) compared to class 3. Furthermore, the higher the bDAS, the less likely is a patient to belong to class 1 (OR 0.41, 95% CI 0.25-0.68) compared to class 2. This means that those with highest bDAS are most likely to belong to class 3, with chronic high-grade disease activity. High bDAS patients are less likely to improve substantially or go into low disease activity states unlike those whose initial bDAS are low to moderate. This may appear different from the results of MRM where high bDAS predicted quicker resolution. In MRM, the whole population was studied together although there was significant heterogeneity within the population. LCTA allows us to group patients into more homogeneous subgroups and then more precisely clarify the effect of potential baseline membership predictors.

Time-varying covariates can also be studied in LCTA and can be formulated in different ways depending on the underlying question [40, 41]. As the computations are very complex and interpretations challenging, we chose to leave out time-varying covariates for this review.

In summary, if a researcher suspects that there are several prognostic subgroups within the study population, the LCTA can be used to identify these subpopulations. Baseline factors may identify patients' memberships in different prognostic subpopulations, thus allowing more individualized management. Time-varying covariates can also be studied but interpretations are more complex (Additional file 1: Appendix).

Question 4a: What are the separate disease activity courses for the skin and musculoskeletal components of JDM and what is the relationship between these two disease components?

In this case, we have two potential outcomes: the modified skin (SDAS) and musculoskeletal (MDAS) components of JDM. We are interested in how the disease courses evolve over time and the correlation of disease activity in the two components of JDM over time. The best way to study how two different outcomes evolve simultaneously over time is a joint model as shown in Fig. 5 (Additional file 1: Appendix) [12–14, 42, 43]. The joint model refers to the concurrent modeling of two outcome trajectories (SDAS and MDAS) in one model. The basic model used here to model the trajectories is also the MRM.

The two disease components of JDM follow different trajectories. The MDAS improves more rapidly (within the first 10 months after diagnosis) to minimal activity. In contrast, the SDAS improves less rapidly and persists at a low activity level for almost 20 months (Fig. 5). The two disease components therefore follow discordant courses, as confirmed by the low correlation between the two trajectories ($r = 0.32$) [13]. This relationship between two or more outcome trajectories can only be studied using the joint model and not by using separate models for the individual components.

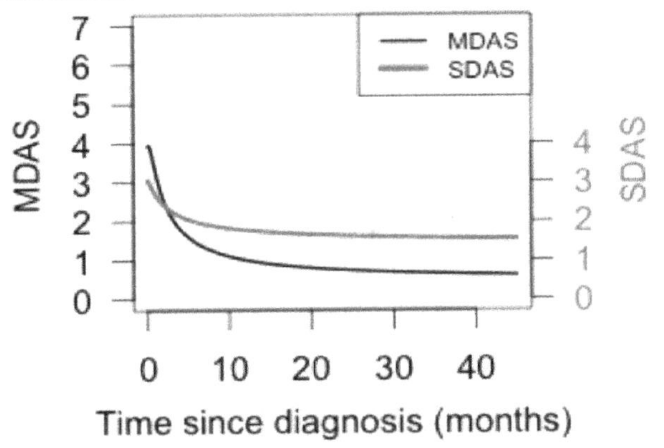

Fig. 5 Musculoskeletal and skin disease activity trajectories in JDM (joint multivariate modeling). Disease Activity Scores, DAS; Musculoskeletal DAS, MDAS; Skin DAS, SDAS. MDAS and SDAS are components of the modified DAS. The left y axis (*black*) represented the MDAS (maximum score = 7) and the right y-axis (*grey*) represented the SDAS (maximum score = 4). The MDAS and SDAS curves are colour coded to match their respective axes

In our example above, both outcomes were treated as continuous outcomes. However, outcomes of different natures can be jointly modeled. We can model a continuous outcome (e.g., DASm), with a time-to-event outcome (e.g., calcinosis), a binary outcome (e.g., nailfold capillary abnormality) or a count (e.g., active joint count). Furthermore, as alluded to previously, more than one outcome can be jointly studied in the LCTA; in this case, members within the same subclass of joint outcomes would have similar trajectories or risk of events [38, 39, 44]. This way of examining outcomes more closely resembles the real world where several clinically relevant outcomes may be considered equally important in clinical decision making.

Question 4b: What factor(s) predicts the joint disease activity courses of the skin and musculoskeletal components of disease in an individual with JDM?

We evaluated the predictive effects of bDAS (time-invariant) on the joint MDAS and SDAS trajectories (Table 1). In this joint model, individuals with higher bDAS have a faster decline in the slope of the MDASm trajectory; but bDAS does not significantly affect the slope of the SDAS trajectory. Prior treatment with methotrexate or steroid (time-varying factors) does not significantly influence the MDAS and SDAS trajectories, perhaps because everyone received the same protocol of treatment. Thus, joint modeling can distinguish the prognostic effects of predictors for the major components of JDM disease activity.

In summary, if a researcher is interested in more than one (or more than one kind of) outcome and wants to evaluate the relationship (i.e., correlation) among these

Table 1 Predictors identified from the joint multivariate model of MDAS and SDAS

Predictor	Outcome	Predictor Estimate	Standard Error	p
bDAS	MDAS	0.0363	0.0316	0.25
	SDAS	0.0214	0.0342	0.53
Time[a]*bDAS	MDAS	1.0140	0.1321	**<0.0001**
	SDAS	0.0362	0.1261	0.77
Steroid[b]	MDAS	-0.0919	0.0753	0.22
	SDAS	0.1211	0.0688	0.08

bDAS Baseline DASm measurement; Time *bDAS denotes the crossing of a time term with bDAS
[a]The shapes of the MDAS and SDAS models are defined using 2 time terms each (fractional polynomials). MDAS and SDAS crossed with their common time form ($p = -1$,) of their respective fractional polynomials (see Additional file 1: Appendix)
[b]Steroid treatment from 3 months before each occasion of DASm measurement, i.e., it is a time-varying predictor. Significant results have been bolded

outcomes over time, the joint model can be used. The joint model can be used in the LCTA context so that latent classes of the different outcomes of interest can be delineated. The joint model also allows direct comparisons of the differing effects of the same predictors on multiple outcomes simultaneously.

Conclusions

In this paper, we have illustrated the use of longitudinal design and analysis in studying prognosis. Longitudinal studies are superior to cross-sectional studies as they use all available data, thereby giving a more complete view of patients' outcomes.

We have presented four different ways of analyzing longitudinal observational data depending on the question(s) of interest. The GEE is best used if a population-level view is preferred and the visit schedule is not related to the outcome studied. This population view may be more relevant to health services researchers addressing population level questions, e.g., healthcare utilization. The MRM should be used if an individual level view is of interest. The LCTA should be used when the researcher wants to identify subgroups of patients within a heterogeneous cohort, with different outcome trajectories, and identify the factors predicting their membership in these subgroups. Joint modeling is best used to study the evolution and correlation among multiple outcome trajectories and the differing effects of predictors on simultaneous multiple outcome trajectories. We have summarized salient points about the four models in an overview table (Table 2). These four methods can also be combined with other methods, e.g., propensity scoring [45] and marginal structural modeling [46], to answer other kinds of questions (e.g., therapeutic) in a longitudinal study [47].

While the methods presented in this paper have the potential to transform our understanding of prognosis, we acknowledge that these methods could be challenging to use without necessary expertise. We therefore recommend consulting with biostatisticians knowledgeable in these methods to help design and analyze longitudinal studies. Our review is not meant to be an exhaustive review of all available longitudinal analytic methods. For example, Markov multistate models can also be used to determine patients' transition between disease states longitudinally [15]. In the interest of simplicity, we tested a minimum number and kind of predictors in these models. In practice, more predictors can be tested in these models, with a far greater confidence in predicting individuals' disease trajectories.

The methods outlined in this paper will allow for a more complete understanding of longitudinal outcomes and a more precise understanding of the effects of

Table 2 Overview of the 4 modern longitudinal analytic methods

Model	Questions	Advantages	Disadvantages
GEE	What is the averaged outcome trajectory for the population? (Trajectory of averages)	Parameter estimates robust to misspecification of the covariance structure. Both time-invariant and time-varying predictors can be studied.	No individual level inference Assumes missing data to be missing completely at random (MCAR), which may not be true for many longitudinal studies.
MRM	What is the outcome trajectory of the individual? What is the average outcome trajectory for the population? (Average of trajectories)	Individual level inference possible with the incorporation of random effects. Both time-invariant and time-varying predictors can be studied. Assumes missing data to be missing at random (MAR), which is more likely in longitudinal studies.	Misspecification of covariance structure may bias parameter estimates[45]
LCTA[a]	Are there distinct subgroups within the study population? What are the trajectories of the identifiable subgroups within the population?	Objectively identifies latent distinct subgroups within a heterogenous population. Able to use time-invariant factors to predict group membership. Able to study effects of time-varying covariates in different ways (depending on question and underlying theoretical framework) Assumes data to be missing at random (MAR).	Complex and time-consuming computing procedures. Interpretation of time-varying covariates can be challenging depending on the formulation.
Joint Model[b]	What are the trajectories of (multiple) outcomes of interest? What is the correlation between the outcome trajectories of interest (i.e., are the trajectories concordant or discordant)?	Multiple outcome trajectories of disparate nature (e.g., continuous with binary, binary-poisson, continuous-survival) can be studied simultaneously. Objective determination of the longitudinal correlation of the trajectories. Joint model with time-to-dropout may be used as a means to adjust for data missing not at random (MNAR).	Modeling procedures can be complex with increasing number and kinds of outcomes modeled jointly.

[a]Usually modeled with MRM as the base model
[b]MRM may be used as the base model for continuous, binary and count data. Proportional hazard is used for time-to-event outcomes

predictors. Combination of these methods with molecular information holds great potential to transform clinical practice towards the ultimate goal of precision medicine.

Abbreviations

bDAS: Baseline disease activity score; DASm: Modified disease activity score; GEE: Generalized estimating equation; JDM: Juvenile dermatomyositis; LCTA: Latent class trajectory analysis; MANOVA: Multivariate analysis of variance; MDAS: Musculoskeletal disease activity score; MRM: Mixed effects regression model; RANOVA: Repeated measures analysis of variance; SDAS: Skin-disease activity score

Acknowledgements

Not applicable.

Funding

The Canadian Institute of Health Research (CIHR) and the SickKids clinician-scientist training program funded Dr Lim's salary and research for this work.

Authors' contributions

LL, RM, EP, BF conceptualized the design of the study. LL and BF acquired the clinical data. LL, RM and EP were involved in the analysis of data. All authors were involved in the interpretation of data, drafting and revision of the manuscript. All authors read and approved the final manuscript.

Competing interests

The authors declared that they have no competing interests.

Consent for publication

Not applicable.

Author details

[1]Children's Hospital Research Institute of Manitoba, University of Manitoba, Winnipeg, Canada. [2]Department of Pediatrics, University of Manitoba, Winnipeg, Canada. [3]Institute of Health Policy Management and Evaluation, University of Toronto, Toronto, Canada. [4]The Child Health Evaluative Sciences Program, SickKids Research Institute, Toronto, Canada. [5]Department of Family and Community Medicine, University of Toronto, Toronto, Canada. [6]Department of Medicine, Toronto Western Research Institute, University of Toronto, Toronto, Canada. [7]Centre for Prognosis Studies, University Health Network, Toronto Western Hospital, Toronto, Canada. [8]Division of Rheumatology, SickKids, Toronto, Canada. [9]Physiology and Experimental Medicine Program, SickKids Research Institute, Toronto, Canada. [10]Department of Pediatrics and Immunology, University of Toronto, Toronto, Canada. [11]The Dalla Lana School of Public Health, University of Toronto, Toronto, Canada.

References

1. Singer JD, Willett JB. Applied Longitudinal Data Analysis- Modeling Change and Event Occurrence. New York: Oxford University Press; 2003.
2. Verkleij SP, Hoekstra T, Rozendaal RM, Waarsing JH, Koes BW, Luijsterburg PA, Bierma-Zeinstra SM. Defining discriminative pain trajectories in hip osteoarthritis over a 2-year time period. Ann Rheum Dis. 2012;71:1517–23.
3. Petri M, Purvey S, Fang H, Magder LS. Predictors of organ damage in systemic lupus erythematosus: the Hopkins Lupus Cohort. Arthritis Rheum. 2012;64:4021–8.
4. Holla JF, van der Leeden M, Heymans MW, Roorda LD, Bierma-Zeinstra SM, Boers M, Lems WF, Steultjens MP, Dekker J. Three trajectories of activity limitations in early symptomatic knee osteoarthritis: a 5-year follow-up study. Ann Rheum Dis. 2014;73:1369–75.
5. Winer B. Statistical Principles in Experimental Design. New York: McGraw-Hill; 1971.
6. Bock R. Multivariate Statistical Methods in Behavioral Research. New York: McGraw-Hill; 1975.
7. Zeger SL, Liang KY, Albert PS. Models for longitudinal data: a generalized estimating equation approach. Biometrics. 1988;44:1049–60.
8. Raudenbush SW, Chan WS. Application of a hierarchical linear model to the study of adolescent deviance in an overlapping cohort design. J Consult Clin Psychol. 1993;61:941–51.
9. Gibbons RD, Hedeker D, DuToit S. Advances in analysis of longitudinal data. Annu Rev Clin Psychol. 2010;6:79–107.
10. Muthen B, Shedden K. Finite mixture modeling with mixture outcomes using the EM algorithm. Biometrics. 1999;55:463–9.
11. Nagin D. Analyzing developmental trajectories: a semiparametric, group-based approach. Psychol Methods. 1999;4:139–57.
12. Diggle PJ, Sousa I, Chetwynd AG. Joint modelling of repeated measurements and time-to-event outcomes: the fourth Armitage lecture. Stat Med. 2008;27:2981–98.
13. Fieuws S, Verbeke G. Joint modelling of multivariate longitudinal profiles: pitfalls of the random-effects approach. Stat Med. 2004;23:3093–104.
14. Tsiatis A, Davidian M. Joint modeling of longitudinal and time-to-event data: an overview. Statistica Sinica. 2004;14:809–34.
15. Commenges D. Multi-state models in epidemiology. Lifetime Data Anal. 1999;5:315–27.
16. Twisk JWR. Applied Longitudinal Data Analysis for Epidemiology. A Practical Guide. New York: Cambridge University Press; 2003.
17. Hedeker D, Gibbons RD. Longitudinal Data Analysis. Hoboken: Wiley; 2006.
18. Cooley WW, Lohnes PR. Multivariate Data Analysis. New York: Wiley; 1971.
19. Muthen B, Asparouhov T, Hunter AM, Leuchter AF. Growth modeling with nonignorable dropout: alternative analyses of the STAR*D antidepressant trial. Psychol Methods. 2011;16:17–33.
20. Bowyer SL, Blane CE, Sullivan DB, Cassidy JT. Childhood dermatomyositis: factors predicting functional outcome and development of dystrophic calcification. J Pediatr. 1983;103:882–8.
21. Bronner IM, van der Meulen MFG, de Visser M, Kalmijn S, van Venrooij WJ, Voskuyl AE, Dinant HJ, Linssen WHJP, Wokke JHJ, Hoogendijk JE. Long-term outcome in polymyositis and dermatomyositis. Ann Rheum Dis. 2006;65: 1456–61.
22. Spencer CH, Hanson V, Singsen BH, Bernstein BH, Kornreich HK, King KK. Course of treated juvenile dermatomyositis. J Pediatr. 1984;105:399–408.
23. Stringer E, Singh-Grewal D, Feldman BM. Predicting the course of juvenile dermatomyositis: significance of early clinical and laboratory features. [Erratum appears in Arthritis Rheum. 2008 Dec;58(12):3950]. Arthritis Rheum. 2008;58:3585–92.
24. Huber AM, Lang B, LeBlanc CM, Birdi N, Bolaria RK, Malleson P, MacNeil I, Momy JA, Avery G, Feldman BM. Medium- and long-term functional outcomes in a multicenter cohort of children with juvenile dermatomyositis. Arthritis Rheum. 2000;43:541–9.
25. Sanner H, Gran J-T, Sjaastad I, Flato B. Cumulative organ damage and prognostic factors in juvenile dermatomyositis: a cross-sectional study median 16.8 years after symptom onset. Rheumatology. 2009;48:1541–7.
26. Ramanan AV, Campbell-Webster N, Ota S, Parker S, Tran D, Tyrrell PN, Cameron B, Spiegel L, Schneider R, Laxer RM, et al. The effectiveness of treating juvenile dermatomyositis with methotrexate and aggressively tapered corticosteroids. Arthritis Rheum. 2005;52:3570–8.
27. Schmeling H, Stephens S, Goia C, Manlhiot C, Schneider R, Luthra S, Stringer E, Feldman BM. Nailfold capillary density is importantly associated over time with muscle and skin disease activity in juvenile dermatomyositis. Rheumatology. 2011;50:885–93.
28. Pachman LM. Imperfect indications of disease activity in juvenile dermatomyositis. J Rheumatol. 1995;22:193–7.
29. Preisser JS, Lohman KK, Rathouz PJ. Performance of weighted estimating equations for longitudinal binary data with drop-outs missing at random. Stat Med. 2002;21(20):3035–54.

30. Lim LS, Lee SJ, Feldman BM, Gladman DD, Pullenayegum E, Uleryk E, Silverman ED. A systematic review of the quality of prognosis studies in systemic lupus erythematosus. Arthritis Care Res. 2014;66:1536–41.
31. Diggle P, Heagerty P, Liang KY, Zeger S. Analysis of Longitudinal Data. 2nd ed. Oxford: Oxford University Press; 2002.
32. Cleveland WS, Devlin SJ, Grosse E. Regression by local fitting. J Econ. 1988;37:87–114.
33. Bryk AS, Raudenbush SW. Hierarchical Linear Models: Applications and Data Analysis Methods. Newbury Park: Sage Publications; 1992.
34. Carrière I, Bouyer J. Choosing marginal or random-effects models for longitudinal binary responses: application to self-reported disability among older persons. BMC Med Res Methodol. 2002;2:15.
35. Fitzmaurice GM, Laird NM, Ware JH. Applied longitudinal analysis. Hoboken: Wiley; 2012.
36. Hu FB, Goldberg J, Hedeker D, Flay BR, Pentz MA. Comparison of population-averaged and subject-specific approaches for analyzing repeated binary outcomes. Am J Epidemiol. 1998;147:694–703.
37. Neelon B, Swamy GK, Burgette LF, Miranda ML. A Bayesian growth mixture model to examine maternal hypertension and birth outcomes. Stat Med. 2011;30:2721–35.
38. Elliott MR, Gallo JJ, Ten Have TR, Bogner HR, Katz IR. Using a Bayesian latent growth curve model to identify trajectories of positive affect and negative events following myocardial infarction. Biostatistics. 2005;6:119–43.
39. Leiby BE. Identification of multivariate responders and non-responders by using Bayesian growth curve latent class models. Appl Statist. 2009;2009:505–24.
40. Proust-Lima C, Letenneur L, Jacqmin-Gadda H. A nonlinear latent class model for joint analysis of multivariate longitudinal data and a binary outcome. Stat Med. 2007;2007:2229–45.
41. Lin H, Han L, Peduzzi PN, Murphy TE, Gill TM, Allore HG. A dynamic trajectory class model for intensive longitudinal categorical outcome. Stat Med. 2014;33:2645–64.
42. Fieuws S, Verbeke G. Pairwise fitting of mixed models for the joint modeling of multivariate longitudinal profiles. Biometrics. 2006;62:424–31.
43. Hogan JW, Laird NM. Increasing efficiency from censored survival data by using random effects to model longitudinal covariates. Stat Methods Med Res. 1998;7:28–48.
44. Proust-Lima C, Sene M, Taylor JM, Jacqmin-Gadda H. Joint latent class models for longitudinal and time-to-event data: a review. Stat Methods Med Res. 2014;23:74–90.
45. Dehejia RH, Wahba S. Propensity score-matching methods for nonexperimental causal studies. Rev Econ Stat. 2002;84(1):151–61.
46. Robins JM, Hernan M, Brumback B. Marginal structural models and causal inference in epidemiology. Epidemiology. 2000;11:550–60.
47. Faries DE, Leon AC, Haro JM, Obenchain RL. Analysis of Observational Health Care Data Using SAS. Cary: SAS Institute Inc; 2010.

5

Health-related quality of life among Swedish children with Juvenile Idiopathic Arthritis: parent–child discrepancies, gender differences and comparison with a European cohort

Veronica Lundberg* and Catharina Eriksson

Abstract

Background: This study investigates gender differences in self-reports and between parent and child reports in Health-related Quality of Life (HRQOL), measured with disease-specific and generic instruments for chronic disease. Comparison of HRQOL results in this Juvenile Idiopathic Arthritis (JIA) sample to a European cohort of children with JIA and one of children with other health conditions are also made.

Methods: Fifty-three children with juvenile idiopathic arthritis (JIA), aged 8–18 years, and their parents completed the condition-specific DISABKIDS for JIA, and the DISABKIDS generic instrument for chronic conditions (DCGM-37) in a cross-sectional study. European reference data were used for comparison of child and parental reports.

Results: Child self-reports in DCGM-37 and DISABKIDS for JIA showed no gender differences. Parental and child reports of the child's HRQOL differed only in DCGM-37; this was among girls who scored their independence ($p = 0.03$), physical limitation ($p = 0.01$), social exclusion ($p = 0.03$), emotions ($p < 0.01$), and general transformed score ($p < 0.01$) higher than did their parents. Our sample of children with JIA reported more physical limitation compared to samples of European children with JIA ($p = 0.01$), European children with chronic conditions ($p < 0.01$), and their parents ($p = 0.01$ and $p < 0.01$). The Swedish children reported more problem with understanding compared to the European JIA sample ($p = 0.03$). Swedish parents perceived their children's independence significantly lower than did the European parents of JIA children ($p < 0.01$), as well as European parents of children with chronic conditions ($p = 0.03$). The Swedish parents also perceived their children to have significantly lower social inclusion ($p < 0.05$) and general transformed score ($p = 0.04$), in comparison to European parents of children with chronic conditions.

Conclusions: Parent–child differences in assessment of quality of life depend on the HRQOL instrument used, especially among girls. In comparison to European cohorts, our sample of children with JIA experienced more physical limitations and less understanding.

Keywords: Gender, Informant discrepancies, Paediatrics, Questionnaire

* Correspondence: veronica.lundberg@vll.se
Department of Clinical Sciences, Pediatrics, Umeå University, SE 901 85 Umeå, Sweden

Background

Juvenile idiopathic arthritis (JIA) encompasses all forms of arthritis that begin before the age of 16 years, persists for more than 6 weeks, and are of unknown cause [1–3]. JIA is classified into seven disease subtypes by to the International League of Associations for Rheumatology (ILAR) [4]. Improvement in functional outcomes has been documented, and is due to progress in disease management [1]. Still, growing up with JIA can be associated with risk for numerous functional limitations, e.g., swollen joints, medication side effects, pain, fatigue [3, 5, 6], and visual impairment [3, 6]. Children with JIA are more likely to report a lower health related quality of life (HRQOL), compared to normative data [2, 3, 7].

HRQOL measures can be divided into condition-specific measures, generic, or generic instruments for chronic conditions. Condition-specific instruments address aspects related to a specific condition, its treatment, or symptoms. Generic instruments are suitable to measure HRQOL across both healthy populations and populations with medical health conditions, while generic instruments for chronic conditions assesses HRQOL only among children with various chronic health conditions. In our previous study, we used the generic HRQOL instrument Pediatric Quality of Life inventory (PedsQL) in the same sample as in this present article, and found that more than half of girls and boys with JIA experienced suboptimal HRQOL compared to a healthy population [7].

Differences between self-report and parent-report (proxy-rater) has been demonstrated in HRQOL measurements of children with and without health conditions [8, 9]. However, there are mixed findings in earlier studies that consider gender differences in parental versus child reports. They suggest that a child's gender may not be related to informant discrepancies, except in specific populations [10]. Our previous study showed gender differences between parent and child self-reports for the child HRQOL in JIA children, measured with the generic PedsQL. The most significant differences were among girls, who rated their HRQOL better in most subdomains compared to their parents [7].

To our knowledge, there have been no studies that evaluate parent–child discrepancies among different types of HRQOL instruments, e.g., disease-specific and generic HRQOL instruments for chronic conditions.

Objectives

The primary aims of the present study were to evaluate child self-reported and parent-reported HRQOL with instruments for chronic conditions, and a condition-specific HRQOL instrument for JIA. We specifically wanted to evaluate for gender differences in HRQOL self-report, and to explore gender differences in parent report of a child's HRQOL. The secondary aims were to compare the HRQOL results in this JIA sample to a European cohort of children with JIA and one of children with other health conditions.

Methods

Study design and study population

This cross-sectional questionnaire survey included children and adolescents registered with a diagnosis of JIA at the Department of Child and Adolescent Medicine, Norrlands University Hospital, Umeå, Sweden. The study population included all eligible children, identified through clinical appointment schedules at routine outpatient appointments, between September 2009 and December 2010.

Participants

Eligibility criteria were children aged 8 to 18 years with a JIA diagnosis defined by the ILAR classification criteria [4]. Of 69 eligible children, 56 children and their parents agreed to participate. The reason for declining participation was unknown in six families, four parents said that their child only had small problems due to JIA, two cited a lack of time, and one child was discharged from the clinic. Three were excluded because of a missing parental report. Therefore, 53 children (38 girls and 15 boys) remained as the study group. Of the participating parents, 37 were mothers, 12 were fathers, and in four families the mothers and fathers completed the questionnaires together. For nine of the girls, at least one additional diagnosis was reported by the child or parent, i.e., uveitis, overweight, attention-deficit/hyperactivity disorder, asthma, dermatitis, Turners syndrome, celiac disease, Crohn's disease, or thyroid gland disease. Among five of the boys, at least one additional diagnosis was reported, i.e., asthma, allergy, panic disorder, Raynaud's syndrome, or lactose intolerance.

Measures

HRQOL

The DISABKIDS generic instrument for chronic conditions (DCGM-37) consists of 37 items assigned to six sub-scales: *independence, emotional, social inclusion, social exclusion, physical limitation,* and *medication.* DCGM-37 was tested in 2002–2003 cross-culturally in seven European countries, including Sweden. The findings with respect to internal consistency (Chronbachs'Alpha: 0.70–0.87 in child version and 0.77–0.90 in proxy version) and test-retest reliability (0.71–0.83) has been demonstrated. The results indicate that DCGM-37 is suitable for HRQOL comparisons in children and adolescents with different diseases and across cultures [11–13]. The condition-specific DISABKIDS for JIA addresses arthritis-specific symptoms and limitations. Its 12 items are assigned to two sub-scales: *impact,* and *understanding.* The internal consistency of each sub-scale was between 0.73 and 0.87, in a field study among children with JIA

[13]. Both the JIA DISABKIDS and DCGM-37 are suitable for use between ages 8 and 16 years. Each item relates to symptoms during the last four weeks, and was answered on a five-point Likert scale between 1 (never) to 5 (always). In our sample, when a child or parent registered an odd number, the score was rounded to the inferior option. The scale scores were transformed with the syntaxes for DISABKIDS scales, to a range of 0 to 100, with higher values indicating better HRQOL [12]. Both self-report and an equivalent parent version was included.

European reference data, obtained from the DISABKIDS manual [12] were used for comparison with the Swedish sample of JIA patients. The reference data, based on a field study, included a European cohort of $n = 148$ children with JIA, and a cohort of $n = 1152$ participants with the following chronic conditions; arthritis, asthma, atopic dermatitis, cerebral palsy, cystic fibrosis, diabetes and epilepsy [12].

Disability was measured by the Childhood Health Assessment Questionnaire (CHAQ) [14], composed of 30 items that measure eight functional areas. Each question was scored on a four-point scale between 0 (no difficulty) and 3 (unable to do). The question with the highest score determined the score for that functional area. The scores for each of the eight functional areas were averaged to calculate a Disability Index (DI) that ranged from 0 (no disability) to 3 (disabled) [14]. Suggested cut-off levels for disability are at medians of 0.13 (mild), 0.63 (mild-to-moderate), and 1.75 (moderate) [15]. The original CHAQ showed internal reliability (Chronbachs'Alpha 0.94) and test-retest reliability with Spearman's correlation coefficient of 0.8 and convergent validity between Kendall's tau; 0.54–.77. The Swedish version of CHAQ showed internal reliability of Cronbach's alpha 0.89, test-retest reliability for the disability index was high (r(S) =0.92, r(P) = 0.97; $p < 0.00001$) [14, 16].

Disease duration in years was calculated from medical record data, based on the date of diagnosis and according to ILAR classification criteria.

Disease activity was measured by a paediatric rheumatologist who assessed global disease activity into categories of no, mild, moderate, or high. Mild disease activity was defined as between no activity and moderate activity, moderate activity meant the child needed changes in medical therapy, and high activity captured severe immunologic and clinical activity. Also erythrocyte sedimentation rate (ESR) in mm/hour was used.

Medications were compiled into four categories: 1) disease modifying anti-rheumatic drugs (DMARDs), e.g., azathioprine, cyclosporine, hydroxychloroquine, methotrexate, and sulfasalazine; 2) non-steroidal anti-inflammatory drugs (NSAIDs); 3) biological medications, e.g., adalimumab, anakinra, etanercept, infliximab and rituximab; and 4) corticosteroid therapy (Table 1).

Procedures

Families who agreed to participate in the study completed a mental health questionnaire; the Strengths and Difficulties Questionnaire and three HRQOL questionnaires, of which the DISABKIDS for JIA and the DCGM-37 were included in this study. The third HRQOL questionnaire, PedsQL is presented in an earlier article [7]. All these questionnaires were answered prior to a scheduled medical visit at the paediatric outpatient clinic. Parents and children completed the questionnaires separately, and a research assistant was available for the child. The CHAQ is used routinely in clinical practice, and was answered by children and their parents at home before the outpatient clinic visit. Estimated time to complete all of the study questionnaires was 20–40 min for each child, plus another ten minutes for the CHAQ to be completed at home. Nor the children or parents were reimbursed for their time participating in this study.

Statistics

Data from girls, boys, and their parents were analysed separately and as one group. Results of the descriptive analysis are presented as median and range, or numbers (n) and percentages (%). HRQOL results are presented as mean, standard deviation (SD), median (Md), and range. Mann Whitney *U* test was used to analyse gender differences in characteristics and to compare the median of HRQOL between boys and girls. The Wilcoxon signed-rank test was used to analyse differences between self-reports and parental reports of HRQOL. Student's one sample *t*-test with hypothesized mean values obtained from the European reference data in tables 4–11, 4–12, 4–15, 4–16 and 4–278 in the DISABKIDS manual were used to evaluate for HRQOL differences between the Swedish JIA sample and European samples [12]. The analyses were performed using Statistical Package for the Social Sciences (SPSS) version 18, 19 and 22. Statistical significance was defined as $P < 0.05$.

Results

Sample characteristics

The 53 children with JIA had a median age of 14 years (range 8–18). The paediatric rheumatologist categorized no or low disease activity among 87% of the girls and 86% of the boys. Girls and boys differed significantly only in JIA sub-diagnosis (Table 1).

Generic HRQOL for chronic disease

There were gender differences between child self-report and parental report in DCGM-37. The girls and their parents differed significantly in the subscales of *independence, physical limitation, social exclusion, emotion*, and *general transformed score*. Among the boys, there were no

Table 1 Characteristics of 53 children with juvenile idiopathic arthritis aged 8–18 years

	Girls (*n* = 38)	Boys (*n* = 15)	*P*-value[a]
Age in years, Md (range)	13 (8–18)	15 (10–18)	0.51
8–12 years, *n* (%)	16 (42)	5 (33)	
13–18 years, *n* (%)	22 (58)	10 (67)	
CHAQ Disability Index[b], Md (range)	0.50 (0–2.75)	0.38 (0–1.38)	0.65
Categories, *n* (%)			0.56
None-mild	12 (32)	5 (33)	
Mild-moderate	9 (24)	5 (33)	
Moderate	13 (34)	5 (33)	
Severe	3 (8)		
Missing	1 (3)		
Pain VAS[c], 0–100 Md (range)	32 (0–93)	50 (0–99)	0.50
Well-being VAS[d], 0–100 Md (range)	22 (0–99)	27 (0–100)	0.75
ILAR diagnosis[e], ***n* (%)**			*0.01*
Systemic arthritis	1 (3)	1 (7)	
Oligoarthritis	16 (42)	3 (20)	
Polyarticular arthritis, RF[f]-negative	2 (5)		
Polyarticular arthritis, RF[f]-positive	8 (21)	1 (7)	
Psoriatic arthritis	6 (16)		
Enthesitis-related arthritis	3 (8)	5 (33)	
Unspecified arthritis	2 (5)	5 (33)	
Physical education participation, *n* (%)			0.08
Always	12 (32)	9 (60)	
Sometimes	16 (42)	4 (27)	
Not at all	6 (16)	2 (13)	
Not relevant	3 (8)		
Missing	1 (3)		
Disease duration in years Md (range)	4.5 (0–16)	3.0 (0–13)	0.09
ESR[g], mm/hour, Md (range)	5 (2–31)	4 (2–35)	0.14
Disease activity categories, *n* (%)			0.37
No	13 (34)	8 (53)	
Low	20 (53)	5 (33)	
Moderate	4 (10)	2 (13)	
High	0	0	
Missing	1 (3)	0	
Medication at study visit[h], *n* (%)			
DMARD	24 (63)	7 (47)	0.70
NSAID	25 (66)	8 (53)	0.42
Biologic medication	4 (10)	0	
Corticosteroid therapy	7 (18)	0	
Eye drops/corticosteroid	2 (5)	0	

[a]Mann Whitney *U* test
[b]Childhood Health Assessment Questionnaire Disability Index
[c]Visual Analogue Scale for pain during the past week; 0 = no pain and 100 = very severe pain
[d]Visual Analogue Scale for assessment of overall well-being; 0 = very good and 100 = very bad
[e]JIA- diagnosis defined by the International League of Associations for Rheumatology (ILAR) classification criteria
[f]Rheumatoid factor
[g]Erythrocyte sedimentation rate
[h]Disease modifying anti-rheumatic drug (DMARD), Non-steroid anti-inflammatory drug (NSAID)

differences between self-reports and parental reports on any subscales or for the total scale score. There were no differences between girls' and boys' self-report for any of the six DCGM-37 subscales, total general transformed score, or the 37 specific questions included in the questionnaire. However, among the parents' answers in the DCGM-37 *social exclusion* dimension, parents of boys reported higher (better) child scores than did parents of girls ($P = 0.05$) (Table 2).

JIA-specific HRQOL

Children reported a mean condition-specific *impact* score of 60.30 (SD 22.21) and an *understanding* mean score of 60.58 (SD 24.15). The parental mean *impact* score was 57.98 (SD 21.34); the *understanding* mean score was 63.83 (SD 25.79). No significant differences between genders were found in the self-report for condition-specific DISABKIDS for JIA questionnaire, or between the children and their parents.

Comparison with the European reference data cohort

On the DCGM-37, the Swedish JIA children scored significantly lower on the *physical limitation* subscale than both the European JIA children ($P = 0.01$) or European children with chronic conditions ($P < 0.01$). The parents reported significantly lower scores on child *physical limitation* compared to European parents of JIA children ($P = 0.01$) or European parents of children with chronic conditions ($P < 0.01$). The Swedish parents perceived their children's *independence* to be significantly lower than the European parents of children with JIA ($P < 0.01$), as well as the European parents of children with a chronic condition ($P = 0.03$). In comparison to the Swedish sample, European parents of children with chronic conditions perceived their children to have significantly better *social inclusion* ($P < 0.05$) and general transformed score ($P = 0.04$) (Table 3).

In the JIA-specific HRQOL instrument, our Swedish JIA children rated the *understanding* scale significantly lower than the European JIA sample: 60.58 (SD 24.15) versus 67.75 (SD 26.73) ($P = 0.03$).

Discussion

We found no differences between parental and child reports with the condition-specific HRQOL instrument DISABKIDS for JIA. Nor did we find a gender difference in children's self-reports. However, there were gender differences between parental and child reporting in DCGM-37; girls reported significantly better scores on several HRQOL sub-scales compared with parental reports. This confirms our previous finding in this same sample when the generic instrument PedsQL was used [7]. In the generic questionnaire PedsQL, the parent–child differences were also evident among the girls, who tended to reported better physical health, psychosocial health, and total HRQOL compared to their parents' reports [7]. Also in accordance with our previous results [7], the boys tended to score lower on several HRQOL sub-scales, in both the conditions-specific DISABKIDS for JIA and the DCGM-37, compared to their parents. Such a scoring difference was not significant in the present study. Some authors found gender differences, with lower parent–child agreement in mental health between girls and their parents [10, 17], while others found inconsistent results [10]. Differences in agreement that depend on whether the mother or father is the proxy-rater were not explored in this study. A review by Upton et al. found a possible interaction of age and gender in parent–child agreement on HRQOL ratings; this depended on the gender of the parental proxy-rater. Fathers and mothers can have different perspectives on child health and behaviour, and sons and daughters might also differ in their relationship with each parents [8]. Mothers' and fathers' ratings correlate moderately, and bigger differences are seen between father/child ratings than for mother/child ratings [9].

Eiser et al. describe in their review, that a parent's own well-being may affect the report of their child's HRQOL and symptoms. If the parents report higher levels of emotional distress, they also report more negative perceptions of their child's HRQOL [9]. However, Haverman et al. found that the parents of children with JIA self-reported their own HRQOL similar to parents of healthy children [18]. Specific HRQOL subdomains are suggested to affect parent–child agreement, with better agreement in observable behaviours such as physical functioning than in internal symptoms such as pain, emotional distress, or fatigue [9]. For example, in the PedsQL the majority of items involve observable items and are suggested to reflect good agreement [8]. However, Upton et al. found divergent findings for parent–child agreement on specific subscales, e.g., observable characteristics such as physical health and social and emotional functioning in healthy children and children with different health conditions [8].

Child self-report may be more reliable for information regarding minor, short-term effects of treatment, moment-to-moment HRQOL and disease-specific symptoms, whereas parents report might reflects overall symptoms occurring over time [9, 19]. Children might also report more symptoms, but less impact of their perceived difficulties than do their parents [19]. In children with a diagnosed medical condition, parental involvement and understanding increases regarding their child's health issues and well-being [8, 9]. Even level of disease activity seems to affect parent–child agreement among children with polyarticular JIA. If the child had active disease, the parent–child agreement was higher than

Table 2 Health related quality of life measured with DISABKIDS generic instrument for chronic conditions (DCGM-37), and differences in self-report and parent-report

	Girls $n = 38$ Mean (SD)	Girls' parents $n = 38$ Mean (SD)		Boys $n = 15$ Mean (SD)	Boys' parents $n = 15$ Mean (SD)		Girls parents versus boys parents	Girls versus boys
	Median (range)	Median (range)	*P*-value[1]	Median (range)	Median (range)	*P*- Value[1]	*P*- Value[2]	*P*- Value[3]
Independence	75.66 (13.55)	69.71 (17.51)		71.11 (21.10)	75.28 (19.51)		0.23	0.67
	75.00 (50.00–100)	70.83 (29.17–100)	*0.03*	75.00 (25.00–100)	79.17 (20.83–100)	0.17		
Physical limitation	65.94 (21.04)	58.66 (22.25)	*0.01*	62.78 (24.42)	66.67 (24.14)	0.21	0.11	0.70
	66.67 (20.83–100)	54.17 (20.83–100)		62.50 (8.33–100)	70.83 (0.00–100)			
Social inclusion	70.94 (17.82)	66.99 (18.82)	0.18	69.72 (23.06)	72.94 (19.55)	0.67	0.19	0.92
	75.00 (37.50–100)	62.50 (37.50–100)		66.67 (20.83–100)	75.00 (20.83–100)			
Social exclusion	83.55 (15.59)	78.24 (19.11)	*0.03*	83.61 (17.64)	87.22 (21.45)	0.26	*0.05*	0.85
	87.50 (33.33–100)	81.25 (33.33–100)		87.50 (33.33–100)	91.67 (16.67–100)			
Emotion	75.99 (23.48)	67.09 (23.08)	*<0.01*	70.00 (22.66)	71.30 (26.02)	0.92	0.48	0.32
	82.14 (7.14–100)	66.07 (10.71–100)		67.86 (14.29–100)	78.57 (7.14–100)			
Medication	71.59 (25.67)	65.62 (2.93)	0.11	84.09 (15.68)	75.32 (18.28)	0.11	0.36	0.19
	77.08 (20.00–100)	75.00 (0.00–100)		87.50 (54.17–100)	79.17 (50.00–100)			
Missing[a]	6	2		4	2			
General transformed score	74.24 (16.13)	67.93 (17.59)	*<0.01*	73.31 (17.99)	74.89 (18.60)	0.90	0.16	0.94
	78.77 (37.50–100)	69.93 (30.41–96.8)		73.65 (29.05–100)	74.19 (23.65–100)			

[a]Missing referring medication
[1]Wilcoxon signed rank test. *P*-value between child and parent report
[2]Mann Whitney *U* test. *P*-value between parents of girls and parents of boys, with JIA
[3]Mann Whitney *U* test. *P*-value between girls and boys with JIA

Table 3 DISABKIDS generic instrument for chronic conditions (DCGM-37) in Swedish children aged 8–18 years, parents and a European sample aged 8–16 years

	Swedish Sample of JIA children $n = 53$ Mean (SD)	European sample of JIA children[1] $n = 148$ Mean	P-value[2]	European sample of children with chronic conditions[3] $n = 1.152$ Mean (SD)	P-value[4]	Swedish sample of parents of children with JIA $n = 53$ Mean (SD)	European sample of parents of children with JIA[5] $n = 141$ Mean	P-value[6]	European sample of parents of children with chronic conditions[7] $n = 1.152$ Mean (SD)	P-value[8]
Independ-ence	74.37 (15.96)	77.58	0.10	76.90 (18.34)	0.24	71.29 (18.09)	79.34	*<0.01*	76.60 (17.25)	*0.03*
Physical limitation	65.05 (21.85)	73.02	*0.01*	73.85 (18.23)	*<0.01*	60.92 (22.85)	68.54	*0.01*	70.19 (18.32)	*<0.01*
Social inclusion	70.60 (19.22)	72.86	0.37	75.25 (17.81)	0.10	68.68 (19.03)	72.59	0.10	74.28 (17.65)	*<0.05*
Social exclusion	83.57 (16.02)	85.79	0.27	85.15 (15.56)	0.52	80.78 (20.01)	82.69	0.42	80.91 (16.79)	0.94
Emotion	74.29 (23.19)	73.02	0.69	76.72 (20.56)	0.40	68.28 (23.78)	70.24	0.60	71.61 (20.49)	0.26
Medication	74.79 (23.98)	67.98	0.07	72.25 (22.71)	0.45	68.20 (25.12)	66.44	0.54	69.90 (22.15)	0.62
Missing[9]	10					4				
General transformed score	73.98 (16.51)	76.13	0.38	76.99 (14.22)	0.19	69.90 (17.98)	74.12	0.10	74.90 (14.55)	*0.04*

[1]European field study sample of children with arthritis (12) table 4–11
[2]One sample *t*-test. *P*-value between samples of Swedish JIA children and European JIA children
[3]European field study sample of children with chronic conditions: asthma, arthritis, dermatitis, diabetes, cerebral palsy, cystic fibrosis, epilepsy (12), table 4–15
[4]One sample *t*-test. *P*-value between Swedish sample of children with JIA and European sample of children with chronic conditions
[5]European field study sample of parents of children with JIA (12) table 4–12
[6]One sample *t*-test. *P*-value between Swedish sample of parents of children with JIA and European sample of parents of children with JIA
[7]European field study sample of parents of children with chronic conditions (12), table 4–16
[8]One sample *t*-test. *P*-value between Swedish parents of children with JIA and European parents of children with chronic conditions
[9]Missing referring medication

among children with inactive disease [20]. Parents of children with JIA might perceive their children as vulnerable, especially when the children have a shorter disease duration, higher degree of functional disability, or greater disease activity [18]. On the other hand, our sample of children did not differ in any of these characteristics. This view would therefore not explain the significant inter-rater differences on the DCGM-37 among girls. ILAR diagnosis was the only variable that differed among girls and boys in our sample. Parents are not in position to observe their children in environments outside the family, or how these influence the child's feelings and function on a daily basis. And this is especially true for school-aged children and adolescents [9]. Interrater agreement can depend on the developmental level and age of the child, as well as the characteristics of the illness [9]. Yet, the authors found divergent results in a review that compared parent–child agreement in relation to child's age. This ranged from no correlation with the child's age to lower concordance between parents and adolescent children [8]. Due to the small sample, we did not evaluate for age differences in our study.

The sub-scales in the condition-specific DISABKIDS for JIA are supposed to be sensitive to treatment and improvement of the condition. The subscales *impact* and *understanding* are related to the invisibility and fluctuation of JIA symptoms [12]. In comparison to the European sample of children with JIA, our Swedish sample rated their *understanding* subscale significantly lower. This implies greater feelings of social exclusion and lack of empathy by peers and teachers. This suggests that Swedish children with JIA need more interventions in health education within school-based services [12].

The Swedish children with JIA and their parents scored significantly lower on the child *physical limitation* DCGM-37 subscale compared to the European children with JIA, European children with chronic conditions, and their parents. This indicates that our sample of children with JIA experience more functional limitations that are caused by JIA, and might need targeting intervention regarding exercise training [12]. Children with JIA have reduced anaerobic capacity and muscle strength. This results in physical, mental, and metabolic disorders. Exercise training is beneficial for JIA children, and leads to improved muscle strength, range of motion, quality of life, and reduced joint stiffness, without affecting disease activity [21]. Therefore, preventing physical limitations and supporting exercise training is essential in JIA. The Swedish parents perceive their children's *independence* to be significantly lower compared to European parents of children with JIA, and European parents of children with a chronic condition. Compared to Swedish parents, European parents of children with chronic conditions perceive their children to have better *social inclusion* and a higher general transformed score. Comparison between these samples should be interpreted with caution since the characteristics and eventual comorbidity of the European samples are not described in detail [12]. A selection bias might therefore be evident, since the participants in the Swedish sample might not be exchangeable to those in the European cohort. The clinical relevance of different HRQOL domains may also vary between subgroups within broader disease groups like JIA. This makes meaningful comparisons difficult [8]. We do not know what demands our sample requires in daily life, or if these requirements differ between European countries; e.g., physical demands in school physical education classes, sports or recreational activities.

Possible bias in the results could be present because DISABKIDS assesses children 8–16 years of age, and we included children 8–18 years of age. The reason for including even 16–18 year old participants for us, were to evaluate for differences in parent–child discrepancies between three different HRQOL instruments; this present study and our previous study with the same sample [7]. Also, in our sample there was a relatively high frequency of comorbidity related to JIA or unrelated conditions. These may have influenced our results. Four children declined participation because they only had minor symptoms of JIA. This might have biased our results towards a lower HRQOL in some subscales. This sample size was small, especially among the boys. Only 15 boys were available for the study, and the comparisons involving the boys might therefore be underpowered. The multiple comparisons might also have resulted in significant results by chance. Other possible confounders such as socioeconomic status or parental education were not measured in this study.

Extensive attention has thus been given to examining informant characteristics that affect parent–child differences. Our results in the present and an earlier study show that the HRQOL instrument used can also influence parent–child differences in HRQOL. Differences, especially among girls, were evident in generic HRQOL measurement in our previous study [7], and in the DISABKIDS generic HRQOL instrument for chronic conditions in this study. But no differences were evident in the conditions specific HRQOL instrument DISABKIDS for JIA. To our knowledge this is the first study investigating parent–child proxy-rate discrepancies in different HRQOL instruments. Inconsistent or no differences exist for many of the child and parent characteristics reviewed in earlier studies (e.g., child's age, gender, problem type, HRQOL subdomains, social desirability, child and parent health, relationship) with regard to parent–child differences in reports of the child's HRQOL. Knowledge of all available research is essential to take into account when evaluating child self-report of HRQOL. Integrating and analysing all such variables into paediatric healthcare might be impractical. However, implementation of routine HRQOL measurements in clinical care is an important goal for assessment of paediatric patients with chronic health conditions like JIA. This is especially the case since JIA involves fluctuating disease-activity, long-term treatment, common medication side effects, social and physical limitations, and comorbidities related or unrelated to JIA. Facilitating child self-report is essential when one considers the many variables that can affect parent–child differences in HRQOL measurement. Child self-report should be complemented by parent-report in order to give a more complete report of the child's health.

We agree with other authors [8, 9], that information from both the child and parent provides a richer picture and invaluable information. Therefore, both need to be included whenever evaluating a child's HRQOL. If the child is unable to self-report, a condition specific HRQOL measurement like DISABKIDS for JIA, might be preferable for proxy-report and best reflect the child's own opinion of their HRQOL at the time of evaluation. Routine HRQOL measurement in the clinic can promote targeted interventions from healthcare professionals. For example, interventions could be directed toward the physical limitations and understanding evident in our sample.

Conclusions

Differences in parent vs. child self-report were evident among girls with JIA when measured with the generic instrument for chronic disease, DCGM-37. These results may indicate that parent–child differences depend on the type of HRQOL instrument used. There was no gender differences among children's self-report on any of the HRQOL instruments used in this study. In comparison to a European cohort, Swedish children with JIA experience more physical limitation and problems with understanding.

Acknowledgements
The authors wish to thank all of the children and families who participated in the study and Viveca Lindh for supporting the initial work and data collection.

Funding
This work was financially supported by the Majblomman Foundation.

Authors' contributions
VLU participated in conception and design of the study, in acquisition of data, analysis and interpretation of data, and in drafting of the manuscript. CEI contributed in conception and design of the study, in the analysis and interpretation of data, and in editing the manuscript. Both authors provided critical revision of the manuscript, read and gave final approval of the manuscript to be published.

Competing interests
The authors declare they have no competing interests.

Consent for publication
Not applicable.

References

1. Ravelli A, Martini A. Juvenile idiopathic arthritis. Lancet. 2007;369(9563):767–78.
2. Prince FH, Otten MH, van Suijlekom-Smit LW. Diagnosis and management of juvenile idiopathic arthritis. BMJ. 2010;341:c6434.
3. Moorthy LN, Peterson MG, Hassett AL, Lehman TJ. Burden of childhood-onset arthritis. Pediatr Rheumatol Online J. 2010;8:20.
4. Petty RE, Southwood TR, Baum J, et al. Revision of the proposed classification criteria for juvenile idiopathic arthritis: Durban, 1997. J Rheumatol. 1998;25(10):1991–4.
5. Eyckmans L, Hilderson D, Westhovens R, et al. What does it mean to grow up with juvenile idiopathic arthritis? A qualitative study on the perspectives of patients. Clin Rheumatol. 2011;30(4):459–65.
6. Miller-Hoover S. Juvenile idiopathic arthritis: why do I have to hurt so much? J Infus Nurs. 2005;28(6):385–91.
7. Lundberg V, Lindh V, Eriksson C, et al. Health-related quality of life in girls and boys with juvenile idiopathic arthritis: self- and parental reports in a cross-sectional study. Pediatr Rheumatol Online J. 2012;10(1):33.
8. Upton P, Lawford J, Eiser C. Parent–child agreement across child health-related quality of life instruments: a review of the literature. Qual Life Res. 2008;17(6):895–913.
9. Eiser C, Varni JW. Health-related quality of life and symptom reporting: similarities and differences between children and their parents. Eur J Pediatr. 2013;172(10):1299–304.
10. De Los Reyes A, Kazdin AE. Informant discrepancies in the assessment of childhood psychopathology: a critical review, theoretical framework, and recommendations for further study. Psychol Bull. 2005;131(4):483–509.
11. Simeoni M, Schmidt S, Muehlan H, et al. Field testing of a European quality of life instrument for children and adolescents with chronic conditions: the 37-item DISABKIDS Chronic Generic Module. Qual Life Res. 2007;16(5):881–93.
12. Schmidt S, Peterson C, Muhlan H, et al. The DISABKIDS Questionnaires-Handbook incl. CD-Rom. Lengerich: Pabst Science Publishers; 2006.
13. Baars R, Atherton C, Koopman H, et al. The European DISABKIDS project: development of seven condition-specific modules to measure health related quality of life in children and adolescents. Health Qual Life Outcomes. 2005;3:70.
14. Singh G, Athreya B, Fries J, Goldsmith D. Measurement of health status in children with juvenile rheumatoid arthritis. Arthritis Rheum. 1994;37(12): 1761–9.
15. Dempster H, Porepa M, Young N, Feldman BM. The clinical meaning of functional outcome scores in children with juvenile arthritis. Arthritis Rheum. 2001;44(8):1768–74.
16. Andersson Gäre B, Fasth A, Wiklund I. Measurement of functional status in juvenile chronic arthritis: evaluation of a Swedish version of the Childhood Health Assessment Questionnaire. Clin Exp Rheumatol. 1993;11(5):569–76.
17. Waters E, Stewart-Brown S, Fitzpatrick R. Agreement between adolescent self-report and parent reports of health and well-being: results of an epidemiological study. Child Care Health Dev. 2003;29(6):501–9.
18. Haverman L, van Oers HA, Maurice-Stam H, et al. Health related quality of life and parental perceptions of child vulnerability among parents of a child with juvenile idiopathic arthritis: results from a web-based survey. Pediatr Rheumatol Online J. 2014;12:34.
19. Van Roy B, Groholt B, Heyerdahl S, Clench-Aas J. Understanding discrepancies in parent–child reporting of emotional and behavioural problems: Effects of relational and socio-demographic factors. BMC Psychiatry. 2010;10:56.
20. Ringold S, Wallace CA, Rivara FP. Health-related quality of life, physical function, fatigue, and disease activity in children with established polyarticular juvenile idiopathic arthritis. J Rheumatol. 2009;36(6):1330–6.

6

Muscle MRI at the time of questionable disease flares in Juvenile Dermatomyositis (JDM)

Rabheh Abdul-Aziz[1,2*], Chack-Yung Yu[1], Brent Adler[1], Sharon Bout-Tabaku[1], Katherine E. Lintner[1], Melissa Moore-Clingenpeel[1] and Charles H. Spencer[1]

Abstract

Background: The course of JDM has improved substantially over the last 70 years with early and aggressive treatments. Yet it remains difficult to detect disease flares as symptoms may be mild; signs of rash and muscle weakness vary widely and are often equivocal; laboratory tests of muscle enzyme levels are often normal; electromyography and muscle biopsy are invasive. Alternative tools are needed to help decide if more aggressive treatment is needed. Our objective is to determine the effectiveness of muscle Magnetic Resonance Imaging (MRI) in detecting JDM flares, and how an MRI affects physician's decision-making regarding treatment.

Methods: This study was approved by the Institutional Review Board of Nationwide Children's Hospital. JDM patients were consulted between 1/2005 and 6/2015. MRIs were performed on both lower extremities without contrast sequentially: axial T1, axial T2 fat saturation, axial and coronal inversion recovery, and axial diffusion weighted. The physician decision that a JDM patient was in a flare was considered the gold standard. MRI results were compared with physician's decisions on whether a relapse had occurred, and if there was a concordance between the assessment methods.

Results: Forty-five JDM patients were studied. Eighty percent had weakness at diagnosis, 100% typical rash, and 73% typical nail-fold capillary changes. At diagnosis, muscle enzymes were compatible with JDM generally (CK 52%, LDH 62%, aldolase 72%, AST 54% abnormal). EMG was abnormal in 3/8, muscle biopsy typical of JDM in 10/11, and MRI abnormal demonstrating myositis in 31/40. Thirteen patients had a repeat MRI for possible flares with differing indications. Three repeat MRI's were abnormal, demonstrating myositis. There was moderate agreement about flares between MRI findings and physician's treatment decisions (kappa = 0.59). In each abnormal MRI case the physician decided to increase treatment (100% probability for flares). MRI was negative for myositis in 10 patients, by which 7/10 the physicians chose to continue or to taper the medications (70% probability for non-flares).

Conclusion: A muscle MRI would facilitate objective assessments of JDM flares. When an MRI shows myositis, physicians tend to treat 100% of the time. When an MRI shows no myositis, physicians continued the same medications or tapered medications 70% of the time. Further studies would help confirm the utility and cost-effectiveness of MRI to determine JDM flares.

Keywords: MRI, Juvenile dermatomyositis

* Correspondence: raziz@upa.chob.edu
[1]Nationwide Children's Hospital, 700 Children's Dr, Columbus, OH 43205, USA
[2]Women & Children's Hospital of Buffalo, 219 Bryant Street, Buffalo, NY 14222, USA

Background

Juvenile dermatomyositis (JDM) is a chronic multisystem disease of presumed autoimmune origin. JDM is the most common of the idiopathic inflammatory myopathies of childhood, comprising 85% of cases [1]. It affects primarily skin and muscle, with less frequent involvement of other organs, including cardiovascular system, gastrointestinal tract, and lungs [2]. Although the outcomes of JDM have improved over the last few decades, the disease is still associated with significant morbidity [3].

The significant morbidity of JDM necessitates earlier treatment, earlier identification of flares and optimal treatment to prevent the associated morbidity.

Traditionally, the diagnosis of JDM was based on the Bohan and Peter criteria [4, 5]. Definite JDM consists of classic skin involvement and at least three of the following: 1) proximal muscle weakness, 2) elevation of muscle enzyme (s), 3) myopathic changes on electromyography (EMG) and 4) abnormal muscle biopsy suggestive of inflammatory myopathy [4, 5]. Probable JDM is defined as patients who have the characteristic rash and fulfill only two of the above criteria.

An expanded definition with more criteria was proposed in 2006 using an international consensus survey [2]. These new criteria include: 1) typical findings on muscle magnetic resonance imaging (MRI) and ultrasonography, 2) nailfold capillaroscopy abnormalities, 3) calcinosis, and 4) dysphonia [2].

Disease course was divided into three groups according to patterns of active and inactive disease: monocyclic, polycyclic, and chronic continuous, based on previous descriptions in the literature [6, 7]. One of the determining factors in patient response to treatment is whether the patient develops a disease flare after treatment is begun. In some patients it is difficult to determine a flare. JDM patients are usually treated with prednisone for one year according to Consensus Treatments for moderate JDM (CTP protocol) [8]. However, one possible side effect of prednisone is muscle weakness, which could confound detection of muscle weakness caused by flare during treatment. This means that deciding whether the new muscle weakness is due to JDM flare, side effects of steroids, or other causes may be a clinical puzzle. Usually in such cases we perform muscle enzymes assays, but results for tests may be normal despite a disease flare [9]. In these cases MRI results can help confirm the presence of muscle inflammation. Judicious use of MRI may offer the potential for further improving the management of JDM as it can aid in the assessment of occult active disease and muscle damage.

MRI is a non-invasive and well-tolerated examination. It is radiation free, painless, and can be repeated and compared with the initial MRI at diagnosis. MRI is preferred over EMG for evaluation and diagnosis of JDM. MRI is sensitive in detecting muscle inflammation, but it is not specific to a diagnosis of myositis because muscular dystrophies and other myopathies may have associated edema on MRI [2]. The signal changes on imaging need to be interpreted in the context of the clinical setting.

There is limited data about the role of MRI to determine disease flares when the clinical assessment and muscle enzymes are equivocal. Malattia et al., compared whole-body MRI (WB-MRI) with clinical examination to assess disease activity in 41 JDM patients at presentation, which they repeated in 18 patients at a median follow-up of 9 months [10]. They concluded that WB-MRI provides additional information to clinical evaluation and represents a promising tool to estimate total inflammatory burden, tailor treatment, and monitor its efficacy. Follow-up WB-MRI showed resolution of inflammation in nine patients whereas clinical criteria for remission were satisfied in five [10]. Our objective here is to determine if lower extremity muscle MRI assists in determining whether patients with JDM are in a disease flare. We hypothesize that MRI of the muscles may facilitate diagnose if a patient is having a disease flare when clinical assessment and laboratory markers are equivocal.

Methods

This study protocol was approved by the Nationwide Children's Hospital (NCH) Institutional Review Board (IRB). Written parental consent and patient assent were obtained. Patients were identified by diagnostic codes of Juvenile Dermatomyositis (ICD 10 code M33.90 and ICD9 code 710.3). Patients were included in the study if they met the modified Bohan and Peter criteria including MRI evidence of myositis (modification introduced by the Childhood Arthritis and Rheumatology Research Alliance (CARRA) Registry investigators) (2, 5), and characterized in a recent publication [11]. We included two JDM-like patients with predominant skin manifestations. Both patients have typical JDM rash and capillary dilatation, but never had any clinical muscle weakness. We included these patients as they could present with rash and then develop weakness later. We excluded patients with myositis in association with other connective tissue diseases, such as scleroderma and the overlap syndromes. A flare is considered when patients have a recurrence of active disease after a definite remission.

We analyzed the medical records retrospectively of children with JDM at NCH from January 2005 to June 2015. The data were collected using the NCH electronic medical record for the patients followed after 2007 and the paper chart for the patients followed from 2005 to 2007. Data were entered into an electronic database and were stored using linked anonymous codes. We recorded the following data: demographics, clinical presentation at the onset and at the time of repeat MRI, laboratory and images results, and therapeutics used. We specifically recorded the result of initial MRI and the corresponding muscle enzyme levels at the time of initial MRI. We also recorded the result of follow-up MRI and the corresponding muscle enzyme levels at the time. Additionally, we recorded the patient's current treatment before and after the follow-up MRI. We looked at the sequence of following patients with flares including history, physical examination, levels of muscle enzymes, and we reviewed the physician assessment before and after the muscle MRI based on available chart information from the patient visits.

In our study, the MRI of both lower extremities was performed without gadolinium contrast utilizing the following sequences: axial T1, axial T2 fat saturation, axial and coronal inversion recovery, and axial diffusion weighted sequences.

Physician decisions to identify flares were considered the gold standard. Evidence of flare was noted by the presence of an active rash, a reduced childhood myositis assessment scale (CMAS) score for muscle weakness, and elevated levels of muscle enzymes after a remission lasting 6 months or more. We compared the MRI result for the presence of myositis or not with physician decisions and determined the concordance/discordance for flares or remission. Concordance occurred when MRI showed myositis and the physician's decision was to treat the patient for a flare, either by increasing the current medications or by starting new medications. Concordance was also present if the MRI did not show active myositis and the physician did not treat the patient for a flare and continued the same medication, continued off medication if the patient was not on treatment, or tapered the current treatment. Cohen's kappa was used to evaluate the chance-corrected agreement between physician decisions and MRI findings. Bayes' rule was used to determine the conditional probability that the physician would decide to treat for flare or remission given the MRI findings. McNemar tests for paired proportions were also used to examine the agreement of MRI and elevated levels of muscle enzymes. All tests were 2-sided and p-values less than 0.05 were considered statistically significant.

Results

Forty-five patients were identified and demographic and disease characteristics are shown in Tables 1 and 2.

The MRI was used at the initial presentation to determine the diagnosis of JDM in 40/45 patients. The repeat MRI was done in 13 patients. Two of the thirteen patients who had repeat MRI did not have an MRI performed at presentation. We stratified the patients with repeat MRI results according to the reason for repeating the MRI. All patients had history, physical examination, and muscle enzymes determined before the physician made a decision to follow up with MRI due to equivocal flare findings (Additional file 1). Reasons for repeating the MRI include thigh pain in one patient, calf pain in one patient (Fig. 1), hip pain in one patient, to determine remission in one patient, weakness in 4 patients, worsening nail fold capillary dilation without other signs of flare in one patient, rash in 3 patients, and an elevated muscle enzyme level without any other signs of flare in one patient.

MRI was performed in two patients (DM # 2 and DM # 7) for a third time. The reason for repeating the MRI again was to determine remission and whether or not to discontinue treatment. In DM # 2, the MRI showed no abnormality and a decision was made to continue tapering the medication. The patient did well without any flare thereafter. In DM # 7, the MRI showed bright T2 signal within the patellar tendons and superficial fasciae bilaterally. This patient continued on medications based on

Table 1 Demographic Features and Disease Characteristics of 45 Patients with Juvenile Dermatomyositis

Female/male	2.5: 1 (32 F/13 M)
Median age in years	5.8 (1.7–17.9)
Weakness	36/45 (80%)
Rash	45/45 (100%)
Nail fold capillary changes	33/45 (73%)
Calcinosis	5/45 (11%)
Monocyclic disease	12/39 (31%)
Polycyclic disease	12/39 (31%)
Chronic continuous	15/39 (38%)
Not classified (followed less than 2 years)	6

Table 2 Disease characteristics of 45 patients with juvenile dermatomyositis

Test name	Patients with completed test N (%)	Patients with abnormal results N (%)
CK	44/45 (98%)	23/44 (52%)
LDH	37/45 (82%)	23/37 (62%)
Aldolase	43/45 (95%)	31/43 (72%)
AST	44/45 (98%)	24/44 (54%
MRI at diagnosis	40/45 (89%)	31/40 (77%)
EMG	8/45 (18%)	3/8 (38%)
Muscle biopsy	11/45 (24%)	10/11 (90%)
Skin biopsy	2/45 (4%)	2/2 (100%)

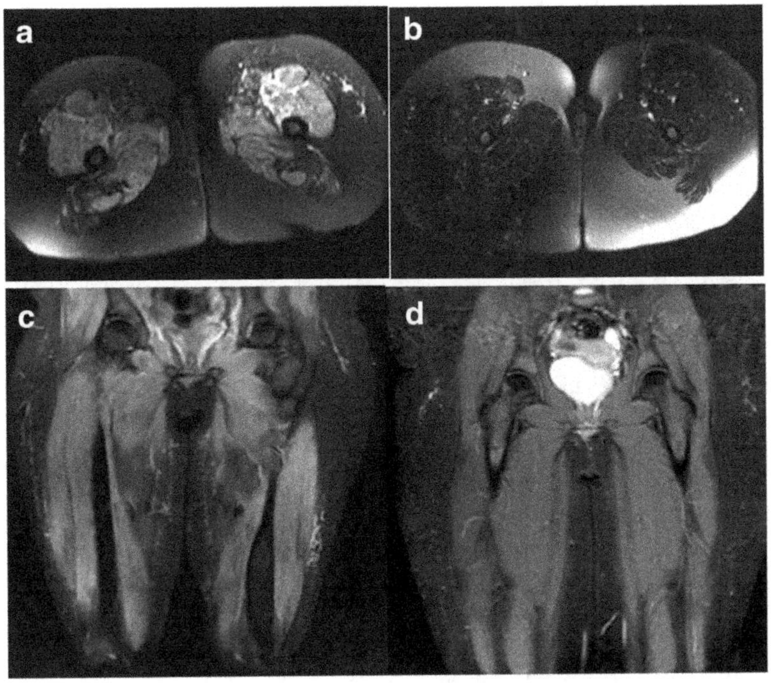

Fig. 1 MRI at time of diagnosis and flares. **a** and **c** showed the axial and coronal section of the first MRI at the time of diagnosis. It showed diffusely increased T2 signal throughout all the muscles of the thigh as well as of the pelvis and hip girdle region with symmetrical involvement except for more patchy involvement in the adductors and in semi-membranous and semi-tendinous muscles. **b** and **d** showed the axial and coronal section of the second MRI at the time of flare. It showed: bilateral increased intramuscular T2 signal within both posterior calves including the lateral head of the gastrocnemius, soleus, and medial head of gastrocnemius and plantaris muscles with corresponding areas of restricted diffusion. The degree of restricted diffusion and T2 prolongation has markedly decreased compared with initial MRI A and C. There is subtle T2 prolongation with corresponding restricted diffusion diffusely within the anterior thigh musculature involving the bilateral vastus lateralis, rectus femoris and subtly within the vastus medialis muscles

findings suggestive of active myositis in MRI. We did not include the third MRI in our data analysis to avoid bias.

Overall, there was moderate agreement between the second MRI findings and physician's decision about flares (kappa = 0.519). However, based on conditional probability of treatment given MRI findings, the agreement is revealed to be more substantial. When the MRI findings show myositis, physicians tend to treat for myositis 100% of the time, while when MRI findings show no myositis, physicians tapered treatment 70% of the time.

As shown in Table 3, in two of the cases where MRI revealed myositis, the patients had no elevated enzymes. Conversely, in three of the patients with elevated enzymes, MRI did not show myositis. As expected, there was no statistically significant association between elevated muscle enzymes and MRI findings (McNemar's test p-value = 1.0000) (Table 3).

Table 3 Association Between Elevated Muscle Enzymes and MRI Findings

	Myositis by MRI	No myositis by MRI	p-value (McNemar's test)
Elevated enzyme(s)	1	3	1.0000
No elevated enzyme(s)	2	7	

Discussion

In recent years, muscle magnetic resonance imaging (MRI) has played an increasingly important role in the diagnosis of inflammatory muscle disease. In many situations, MRIs have decreased the need for invasive procedures such as EMG and muscle biopsy [12, 13]. In our short report the muscle MRI was used in 89% at the time of diagnosis, while EMG and muscle biopsy were used in 17 and 24%, respectively. MRI could also be used in the selection of active disease sites for muscle biopsy as well [14]. In our study, we determined if the MRI assists in assessing whether patients with JDM are having a disease flare and how MRI might be affecting physician's decision-making regarding treatment.

We showed that muscles MRI help decide if a patient is having a disease flare when the clinical assessment and laboratory markers are equivocal. When an MRI shows myositis at the time of questionable flares, physicians tend to treat 100% of the time and when an MRI shows no myositis, physicians in this study continued the same medications or tapered medications 70% of the time.

Previous studies showed that serum muscle enzyme values could be unreliable as markers for monitoring disease activity [15, 9]. Our study supported this conclusion as in 75% of the cases in which the MRI showed myositis, the patient had no abnormal enzymes. No statistically significant association were found between abnormal muscle enzymes and MRI findings (McNemar's test p-value = 1.0).

There are limited previous studies on the use of the MRI to guide the decision of flares in JDM. Keim et al. reported the benefit of using the MRI at time of flare in one case [15]. Maillard et al. studied the finding of T2-weighted MRI scans of the thigh muscles in children with active JDM, inactive JDM and healthy children [16]. We showed the effective role of MRI in guiding the diagnosis of flares. Future direction of research may need to investigate this on a larger scale, study the cost effectiveness, and the role of MRI in definition of JDM remission. Disease remission is another questionable area and in many situations it is difficult to determine if the patient has an active or inactive JDM. The Pediatric Rheumatology International Trials Organization (PRINTO) established data-driven criteria with clear evidence-based, cut-off values to identify JDM patients with clinically inactive disease. The best combination of variables to classify a patient as being in a state of inactive disease on or off therapy were at least three of four of the following criteria: creatine kinase ≤150, Childhood Myositis Assessment Scale ≥48, manual muscle testing ≥78, and Myositis Disease Activity Assessment Visual Analogue Scale ≤0.2 [17]. Despite the use of these criteria, we still have some cases where it is difficult to define active or inactive disease similar to our 4-year-old patient (DM #6) where the judgment of CMAS was difficult due to her lack of cooperation with doing the CMAS evaluation. Including MRI findings may offer a better test to distinguish active or inactive JDM disease.

Our study should be interpreted in the light of its limitations; these include the retrospective nature of the study, the small sample size, and subjective definition of flares by using the physician's decision as a gold standard. In addition, we did not attempt to evaluate the cost effectiveness of an MRI in this clinical situation.

Conclusion

Our study suggested that a muscle MRI might be valuable as a test to inform a physician's decision about whether a child with JDM is having a disease flare when other findings or tests may not be helpful. There was a high concordance with physician decision making and the MRI. Further multicenter studies may be needed to confirm the utility and cost-effectiveness of MRI in detecting muscle flares in patients with JDM.

Abbreviations

AST: Aspartate aminotransferase; CARRA: Childhood Arthritis and Rheumatology Research Alliance; CK: Creatine kinase; CMAS: Childhood myositis assessment scale; CTP protocol: Consensus Treatments Protocol for moderate JDM; EMG: Electromyography; JDM: Juvenile dermatomyositis; LDH: Lactate dehydrogenase; MRI: Magnetic resonance imaging; NCH: Nationwide Children's Hospital; PRINTO: Pediatric Rheumatology International Trials Organization; WB-MRI: Whole-body MRI

Acknowledgements

Not applicable

Funding

CY and CH are supported by a grant from the CureJM Foundation.

Authors' contributions

RA, CY, SB, KL, and CS: involvement in retrospective review of cases, interpret the findings, writing the manuscript, and equally contributed as first writers RA of the manuscript. BrA: reviewed each MRI study separately, discussed the findings with first author RA, and involved in writing and reviewing the manuscript. MC, performed all the statistical methods and involved in writing and reviewing the manuscript. All authors read and approved the final manuscript.

Competing interests

The authors declare that they have no competing interests.

References

1. Rider LG, Katz JD, Jones OY. Developments in the classification and treatment of the juvenile idiopathic inflammatory myopathies. Rheum Dis Clin North Am. 2013;39(4):877–904.
2. Brown VE, et al. An international consensus survey of the diagnostic criteria for juvenile dermatomyositis (JDM). Rheumatology (Oxford). 2006;45(8):990–3.
3. Ramanan AV, et al. The effectiveness of treating juvenile dermatomyositis with methotrexate and aggressively tapered corticosteroids. Arthritis Rheum. 2005;52(11):3570–8.
4. Bohan A, Peter JB. Polymyositis and dermatomyositis (first of two parts). N Engl J Med. 1975;292(7):344–7.
5. Bohan A, Peter JB. Polymyositis and dermatomyositis (second of two parts). N Engl J Med. 1975;292(8):403–7.
6. Constantin T, et al. National registry of patients with juvenile idiopathic inflammatory myopathies in Hungary–clinical characteristics and disease course of 44 patients with juvenile dermatomyositis. Autoimmunity. 2006; 39(3):223–32.
7. Spencer CH, et al. Course of treated juvenile dermatomyositis. J Pediatr. 1984;105(3):399–408.
8. Huber AM. Consensus treatments for moderate juvenile dermatomyositis: beyond the first two months. Results of the second Childhood Arthritis and Rheumatology Research Alliance consensus conference. Arthritis Care Res. 2012;64(4):546–53.
9. Naim MY, et al. Enzyme elevation in patients with juvenile dermatomyositis and steroid myopathy. J Rheumatol. 2006;33(7):1392–4.
10. Malattia C, et al. Whole-body MRI in the assessment of disease activity in juvenile dermatomyositis. Ann Rheum Dis. 2014;73(6):1083–90.
11. Lintner KE, et al. Gene copy-number variations (CNVs) of complement C4 and C4A deficiency in genetic risk and pathogenesis of juvenile dermatomyositis. Ann Rheum Dis. 2016;75(9):1599–606.
12. Gowdie PJ, et al. Clinical features and disease course of patients with juvenile dermatomyositis. Int J Rheum Dis. 2013;16(5):561–7.
13. Huppertz HI, Kaiser WA. Serial magnetic resonance imaging in juvenile dermatomyositis–delayed normalization. Rheumatol Int. 1994;14(3):127–9.

14. Pitt AM, et al. MRI-guided biopsy in inflammatory myopathy: initial results. Magn Reson Imaging. 1993;11(8):1093–9.
15. Keim DR, Hernandez RJ, Sullivan DB. Serial magnetic resonance imaging in juvenile dermatomyositis. Arthritis Rheum. 1991;34(12):1580–4.
16. Maillard SM, et al. Quantitative assessment of MRI T2 relaxation time of thigh muscles in juvenile dermatomyositis. Rheumatology (Oxford). 2004; 43(5):603–8.
17. Lazarevic D, et al. The PRINTO criteria for clinically inactive disease in juvenile dermatomyositis. Ann Rheum Dis. 2013;72(5):686–93.

7

Ultrasound-guided steroid tendon sheath injections in juvenile idiopathic arthritis

Shannon E. Peters[1], Ronald M. Laxer[2], Bairbre L. Connolly[3] and Dimitri A. Parra[3*]

Abstract

Background: The aims of this study were to: (a) Identify tendon sheaths most commonly treated with steroid injections in a pediatric patient population with Juvenile Idiopathic Arthritis (JIA); (b) Describe technical aspects of the procedure; (c) Characterize sonographic appearance of tenosynovitis in JIA; (d) Assess agreement between clinical request and sites injected.

Methods: This was a 10 year single-center retrospective study (May 2006-April 2016) of patients with JIA referred by Rheumatology for ultrasound-guided tendon sheath injections. Patient demographics, clinical referral information, sonographic appearance of the tendon sheaths and technical aspects of the procedure were analyzed.

Results: There were 308 procedures of 244 patients (75% female, mean age 9.6 years) who underwent a total of 926 tendon sheath injections. Ankle tendons were most commonly injected (84.9%), specifically the tendon sheaths of tibialis posterior (22.3%), peroneus longus (20%) and brevis (19.7%). The majority of treated sites (91.9%) showed peritendinous fluid and sheath thickening on ultrasound. There were 2 minor intra-procedure complications without sequelae. A good agreement between clinical request and sites injected was observed.

Conclusions: Ultrasound-guided tendon sheath injections with steroids are used frequently to treat patients with JIA. It is a safe intervention with a high technical success rate. The ankle region, specifically the medial compartment, is the site most commonly injected in this group of patients. The most common sonographic finding is peritendinous fluid and sheath thickening. These findings might assist clinicians and radiologists to characterize and more effectively manage tenosynovitis in patients with JIA.

Keywords: Tenosynovitis in children, Steroid injections, Tendon sheath, US-guidance, JIA

Background

Juvenile Idiopathic Arthritis (JIA) is the most common chronic rheumatic disease in childhood with an incidence ranging from 1 to 22 per 100,000 [1]. JIA is defined as persistent arthritis for more than 6 weeks with an onset at less than 16 years of age, after excluding other causes of joint inflammation [2]. The etiology of JIA appears to be multi-factorial, and may be related to genetic factors associated with triggering events such as psychological stress, abnormal hormone levels, trauma or infections [1]. JIA includes seven subtypes of arthritis, according to the clinical features during the first 6 months of disease, and with the following frequencies: oligoarticular JIA (50–60%), polyarticular JIA—both rheumatoid factor positive and negative—(30–35%), systemic JIA (10–20%), juvenile psoriatic arthritis (2–15%), enthesitis-related arthritis (1–7%) and undifferentiated arthritis [1]. The knee is the joint most commonly involved in JIA (77%), followed by the ankle (58%) [3], however, many other joints can be affected and become symptomatic including those in the hands, wrists, feet as well as the hips and temporomandibular joints.

Tenosynovitis is one of the manifestations of JIA, and its persistence after adjacent joint injections can explain a lack of clinical response to intra-articular injections.

* Correspondence: dimitri.parra@sickkids.ca
[3]Image Guided Therapy, Department of Diagnostic Imaging, The Hospital for Sick Children and University of Toronto, Toronto, ON, Canada
Full list of author information is available at the end of the article

The histopathology of tenosynovitis is indistinguishable from joint synovitis in rheumatoid arthritis (RA). Both are characterized by synovial cell hyperplasia, infiltration by inflammatory cells including lymphocytes and plasma cells, and increased vascularity [4]. Tenosynovitis has been found in up to 71% of JIA patients with symptomatic ankle inflammation [5]. A recent study using MRI found that the most common ankle tendon involved in patients with JIA was the tibialis posterior and an average of 3.5 tendons were involved when tenosynovitis was present [6].

Clinically, tenosynovitis can be suspected by swelling, pain or tenderness along the length of the tendon. On ultrasound (US), an increase of fluid within the synovial sheath, hyperemia and sheath thickening are the most characteristic features of tenosynovitis [7]. The OMERACT Ultrasound Task Force defined tenosynovitis in RA and other inflammatory arthritis as hypoechoic or anechoic thickened tissue with or without fluid in the tendon sheath [8]. This definition is utilized in the RA literature; however to the best of our knowledge, there is little literature reporting the sonographic findings of tenosynovitis in JIA.

Tendon sheath steroid injections are one of the treatment options for tenosynovitis and can be performed in conjunction with intra-articular injections. Utilizing US guidance for steroid injections into tendon sheaths has shown clinical advantage to conventional blind injections in the adult RA population [9], and this may be true in the pediatric population.

In our practice, a large population of patients with JIA is referred to interventional radiology (IR) for joint and tendon sheath injections. However, not uncommonly tendon sheath abnormalities are not seen on US at the time of the procedure. This is consistent with other studies that report discordance between clinical examination of the tendons and imaging findings of tenosynovitis [10, 11]. One study reported tenosynovitis on MRI in more than half of their patient population, whereas no tendon involvement had been detected clinically [6]. This is significant as without the presence of peritendinous fluid, safe tendon sheath injections are difficult to perform.

To the best of our knowledge there is limited literature reviewing the incidence, appearance and management of tenosynovitis in children with JIA. This prompted us to review our experience in the management of patients with JIA and tenosynovitis, referred for tendon sheath steroid injections. The aims of the study were to identify the tendon sheaths most commonly injected in our patient population with JIA, describe the technical aspects of the procedure, characterize the sonographic appearance of tenosynovitis in JIA, and assess the agreement between the clinical request and sites injected.

Methods

Institutional Research Ethics Board approval was obtained for this study. A 10-year single center retrospective review was completed for all cases of US-guided tendon sheath injections between May 2006 and April 2016. Patients were identified through the Picture Archiving and Communication System (PACS) (General Electric Centricity, GE Healthcare Canada, Mississauga, Ontario). Patients were included if they had a confirmed diagnosis of JIA and if one or more tendon sheath injections were requested by a rheumatologist, with or without joint injections. Patients were excluded if referral or procedural information was incomplete.

Patient demographics and referral information were collected which included the tendon sheaths and steroid dose requested. Each procedural visit to the IR suite was identified as a separate patient encounter, irrespective of the number of tendons and joints injected, and was counted as a "procedure". The number of prior procedures was also recorded. The procedural data included the type of sedation, the joints and/or tendon sheaths injected and the respective dose of steroid. Each tendon sheath injected was counted individually (i.e. bilateral tibialis posterior injections counted as two injections). If a requested tendon sheath was not injected, the reason was recorded. The number of joints injected was also recorded for each procedure. The procedural imaging and radiological reports were retrospectively reviewed by two investigators (S.P. and D.P.). The sonographic appearance of the tendon sheaths prior to injection was recorded as containing fluid, fluid with thickening of the tendon sheath, echogenic fluid, increased color-Doppler signal, a combination of characteristics, or no fluid or thickening. The injection approach was recorded as either in or out of plane based on the sonographic images reviewed. All quantitative data was analyzed with descriptive statistics using Excel 2011.

To assess the agreement between the clinical request and injected sites, an injection index (InIx) was developed. InIx was defined as the number of tendons injected divided by the number of tendons requested and was calculated for each procedure.

The procedural records were examined for intra-procedure complications including pain, swelling and bruising. Complications were classified as minor or major according to the Society for Interventional Radiology (SIR) guidelines [12]. The focus of this study was procedural and therefore no long-term follow-up for complications such as subcutaneous atrophy was done.

Technique

Sonographic guidance is performed on Philips (ATL 5000, iU 22 and Epic) or Siemens (S2000) equipment using linear transducers (14, 15 or 20-MHz). Procedures are performed by staff pediatric interventional radiologists and/or supervised interventional fellows.

Informed consent is obtained and patient pain and anxiety is controlled by either nurse-administered intravenous sedation (fentanyl (Sandoz Inc., Quebec, Canada), midazolam (Sandoz Inc., Quebec, Canada) with possible ketamine (Sandoz Inc., Quebec, Canada)), by an anesthesiologist, or occasionally with no sedation. The sites to be injected are prepared and draped in a sterile fashion. The US transducer is swept along the length of the tendon in both longitudinal and transverse planes to identify a site of peritendinous fluid or signs of inflammation. After identifying a location along the tendon sheath that permits safe injection, a 25-gauge needle is advanced under direct US visualization into the tendon sheath in either the transverse (out of plane) or longitudinal (in plane) approach. In both approaches the needle tip is directly visualized, and it is ensured that it the needle tip is located within the peritendinous space prior to injection. The "out of plane" approach is favored, as it permits to direct and place the needle tip away from the tendon itself, a technique frequently used in interventional radiology when directing needles in limited spaces with vital structures close by (e.g. neonatal brachial vein access). Triamcinolone hexacetonide (20 mg/ml), the preferred steroid (triamcinolone acetonide if former not available, 40 mg/ml), is injected at the dose prescribed by the referring rheumatologist (usually between 5 and 10 mg = 0.25-0.5 ml). This is followed by injection of a similar volume of local anesthetic to clear the needle track and help prevent subcutaneous atrophy (1% lidocaine; Xylocaine, AstraZeneca Canada Inc., Mississauga, Ontario).

Results

Between May 2006 and April 2016, there were 1275 procedures for joint and/or tendon sheath injections, 350 of which included referrals for tendon sheath injections in 270 patients. In 42/350 procedures the sheaths were not injected due to lack of fluid or inflammatory signs in the tendon sheaths at the time of the procedure. In the remaining 308/350 procedures tendon sheaths were injected in 244 patients. There were 184 females (75.0%) and 60 males (25.0%). Patients ranged in age from 10 months to 17 years and the mean age at time of the procedure was 9 years and 8 months. All patients had a reported diagnosis of JIA.

A total of 926 tendon sheaths were injected, the distribution of which is presented in Table 1. The most commonly injected anatomical site was the ankle. Specific tendon sheaths are shown in Fig. 1 and average steroid dose injected are presented in Table 2. Procedures involved both tendon sheath and joint injections in 296/308 visits (96.1%), compared to tendon sheaths only in 12 visits (3.9%). On average 3 tendon sheaths were injected per procedure (SD: 2.0, 95% CI: 2.78, 3.22) with 2 tendon sheaths injected most frequently (29.6%). On average 3.4 joints were injected per procedure (SD: 2.5, 95% CI: 3.13, 3.67) with 2 joints injected most often (21.8%).

Table 1 Tendon sheaths injected by anatomical site

	Number of tendon sheaths injected	% of Total tendon sheaths
Medial Ankle	412	44.5
Lateral Ankle	367	39.6
Anterior Ankle	7	0.8
Hand	113	12.2
Wrist	23	2.5
Foot	2	0.2
Arm	2	0.2
TOTAL	926	

The majority of patients (78.3%) underwent one procedure during the study period, 17.6% had two, and 4.1% had three or more; 160/244 (51.9%) patients had no prior joint or tendon sheath injections in IR. Of the 53/244 patients who underwent more than one procedure, patients received injections in the same tendon sheaths in 31 instances in a total of 58 tendon sheaths. The ankle region required subsequent injections in the same tendon sheath most often, and an average of 2 tendon sheath injections were required when repeat injections were needed in this region.

Overall, the mean InIx was 0.765; 148 procedures (48.1%) had an InIx of 1.0, indicating that all tendon sheaths were injected as requested, 98 procedures (31.8%) had an InIx between 0.5 and 1.0, 59 procedures (19.2%) had an InIx < 0.5, and in 3 procedures (1%) the InIx was >1.0. The InIx index was 0 in 42 procedures, indicating that no tendon sheaths were injected, due to a lack of peritendinous fluid or signs of inflammation on US (Fig. 2a).

On US, the tendon sheaths in 283/308 (91.9%) procedures showed peritendinous fluid and synovial sheath thickening (Fig. 2b). Accumulation of peritendinous fluid on its own was seen in 19/308 (6.2%). Echogenic peritendinous fluid was seen in 6/308 (1.9%) (Fig. 2c). Increased color-Doppler signal was seen in combination with peritendinous fluid and synovial sheath thickening in 9 procedures (Fig. 2d), and with echogenic peritendinous fluid in 1 procedure.

Approximately two thirds of patients underwent general anesthesia (63.1%), one third had nurse-administered IV sedation (36.0%), and 0.9% received no pain or anxiety management. The average age of patients was 8.6, 11.3 and 16.7 years requiring general anesthesia, IV sedation and no pain management, respectively. Triamcinolone

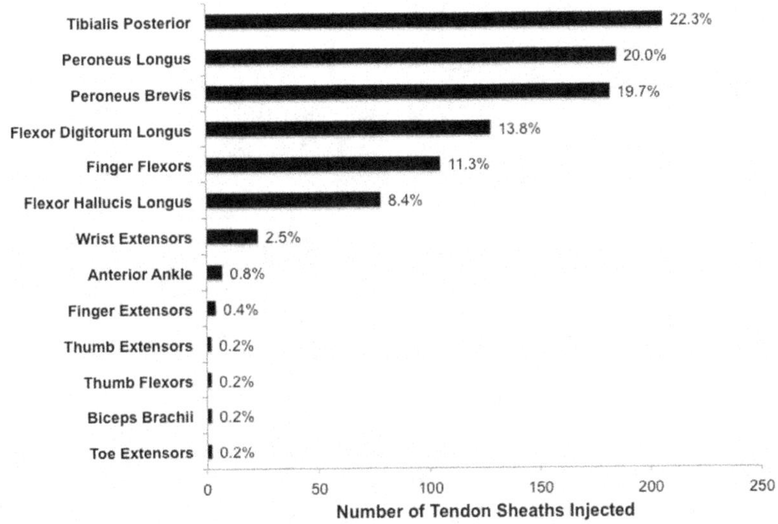

Fig. 1 Distribution of specific tendon sheaths injected

hexacetonide was used in 298 procedures (96.8%), whereas triamcinolone acetonide was used in 10 procedures (3.2%). A 15-MHz linear US probe was used for most procedures ($n = 265$, 86.0%), 14-MHz linear US probe was used in 42 procedures (13.7%) and a 20-MHz linear US probe was used in one procedure (0.3%). An out of plane approach was used in 266 procedures (86.3%) (Fig. 3a), an in plane approach in 32 procedures (10.4%) (Fig. 3b) and a combination of in and out of plane approach was used in 10 procedures (3.3%).

Table 2 Average dose of steroid injected

	Average dose, mg (TH)	Average dose, mg (TA)
Medial Ankle		
• Tibialis Posterior ($n = 206$)	7.20	16.43
• Flexor Digitorum Longus ($n = 128$)	6.76	15.00
• Flexor Hallucis Longus ($n = 78$)	6.89	15.00
Lateral Ankle		
• Peroneus Longus ($n = 185$)	7.01	15.00
• Peroneus Brevis ($n = 182$)	6.96	15.00
• Anterior Ankle ($n = 7$)	7.80	12.50
Hand		
• Finger Flexors ($n = 105$)	5.28	10.00
• Finger Extensors ($n = 4$)	7.75	—
• Thumb Extensor ($n = 2$)	8.50	—
• Thumb Flexor ($n = 2$)	7.50	—
Wrist Extensors ($n = 23$)	8.18	20.00
Biceps Brachii ($n = 2$)	20.00	—
Toe Extensors ($n = 2$)	5.00	—

TH Triamcinolone hexacetonide ($n = 298$); *TA* Triamcinolone acetonide ($n = 10$)

Peritendinous fluid was aspirated in 2 procedures. In one case, fluid suspicious of infection by its echogenic appearance was aspirated from the right biceps brachii tendon sheath (Fig. 4), and sent for culture. In the second case, echogenic peritendinous fluid was similarly aspirated from the tibialis posterior tendon sheath followed by injection of steroid.

Two minor intra-procedure complications were reported. Following one procedure bruising around the medial malleolus arose after injection of the medial ankle tendons (SIR A). In another, peritendinous fluid suspicious of infection was seen on US and injection of steroid was deferred (same patient as above). This necessitated another patient visit after subsequent cultures of the fluid were negative. No major complications were reported.

Discussion

US-guided steroid tendon sheath injections are frequently requested by pediatric rheumatologists to manage children with JIA. The most commonly injected tendon sheaths are the tibialis posterior, peroneus longus and peroneus brevis. In this cohort, the procedure was most commonly performed under general anesthesia, using a 15-MHz linear US probe and 25-gauge needle injecting triamcinolone hexacetonide. The most common sonographic appearance of tenosynovitis in this cohort was accumulation of peritendinous fluid and synovial sheath thickening. There was good agreement between the clinical request and the sonographic signs of inflammation of the tendon sheath.

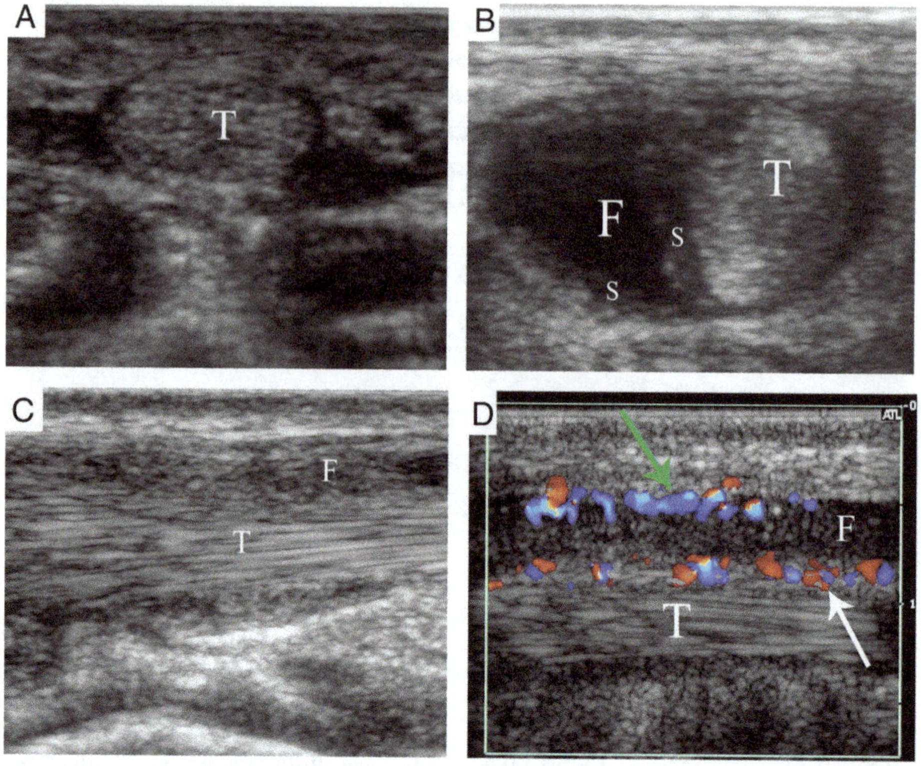

Fig. 2 Sonographic findings of tenosynovitis in JIA. **a** 13 years 5 months old female referred for injection of the 4th flexor tendon sheath of the right hand. Ultrasound showed no fluid or signs of inflammation around the tendon in the transverse view. **b** 9 years 11 months old female referred for injection of the tibialis posterior tendon sheath. Ultrasound showed accumulation of peritendinous fluid and thickening of the synovial sheath in the transverse view. **c** 8 years 1 month old female referred for injection of the tibialis posterior tendon sheath. Ultrasound showed accumulation of echogenic peritendinous fluid in the longitudinal view. **d** 15 years 8 months old male referred for injection of the tibialis posterior tendon sheath. Ultrasound showed peritendinous fluid, synovial thickening with increased color-Doppler signal on the synovium covering the tendon (*white arrow*) and lining the cavity (*green arrow*). T = Tendon, S = Synovial sheath thickening, F = Peritendinous fluid

Tenosynovitis is recognized to occur commonly in the ankle region of children with JIA, with up to 71% of clinically swollen ankles exhibiting sonographic signs of tendon sheath inflammation [5]. Young et al. [13] reported that 75% of the 104 tendon sheath injections were performed in the foot/ankle region in their cohort of patients with JIA. Javadi et al. [6] studied 45 patients with a confirmed diagnosis of JIA and determined using MRI that tenosynovitis was present in 59% of wrists and in 33% of ankles with synovitis respectively, with the tibialis posterior being the most commonly involved. The results of this current study are consistent with previous reports in that tenosynovitis was present in 24% of the referred population and approximately 85% of tendon sheaths injected were in the ankle region, with the tibialis posterior contributing to 22% of all tendon sheaths injected. These current results differ from other studies in that the vast majority of tendon sheath injections were performed in conjunction with intra-articular injections and isolated tendon sheath injections were only performed in 3.9% of procedures, compared to other studies which have reported isolated tenosynovitis in up to 39% of ankles [5]. Of note, isolated tenosynovitis in this patient group was encountered most frequently in the ankle region, with 9/12 procedures involving tendons in this location.

The most frequently employed injection approach was out of plane. This approach provides better visualization of the needle tip within the peritendinous fluid, in the space between the synovial sheath and tendon itself (Fig. 3a). Clear visualization of the needle tip prevents accidental needle entry into the tendon fibers and permits a safe injection.

To the best of our knowledge no large series of US-guided tendon sheath injections in children has been reported, and the sonographic appearance of tenosynovitis in JIA has yet to be described in the literature. Lambot et al. [14] proposed a MRI scoring system for the assessment of tenosynovitis in clinically involved wrists in patients with JIA. In this study, peritendinous fluid accumulation and synovial sheath thickening was observed in the majority of patients with JIA, which is consistent with the OMERACT Ultrasound Task Force's definition of tenosynovitis in other conditions [8].

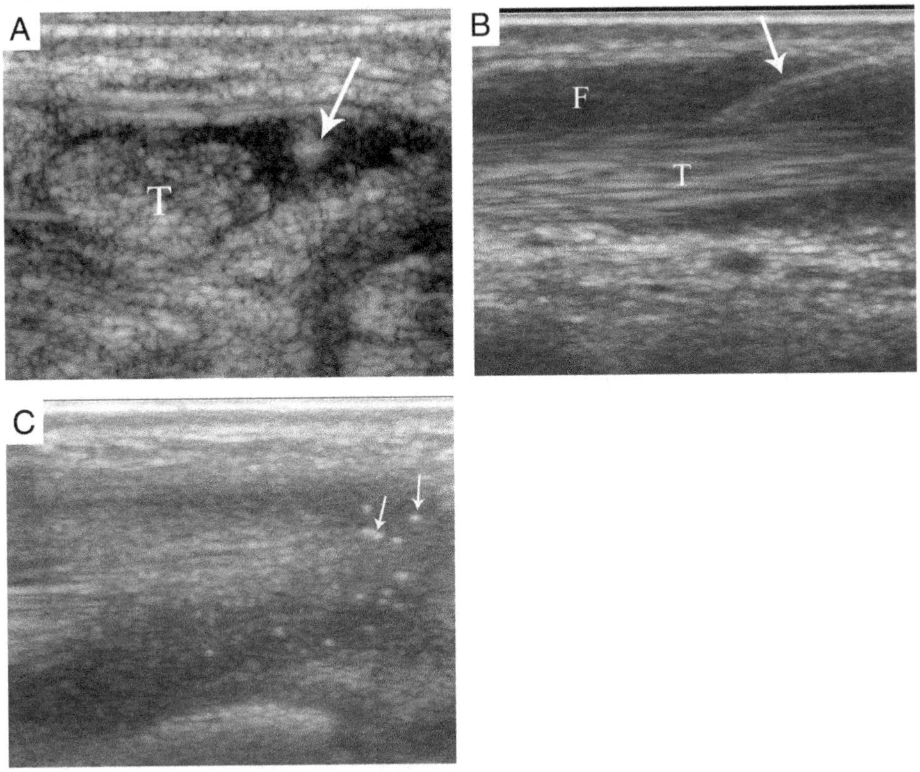

Fig. 3 Sonographic images of tendon sheath injection approach. **a** An out of plane injection of the tibialis posterior tendon sheath of a 13 years 8 months old male. **b** An in plane injection of the tibialis posterior tendon sheath of a 9 years 11 months old female. *Arrows* point to the needle. **c** Steroid solution (*small arrows*) surrounding the tibialis posterior tendon of a 9 year 4 months old male after injection. T = Tendon, F = Peritendinous fluid

Furthermore, a semi-quantitative scoring system in grey-scale and colour Doppler mode US has been developed by the OMERACT US group to assess tenosynovitis [15, 16]. Several studies evaluating this scoring system on patients with RA have shown excellent intra- and inter-reader agreement as well as good ability to detect response to systemic treatment [17, 18]. Moreover, studies evaluating synovitis and tenosynovitis on US in JIA have emerged which outline the usefulness of US in monitoring disease progression, however an US scoring system has yet to be proposed [19, 20].

In this study population there was good agreement between the clinical request and the sites injected. Previous studies have reported a poor inter-observer agreement for clinical examination versus US of the foot in JIA [10]. Pascoli et al. [11] found that clinical examination was inadequate in detecting tenosynovitis in the ankle region, as among 19 lateral ankle tendons thought

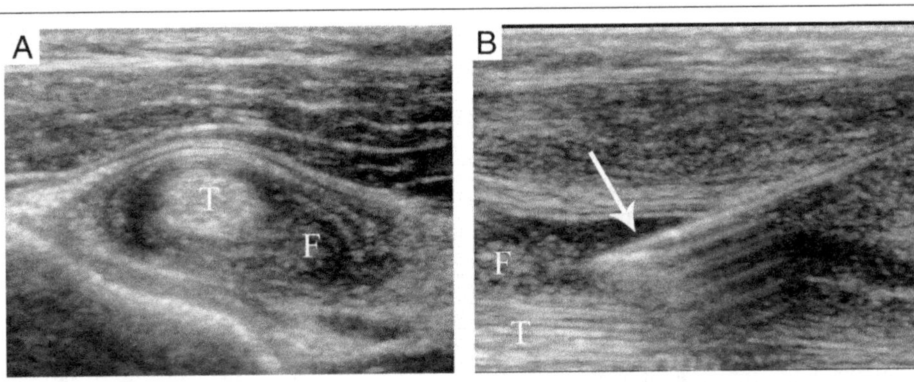

Fig. 4 6 years 8 months old male referred for injection of biceps brachii tendon bilaterally. **a** Ultrasound showed echogenic peritendinous fluid and thickening of the sheath around the tendon (T). **b** The fluid was aspirated with a 20-gauge angiocath™ (*arrow*) and sent for culture

to be clinically involved, less than 50% had sonographic signs of involvement. As previously stated, a tendon sheath may not be injected safely if sufficient peritendinous fluid is not seen on US. As such, good agreement between the clinical signs of and sonographic signs of tenosynovitis may avoid unnecessary referrals and improve hospital efficiency. In this cohort the average InIx was 0.765, indicating that for every 100 tendon sheath injections referred, 77 are performed. Furthermore, the InIx was equal to 1.0 in 148 procedures, indicating that 48% of the clinical referrals were completed as requested. These results demonstrate that tenosynovitis was adequately detected on clinical exam, and that interventionists can expect to inject exactly as requested approximately half of the time.

This study has several limitations. This was a retrospective single-center study. Occasionally images stored in PACS were suboptimal and images may not have been stored for all tendon sheaths treated. Injections occurring in the Rheumatology clinic were not included in the denominator of 1275 procedures. In this institution tendon sheath injections without ultrasound guidance are occasionally performed in isolated treatment of the flexor compartment of the hand.

The focus of this study was procedural and therefore we did not complete a long-term follow-up of patient outcomes. Additionally, patients' medical records were not completed with the level of accuracy required to assess the correlation between the intervention and patient outcomes. Furthermore, it was difficult to assess the impact of the intervention compared to a change in the patient's medical treatment. Most patients required only one procedure and thus we believe this is an indicator of effectiveness in conjunction with the management by the rheumatology team. Additionally, only 31/244 patients (12.7%) required repeat injections into the same tendon sheath and only 58/926 (6.3%) tendon sheaths required a repeat injection. Only 2 minor and no major complications were observed, and thus the procedure was deemed to be safe and exhibit a high technical success rate.

Conclusions

In conclusion, US-guided tendon sheath injections are a frequent procedure in patients with JIA. It is a safe intervention with a high technical success rate. The ankle region, specifically the medial ankle, is most commonly injected. The most frequent US finding of tenosynovitis in JIA is accumulation of peritendinous fluid and synovial sheath thickening. There is good agreement between the clinical request and the sites injected. These findings might assist rheumatologists, radiologists and other health care professionals involved in the care of patients with JIA, to characterize and more effectively manage tenosynovitis in their patients.

Abbreviations

InIx: Injection index; IR: Interventional radiology; JIA: Juvenile idiopathic arthritis; RA: Rheumatoid arthritis; US: Ultrasound

Acknowledgments

To the Rheumatology division at the Hospital for Sick Children for referring the patients to the Interventional Radiology division for image guided injections.

Funding

This was an unfunded study.

Authors' contributions

SP collected, analyzed and interpreted data, and was major contributor in writing the manuscript. DP contributed to the design of the study, collected, analyzed and interpreted data, and contributed in writing the manuscript. RL and BC were involved in revising the manuscript critically for its intellectual content. All authors read and approved the final manuscript.

Competing interests

The authors declare that they have no competing interests.

Consent for publication

Not applicable.

Author details

[1]School of Medicine and Medical Sciences, University College Dublin, Dublin, Ireland. [2]Division of Rheumatology, Department of Pediatrics and Medicine, The Hospital for Sick Children and University of Toronto, Toronto, ON, Canada. [3]Image Guided Therapy, Department of Diagnostic Imaging, The Hospital for Sick Children and University of Toronto, Toronto, ON, Canada.

References

1. Weiss JE, Ilowite NT. Juvenile idiopathic arthritis. Pediatr Clin North Am. 2005;52:413–42. vi.
2. Hashkes PJ, Laxer RM. Medical treatment of juvenile idiopathic arthritis. JAMA. 2005;294:1671–84.
3. Selvaag AM, Flato B, Dale K, Lien G, Vinje O, Smerdel-Ramoya A, Forre O. Radiographic and clinical outcome in early juvenile rheumatoid arthritis and juvenile spondyloarthropathy: a 3-year prospective study. J Rheumatol. 2006;33:1382–91.
4. Kaibara N, Yamada H, Shuto T, Nakashima Y, Okazaki K, Miyahara H, Esaki Y, Hirata G, Iwamoto Y. Comparative histopathological analysis between tenosynovitis and joint synovitis in rheumatoid arthritis. Histopathology. 2008;52:856–64.
5. Rooney ME, McAllister C, Burns JF. Ankle disease in juvenile idiopathic arthritis: ultrasound findings in clinically swollen ankles. J Rheumatol. 2009; 36:1725–9.
6. Javadi S, Kan JH, Orth RC, DeGuzman M. Wrist and ankle MRI of patients with juvenile idiopathic arthritis: identification of unsuspected multicompartmental tenosynovitis and arthritis. AJR Am J Roentgenol. 2014;202:413–7.
7. Grassi W, Filippucci E, Busilacchi P. Musculoskeletal ultrasound. Best Pract Res Clin Rheumatol. 2004;18:813–26.
8. Wakefield RJ, Balint PV, Szkudlarek M, Filippucci E, Backhaus M, D'Agostino MA, Sanchez EN, Iagnocco A, Schmidt WA, Bruyn GA, et al. Musculoskeletal ultrasound including definitions for ultrasonographic pathology. J Rheumatol. 2005;32:2485–7.

9. Gutierrez M, Di Matteo A, Rosemffet M, Cazenave T, Rodriguez-Gil G, Diaz CH, Rios LV, Zamora N, Guzman Mdel C, Carrillo I, et al. Short-term efficacy to conventional blind injection versus ultrasound-guided injection of local corticosteroids in tenosynovitis in patients with inflammatory chronic arthritis: A randomized comparative study. Joint Bone Spine. 2016;83:161–6.
10. Hendry GJ, Gardner-Medwin J, Steultjens MP, Woodburn J, Sturrock RD, Turner DE. Frequent discordance between clinical and musculoskeletal ultrasound examinations of foot disease in juvenile idiopathic arthritis. Arthritis Care Res (Hoboken). 2012;64:441–7.
11. Pascoli L, Wright S, McAllister C, Rooney M. Prospective evaluation of clinical and ultrasound findings in ankle disease in juvenile idiopathic arthritis: importance of ankle ultrasound. J Rheumatol. 2010;37:2409–14.
12. Omary RA, Bettmann MA, Cardella JF, Bakal CW, Schwartzberg MS, Sacks D, Rholl KS, Meranze SG, Lewis CA. Quality improvement guidelines for the reporting and archiving of interventional radiology procedures. J Vasc Interv Radiol. 2003;14:S293–295.
13. Young CM, Shiels 2nd WE, Coley BD, Hogan MJ, Murakami JW, Jones K, Higgins GC, Rennebohm RM. Ultrasound-guided corticosteroid injection therapy for juvenile idiopathic arthritis: 12-year care experience. Pediatr Radiol. 2012;42:1481–9.
14. Lambot K, Boavida P, Damasio MB, Tanturri de Horatio L, Desgranges M, Malattia C, Barbuti D, Bracaglia C, Muller LS, Elie C, et al. MRI assessment of tenosynovitis in children with juvenile idiopathic arthritis: inter- and intra-observer variability. Pediatr Radiol. 2013;43:796–802.
15. Naredo E, D'Agostino MA, Wakefield RJ, Moller I, Balint PV, Filippucci E, Iagnocco A, Karim Z, Terslev L, Bong DA, et al. Reliability of a consensus-based ultrasound score for tenosynovitis in rheumatoid arthritis. Ann Rheum Dis. 2013;72:1328–34.
16. Bruyn GA, Hanova P, Iagnocco A, d'Agostino MA, Moller I, Terslev L, Backhaus M, Balint PV, Filippucci E, Baudoin P, et al. Ultrasound definition of tendon damage in patients with rheumatoid arthritis. Results of a OMERACT consensus-based ultrasound score focussing on the diagnostic reliability. Ann Rheum Dis. 2014;73:1929–34.
17. Ammitzboll-Danielsen M, Ostergaard M, Naredo E, Terslev L. Validity and sensitivity to change of the semi-quantitative OMERACT ultrasound scoring system for tenosynovitis in patients with rheumatoid arthritis. Rheumatology (Oxford). 2016;55:2156–66.
18. Vlad V, Berghea F, Micu M, Varzaru L, Bojinca M, Milicescu M, Ionescu R, Naredo E. Tenosynovitis US scoring systems follow synovitis and clinical scoring systems in RA and are responsive to change after biologic therapy. Med Ultrason. 2015;17:352–60.
19. Collado P, Malattia C. Imaging in paediatric rheumatology: Is it time for imaging? Best Pract Res Clin Rheumatol. 2016;30:720–35.
20. Roth J, Ravagnani V, Backhaus M, Balint P, Bruns A, Bruyn GA, Collado P, De la Cruz L, Guillaume-Czitrom S, Herlin T, et al: Preliminary definitions for the sonographic features of synovitis in children. Arthritis Care Res (Hoboken) 2016. doi: 10.1002/acr.23130.

8

Pilot study comparing the Childhood Arthritis & Rheumatology Research Alliance (CARRA) systemic Juvenile Idiopathic Arthritis Consensus Treatment Plans

Yukiko Kimura[1*], Sriharsha Grevich[2], Timothy Beukelman[3], Esi Morgan[4], Peter A. Nigrovic[5], Kelly Mieszkalski[6], T Brent Graham[7], Maria Ibarra[8], Norman Ilowite[9], Marisa Klein-Gitelman[10], Karen Onel[11], Sampath Prahalad[12], Marilynn Punaro[13], Sarah Ringold[2], Dana Toib[14], Heather Van Mater[15], Jennifer E. Weiss[1], Pamela F. Weiss[16], Laura E. Schanberg[15] and for the CARRA Registry Investigators

Abstract

Objectives: To assess the feasibility of studying the comparative effectiveness of the Childhood Arthritis and Rheumatology Research Alliance (CARRA) consensus treatment plans (CTPs) for systemic Juvenile Idiopathic Arthritis (JIA) using an observational registry.

Methods: Untreated systemic JIA patients enrolled in the CARRA Registry were begun on one of 4 CTPs chosen by the treating physician and patient/family (glucocorticoid [GC] alone; methotrexate [MTX] ± GC; IL1 inhibitor [IL1i] ± GC; IL6 inhibitor [IL6i] ± GC). The primary outcome of clinical inactive disease (CID) without current GC use was assessed at 9 months. Trial registration: clinicaltrials.gov NCT01697254; first registered 9/28/12 (retrospectively enrolled).

Results: Thirty patients were enrolled at 13 sites; eight patients were started on a non-biologic CTP (2 GC, 6 MTX) and 22 patients on a biologic CTP (12 IL1i, 10 IL6i) at disease onset. Demographic and disease features were similar between CTP groups. CTP choice appeared to segregate by site preference. CID off GC was achieved by 37% (11 of 30) including 11/22 (50%) starting a biologic CTP compared to 0/8 starting a non-biologic CTP ($p = 0.014$). There were four serious adverse events: two infections, one appendicitis and one macrophage activation syndrome.

Conclusions: The CARRA systemic JIA CTP pilot study demonstrated successful implementation of CTPs using the CARRA registry infrastructure. Having demonstrated feasibility, a larger study using CTP response to better determine the relative effectiveness of treatments for new-onset systemic JIA is now underway.

Keywords: Systemic Juvenile Idiopathic Arthritis, Still's disease, Biologic response modifiers, Comparative effectiveness, Pediatric rheumatology, Registries

Background

Systemic Juvenile Idiopathic Arthritis (JIA) is a rare childhood inflammatory disease associated with significant morbidity, and characterized by arthritis accompanied by high spiking fevers, plus additional features such as rash, generalized lymphadenopathy, hepatosplenomegaly, and serositis [1]. There is considerable variation in systemic JIA treatment, due in part to a heterogeneous and somewhat unpredictable disease course, differences in physician practices, and until very recently, a lack of clinical trial data [2–5] and evidence based guidelines [6, 7]. Recent trials of IL-1 and IL-6 inhibitors (IL1i and IL6i) which demonstrated striking efficacy in systemic JIA were conducted in children with established chronic disease, so little evidence exists for use of biologic agents in new-onset or untreated systemic JIA. Nevertheless, many pediatric rheumatologists currently treat with IL1i and/or IL6i

* Correspondence: Yukiko.Kimura@HackensackMeridian.org
[1]Pediatric rheumatology, Joseph M. Sanzari Children's Hospital, Hackensack University Medical Center, 30 Prospect Ave, Hackensack, NJ 07601, USA
Full list of author information is available at the end of the article

early in the course of disease [8–10]. Intriguing data from several uncontrolled case series suggest that early use of these biologic agents might favorably alter the potentially devastating outcomes of chronic persistent systemic JIA [10, 11]. On the other hand, as many as 10–40% of patients may have a monocyclic course which remits spontaneously within the first year [12, 13], complicating the evaluation of treatment effectiveness in early disease. An additional consideration is the question of whether rare, potentially fatal cardiopulmonary complications may be associated with the increased use of these agents specifically in systemic JIA [14].

With new options for treatment now commercially available and FDA approved, there is an urgent need to determine the relative effectiveness, safety and tolerability of commonly used treatments in systemic JIA. While a blinded randomized multi-arm controlled clinical trial would be ideal, it would be cost-prohibitive, require a very large sample size and likely not be feasible to perform in such a rare disease of childhood. Comparative effectiveness research (CER) studies in an observational, routine care setting are therefore a more practical approach to examine which treatments are effective and most appropriate for an individual child [15, 16]. In such a study, physician choice (together with patient/caregiver preferences) would be the primary determining factor for treatment selection. Such a study could be successful if there were equipoise between most common treatments and if the treatments and data collection were standardized and captured at predetermined intervals. The development of Consensus-derived standardized Treatment Plans (CTPs) for systemic JIA funded by a National Institute of Arthritis and Musculoskeletal and Skin Diseases (NIAMS) Challenge Grant (1RC1AR058605-01) to the Childhood Arthritis and Rheumatology Research Alliance (CARRA) was a key step in this process and in improving outcomes for patients with systemic JIA [17, 18]. The methods by which the CARRA CTPs were developed using CARRA-wide surveys to identify the current most commonly used treatments for systemic JIA and the standardization process using consensus methodology are outlined in a previously published article [17].

A pilot study comparing the published CARRA systemic JIA CTPs was funded by an Arthritis Foundation Innovative Research Grant and conducted in a limited number of sites in order to test the acceptance and usability of these CTPs in preparation for a future large comparative effectiveness study that would utilize the broader CARRA Registry network. This pilot study was conducted to assess the feasibility of conducting a larger more definitive CER study and to identify possible issues that could arise in such a study [19].

Methods

Patients were enrolled in the CARRA Registry and treated with one of the systemic JIA CTPs at 13 CARRA Registry sites for 9 months during the period from 2011 to 2014. Funding from NIAMS via the American Recovery and Reinvestment Act (ARRA) in 2010 enabled the CARRA Registry, a multi-center prospective observational study of children with pediatric rheumatic diseases including JIA. Altogether, investigators enrolled over 9,500 patients in what is now called the CARRA Legacy Registry, including more than 7,000 with JIA (>500 with systemic JIA) at 60 sites over 3 years [9]. The CARRA Registry general protocol and consent was approved by the Duke University IRB (#Pro00054616) and at all participating site IRBs. Because the CTP study is not interventional and patients received standard-of-care therapy at the discretion of their treating physician, additional consent for participation beyond this standard consent for the CARRA Registry was not required.

The entry criteria used were a CARRA-modified version of the International League of Associations of Rheumatology (ILAR) criteria [20], as published in the original article describing the development of the systemic JIA CTPs [17]. In order to capture as many children with systemic JIA as possible while avoiding inclusion of children with self-limited febrile illnesses or alternative diagnoses, it was decided by consensus of the pediatric rheumatologists in the CARRA JIA Research Committee to adapt the ILAR criteria for new-onset patients. The modifications were to require at least 2 weeks of fever (but not necessarily on continuous days), at least one joint with physician-documented arthritis for at least a week, along with at least one other ILAR systemic JIA feature. No prior treatment for systemic JIA aside from NSAIDs or short-term (less than 2 weeks) GC were allowed. There was no randomization or blinding of treatment assignment; instead, a CTP was chosen for each child by the treating pediatric rheumatologist after discussion with the child and family as part of customary clinical decision making process. The CTP choices were: (1) GC only; (2) Methotrexate ± GC; (3) IL1i (either anakinra or canakinumab) ± GC [18]; and (4) IL6i (tocilizumab) ± GC.

Follow-up visits occurred at intervals defined by the CTPs and consistent with routine care: 2 weeks, 1, 3, 6 and 9 months after baseline. Unscheduled visits were conducted if there was a change in CTP medication. Clinical and laboratory data, determined previously by consensus-based process and also consistent with routine care, were collected at these time points through the CARRA Registry as outlined in the CTPs [17]. The CTPs recommended that if patients worsened or failed to improve sufficiently as determined by the physician's assessment of disease activity, GC could be added or increased, or the treatment (CTP) changed. Suggested GC tapering schedules corresponding to very rapid, rapid, moderate, and slow tapering schedules were provided to be used by the treating physician but were not compulsory. By 3 months after CTP initiation, if the child was still receiving ≥50% of the starting dose of GC, it was recommended that the treatment (CTP) should be changed anticipating a better outcome. The treating physicians were asked why a particular initial CTP was chosen, and to provide the reason if the treating CTP was changed. Serious adverse events, including macrophage activation syndrome (MAS), and side effects of medications, were collected.

Outcomes included the primary endpoint of the study: clinical inactive disease (CID) off glucocorticoids at 9 months. CID was defined using the ACR provisional criteria for defining clinical inactive disease which specifies all the following: no active arthritis, a physician's global assessment of disease activity score of 0, ESR and/or CRP in the normal range, no features of systemic JIA (fever, rash, serositis, splenomegaly, or generalized lymphadenopathy), no uveitis and duration of morning stiffness for <15 min [21]. All inactive disease criteria [22] were available for all children who had a documented 9 month visit. For the primary endpoint analysis, all patients were included even if lost to follow-up. The GC and methotrexate CTP-initiated patients were combined as the non-biologic CTP group, while the IL1i and IL6i CTP initiated patients were combined as the biologic CTP group. Secondarily, all 4 CTPs were analyzed separately assessing achievement of the primary endpoint, as well as the ability to lower GC doses.

Safety assessments included reporting of serious adverse events (SAEs), defined as an adverse event that results in death, is life-threatening, requires hospitalization or prolongation of a hospitalization, persistent or significant disability or in capacity, or a congenital anomaly or birth defect; and adverse events (AEs). AEs were graded using Common Terminology Criteria for Adverse Events (CTCAE v4.0). Grade 1 AE was asymptomatic or with mild symptoms and required either clinical or diagnostic observations or no intervention. Grade 2 AE was defined as moderate severity requiring minimal, local or noninvasive intervention. Grade 3 was a severe or medically significant event but not immediately life-threatening and either hospitalization or prolongation of hospitalization were required. Grade 4 AEs were defined as those with life-threatening consequences or requiring urgent intervention. The MedDRA dictionary was not used for safety reporting in this pilot study.

Differences in data collected from the CTPs were compared using chi square, Fisher's exact, and Wilcoxon rank sum tests.

Results

Thirty untreated, mostly newly diagnosed systemic JIA patients were enrolled into the CARRA Registry at 13 sites and started on a CARRA systemic JIA CTP. The children's clinical and demographic characteristics are summarized in Table 1.

Five patients were taking GC prior to starting their respective CTP (median 12 days prior to baseline): of these patients, three patients started on IL6i, and one each started on IL1i and MTX. One patient started on the IL1i CTP was lost to follow-up after the baseline visit.

Figure 1 shows the number of children in each CTP group that eventually switched CTPs or added a DMARD such as methotrexate. Ultimately, 12 of 30 children (40%) switched from their original CTP or added methotrexate. Figure 2 shows initial CTP choice by site. Sites 1–4 exclusively used non-biologic CTPs to start, while sites 6–13 exclusively used biologic CTPs, with site 5 the only site to start both biologic and non-biologic CTPs. Although the majority of sites enrolled few patients (1 to 3), reasons for selecting a particular CTP varied mostly by site rather than CTP. The most common reasons cited were: "treatment works best" in 19/29 (65.5%) (GC, IL1i, IL6i CTPs); "treatment is safer" in 15/29 (51.7%) (MTX, IL1i, IL6i); "treatment is better tolerated" in 14/29 (48.3%) (MTX, IL1i, IL6i); and "always select(s) this treatment" in 10/29 (34.5%) (GC, IL1i, IL6i).

Owing to the reliance on data collection at regular office visits, there was variability in the designated 9 month visit dates with the median being 39.9 weeks after baseline (IQR: 37.3, 43.4, range 29.9–54.7 weeks) Three children did not have a 9 month visit (1 GC and 2 IL1i CTP patients); of these, 1 of the 2 IL1i treated patients and the GC treated patient were lost to follow-up.

While feasibility of the study methodology rather than clinical outcomes was the major purpose of this study, and with the caveat that no attempt was made to adjust for patient characteristics between these very small groups, differences between non-biologic and biologic CTPs were nevertheless observed. The primary endpoint of CID off GC at 9 months was achieved by 50% of biologic CTP initiated children (11 of the 22 children), whereas none of the eight non-biologic CTP initiated children achieved this endpoint ($p = 0.014$) (Table 2).

This failure to achieve CID off GC was not simply due to slow tapering of GC: 6 of 8 (75%) children started on non-biologic CTPs had active disease at 9 months compared with 9 of 22 (41%) of children started on biologic CTPs ($p = 0.407$); and 6 of 8 (75%) of non-biologic CTP treated children were still taking GC at 9 months, compared to 4 of 22 (18%) of biologic CTP treated children ($p = 0.007$). Table 3 also shows the primary endpoint analysis by individual CTP group, as well as of patients who achieved the endpoint without switching/adding

Table 1 Baseline demographic and disease characteristics in all systemic JIA CTP patients

	GC (*N* = 2)	MTX (*N* = 6)	IL1 Inhibitor (*N* = 12)	IL6 Inhibitor (*N* = 10)	Total (*N* = 30)	*P*-value
Age in years[a]	12.8	3.4	4.0	9.8	5.7	0.047
Female	50%	67%	92%	90%	83%	0.3
White	0%	83%	33%	80%	57%	0.03
Disease duration (days)[a]	121	38	31	55	42.5	0.2
Polyarthritis	0%	50%	67%	80%	63%	0.18
Number of active joints[a]	1.0	4.5	5.0	5.5	4.0	0.28
ESR >3x ULN	100%	67%	91%	43%	73%	0.27
CRP >3x ULN	100%	83%	91%	40%	79%	0.28
Ferritin (ng/mL)[a]	12,874	1,394	1,062	627	783	0.09
CHAQ score[a]	0.9	1.3	1.9	0.8	1.4	0.6
Pain score (0–10)[a]	3	6.5	6	7.5	6	0.6
Physician global assessment (0–10)[a]	4	7	5	5	5.5	0.12
Parent global assessment well-being (0–10)[a]	0	7	6	6	6	0.103
Initiated GC at baseline	100%	100%	42%	70%	67%	0.029
Initial GC dose (mg/kg)[a]	0.67	0.97	0.00	0.68	0.80	0.548
GC prior to baseline	50%	16.7%	8.3%	30%	20%	0.350
Initial dose of each CTP medication in mg/kg (IQR)[a]	0.67 (0.6–0.73)	0.487 (0.46–0.64)	2.93 (2–3.6)[b]	8.14 (8–12)	Not Applicable	

[a]Median
[b]Anakinra dose (anakinra was used as the initial IL-1i in all patients)

CTP medications. Likely due to the small numbers in each group, statistical significance was not achieved in these groups. All but one provider generally followed the CTP GC tapering recommendations, so that if by Month 3, if GC were not tapered to less than 50% of the initial dose, treatment was intensified or the CTP was changed. There was no significant difference in the median number of days from baseline of the 9 month visit between the biologic (282 days) and non-biologic (271 days) CTP groups ($p = 0.599$), despite the variability in the 9 month visit date discussed above.

Adverse events are listed in Table 3. There was one Grade 4 AE infusion reaction with tocilizumab. There were 4 SAE's: 2 that resulted in hospitalization for intravenous antimicrobial therapy (cellulitis in a child taking canakinumab and GC [Grade 3] and varicella in a child taking anakinra [Grade 3]), 1 hospitalization for

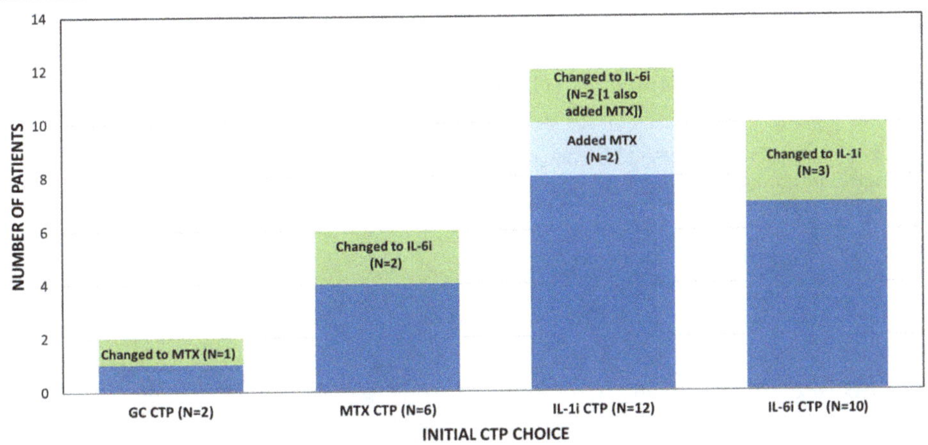

Fig. 1 Initial Consensus Treatment Plan (CTP) Choices and Subsequent Treatment Changes. The total numbers of patients started on each CTP are shown, along with those remaining on the original CTP medication (*dark blue*), switching to a different CTP (*green*) or adding another CTP medication (*light blue*). IL1i: IL1 inhibitor; IL6i: IL6 inhibitor

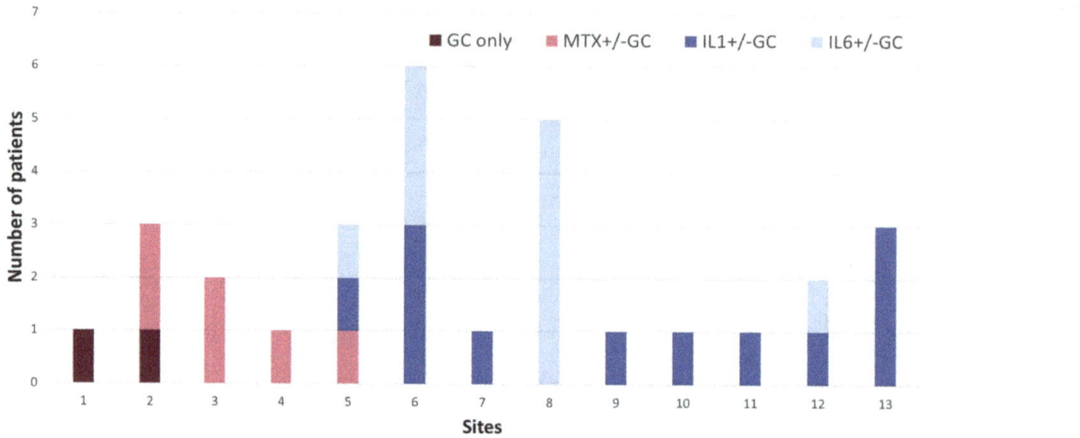

Fig. 2 Initial Consensus Treatment Plan (CTP) Choice By Site. CTP choices distributed by site, showing that 4 sites started only a non-biologic CTP (*red colors*), while 8 sites started only a biologic CTP (*blue colors*), IL1i: IL1 inhibitor; IL6i: IL6 inhibitor

appendicitis and appendectomy on methotrexate and GC, and 1 for macrophage activation syndrome (MAS) in a child on tocilizumab (Grade 3). One additional child who was receiving anakinra developed MAS and was treated with oral prednisone without hospitalization (Grade 2). All patients recovered uneventfully.

Discussion

This pilot study assessed the feasibility of using standardized CARRA CTPs for untreated systemic JIA, 90% of whom had disease onset less than 4 months prior to treatment, to evaluate the comparative effectiveness of commonly used treatment approaches. Importantly, the study established that the CARRA Registry and the coordinating center at the Duke Clinical Research Institute (DCRI) could effectively operationalize and capture the data for such a study, but it also demonstrated that better methods to decrease missing visits and data, and to be able to capture clinical data between visits for the larger study were needed. Interestingly, each plan was used with similar frequency aside from the GC-only plan, confirming community equipoise on treatment selection. The choice of plan varied by site/individual physician rather than disease characteristics of the individual child, with the caveat that at most a few patients were treated at each site. However, plan choice driven by site allows for a "pseudo-block randomization" in the context of a larger observational comparative effectiveness study. The distribution of CTP usage followed results of surveys conducted as part of the development of the original CTPs [17], indicating that there continues to be substantial variability in physician practice with regard to initial treatment choices for systemic JIA.

The results of this pilot study underline the need for a larger definitive comparative effectiveness study assessing all 4 CTPs. The quandary about the safest and most effective treatment of new-onset systemic JIA has been informed by studies of the IL1i anakinra (recombinant IL-1 receptor antagonist). Recent studies looking at early use of anakinra in systemic JIA demonstrated a marked reduction in the development of chronic persistent arthritis from a historical rate of 50–60% to less than 10% [9, 11], a rate of response markedly distinct from that observed in a randomized controlled trial of anakinra in

Table 2 Achievement of Clinical Inactive Disease (CID) off Glucocorticoids (GC) in Non-Biologic and Biologic initiated patients (primary endpoint), as well as in the 4 Consensus Treatment Plan (CTP) groups

							Biologic grouping		
Patient Status at Month 9	Total $N=30$	Gluco-corticoids $N=2$	Methotrex-ate $N=6$	IL1i[a] $N=12$	IL6i[a] $N=10$	*p*-value	Non-Biologic CTP $N=8$	Biologic CTP $N=22$	*p*-value
CID	13/30 (43.3%)	0/2	2/6 (33.3%)	5/12 (41.7%)	6/10 (60.0%)	0.549	2/8 (25.0%)	11/22 (50.0%)	0.407
Off GC	20/30 (66.7%)	1/2 (50.0%)	1/6 (16.7%)	10/12 (83.3%)	8/10 (80.0%)	0.019	2/8 (25.0%)	18/22 (81.8%)	0.007
CID off GC	11/30 (36.7%)	0/2	0/6	5/12 (41.7%)	6/10 (60.0%)	0.079	0/8	11/22 (50.0%)	0.014
CID off GC and no CTP change	8/30 (26.7%)	0/2	0/6	3/12 (25.0%)	5/10 (50.0%)	0.168	0/8	8/22 (36.4%)	0.071

Also shown are all patients who achieved CID (regardless of GC), all patients who were off GC, and all patients who achieved CID off GC and did not change their CTP treatments, at 9 months. Patients lost to follow-up were considered treatment failures
[a]IL1i: IL-1 inhibitor; IL6i: IL-6 inhibitor

Table 3 Adverse events reported in all patients by CTP at time of event

CTP at time of AE	GC	MTX	IL-1 Inhibitor	IL-6 Inhibitor	Total
Grade 2	0	2 (allergic reaction [1], arthritis flare [1])	5 (MAS [1], hepatitis [1], rash [1], Strep pharyngitis [1], injection site reaction [1])	8 (fever [1], rash [1], arthritis flare [2], headache [1], neutropenia [1], viral illness [1], infusion reaction [1])	15
Grade 3	0	0	2 (infections)[b]	0	2
Grade 4	0	0	0	1 (infusion reaction)	1
SAE	0	1[a]	2 (infections)[b]	1 (MAS)	3

[a]Appendicitis and appendectomy
[b]1 varicella (anakinra), 1 cellullitis (canakinumab)

established chronic systemic JIA [2]. These studies raise the possibility of a "window of opportunity" in early systemic JIA during which cytokine blockade could be especially effective [23]. Even though this pilot study included small numbers of children who were followed for only 9 months, the results indicate that untreated systemic JIA patients started on IL-1i or IL-6i biologics achieved the primary endpoint (CID off GC at 9 months) more frequently than children not started on a biologic. Children treated with non-biologic CTPs were more likely to both have continued active disease and continue to be treated with GC compared to those treated with biologic CTPs. Whether this will hold true in a larger population of children followed for a longer period of time remains to be seen, as no attempt was made to correct for baseline clinical features or other potentially confounding variables, rendering the conclusions of this this pilot study far from definitive [19].

Study limitations include the observational design. As noted, no adjustments were made to address confounding by indication (prescriber channeling). The basic CTP approach assumes that treatment choice is determined by physician preferences rather than patient disease characteristics, and further assumes that individual physicians influence disease outcomes only through the CTP choice. We observed evidence in favor of the first assumption in this pilot study, but the latter assumption is difficult to assess given the strong correlations between physician and treatment choice. Missing data points and visits outside of the suggested visit schedule were relatively common, limiting analysis of the results. Children were sometimes started on medications, especially GC, prior to starting the CTP. Short-term use of GC was allowed, which may have changed the baseline disease characteristics of these patients. However, prior treatment with GC is particularly difficult to avoid at presentation of new onset systemic JIA, a phase of the disease in which children are often acutely ill; excluding these children could eliminate significant numbers of children, particularly the sickest children. In addition, patients were followed for a relatively short period of time (9 months), with CID assessed at a single time point that may incompletely reflect the treatment response in this dynamic disease. Evaluation of stably inactive disease, such as clinical inactive disease for 6 consecutive months (i.e., clinical remission) and clinical inactive disease for 12 consecutive months off of all medications (i.e., clinical remission off medication) [21] will be assessed in the larger CTP study informed by this pilot, but was not able to be captured in this study. Data collection through the CARRA Registry will allow assessment of long-term outcomes for decade or more after Registry enrollment, including outcomes such as medication safety and functional status as well as remission. Lastly, the small sample size, differences in the demographics of the study cohort compared to other systemic JIA cohorts, the short follow-up duration and missing data limit the external validity of the results of this pilot study.

The use of modified ILAR criteria for diagnosis may affect the generalizability of the study results. It is recognized that many children with systemic JIA in the earliest stages of disease require treatment, yet may not strictly fulfill ILAR criteria (especially the requirement for 6 weeks of arthritis) [24]. Indeed, the Yamaguchi criteria for Adult Onset Still Disease (the adult correlate of systemic JIA) does not require overt arthritis for diagnosis [25, 26]. It is possible that use of these modified criteria by clinicians other than experienced pediatric rheumatologists may lead to misdiagnosis. We emphasize that it is critical to exclude other diagnoses that may be mistaken for systemic JIA, such as infection, malignancy (in particular acute lymphoblastic leukemia, lymphoma and neuroblastoma) or genetic auto-inflammatory diseases prior to starting treatment for systemic JIA using the CTPs, especially before treatment with GC. In cases where the diagnosis is not based on the triad of characteristic fever, rash and arthritis, the advice of an expert pediatric rheumatologist should be sought.

The larger comparative effectiveness study, implementing the systemic JIA CTP study at 60 or more CARRA Registry sites, will retain the observational study design including non-randomization of treatment allocation. This study, termed the FiRst-line Options in Systemic JIA Treatment (FROST), will address limitations recognized in the pilot study including reducing important potential biases such as confounding by indication by using propensity scoring, as well as instrumental variable and marginal structural model analyses. Bayesian analytic methods will also be utilized for the larger study. Bayesian prior belief exercises needed for the analyses were conducted at a recent CARRA annual meeting. This pilot study was employed to inform the power calculations for FROST, in which we plan to use an intention-to-treat analytic approach (see Additional files 1 and 2). Aggressive efforts to improve data quality are planned, including more rigorous site education and awareness, leveraging various forms of communication. More detailed information about GC use prior to and during treatment will be obtained and analyzed. Children/parents will be queried about symptoms and GC dose on a regular basis using home electronic mobile device reporting. We will collect detailed information about SAEs and important medical events (IME) throughout the CTP study (including MedDRA coding of events). Lastly, important long-term follow up of children started on the CARRA systemic JIA CTPs will be accomplished using existing CARRA Registry infrastructure to follow all enrolled patients for 10 or more years, including use of a call center to contact patients and their families if the child transitions from pediatric to adult care or moves to a non-participating center.

We observed a few unexpected patient characteristics in this small pilot study, such as a female predominance, whereas most large studies of systemic JIA have reported a nearly equal female to male ratio [8, 9]. There were also patients with longer than expected disease duration prior to study enrollment. These differences are anticipated to be minimized by the inclusion of many more patients into the larger FROST CTP study.

Conclusions

This pilot study of the four CARRA standardized CTPs for untreated mostly new-onset systemic JIA successfully demonstrated the feasibility of their implementation in a larger observational comparative effectiveness study using the CARRA Registry for data collection. FROST, the planned follow-on larger, longitudinal study will establish whether biologic medications started early in the disease course will result in better outcomes for children with new onset systemic JIA.

Acknowledgements

The authors wish to thank Thomas A. Phillips, M.A. (DCRI) for statistical assistance and Jane Winsor, B.A. (DCRI) for database programming. PAN was supported by the Fundación Bechara. We also acknowledge the following CARRA Registry site investigators and coordinators:
L. Abramson, E. Anderson, M. Andrew, N. Battle, M. Becker, H. Benham, T. Beukelman, J. Birmingham, P. Blier, A. Brown, H. Brunner, A. Cabrera, D. Canter, D. Carlton, B. Caruso, L. Ceracchio, E. Chalom, J. Chang, P. Charpentier, K. Clark, J. Dean, F. Dedeoglu, B. Feldman, P. Ferguson, M. Fox, K. Francis, M. Gervasini, D. Goldsmith, G. Gorton, B. Gottlieb, T. Graham, T. Griffin, H. Grosbein, S. Guppy, H. Haftel, D. Helfrich, G. Higgins, A. Hillard, J.R. Hollister, J. Hsu, A. Hudgins, C. Hung, A. Huttenlocher, N. Ilowite, A. Imlay, L. Imundo, C.J. Inman, J. Jaqith, R. Jerath, L. Jung, P. Kahn, A. Kapedani, D. Kingsbury, K. Klein, M. Klein-Gitelman, A. Kunkel, S. Lapidus, S. Layburn, T. Lehman, C. Lindsley, M. Macgregor-Hannah, M. Malloy, C. Mawhorter, D. McCurdy, K. Mims, N. Moorthy, D. Morus, E. Muscal, M. Natter, J. Olson, K. O'Neil, K. Onel, M. Orlando, J. Palmquist, M. Phillips, L. Ponder, S. Prahalad, M. Punaro, D. Puplava, S. Quinn, A. Quintero, C. Rabinovich, A. Reed, C. Reed, S. Ringold, M. Riordan, S. Roberson, A. Robinson, J. Rossette, D. Rothman, D. Russo, N. Ruth, K. Schikler, A. Sestak, B. Shaham, Y. Sherman, M. Simmons, N. Singer, S. Spalding, H. Stapp, R. Syed, E. Thomas, K. Torok, D. Trejo, J. Tress, W. Upton, R. Vehe, E. von Scheven, L. Walters, J.E. Weiss, P.F. Weiss, N. Welnick, A. White, J. Woo, J. Wootton, A. Yalcindag, C. Zapp, L. Zemel, and A. Zhu.

Funding

This work was completed with support from an Arthritis Foundation Innovative Research Grant. The National Institute of Arthritis and Musculoskeletal and Skin Disease at the National Institutes of Health (NIH 1RC1AR058605-01) supported the development of the consensus treatment plans. The CARRA Registry was supported by grants from the National Institute of Arthritis and Musculoskeletal and Skin Diseases, Friends of CARRA, the Arthritis Foundation, and the NIH (RC2AR058934).

Authors' contributions

YK, TB, EM, PAN, LES conceived and designed the study, analyzed and interpreted the data, and drafted the manuscript and revisions. SG made substantial contributions to the analysis and interpretation of data and helped to draft the manuscript and revisions. KM, TBG, MI, NI, MKG, KO, SP, MP, SR, DT, HVM, JEW, PFW: made substantial contributions to acquisition of data, and was involved in revising the manuscript critically for important intellectual content. All authors have given final approval of the version to be published and agreed to be accountable for all aspects of the work in ensuring that questions related to the accuracy of integrity of any part of the work are appropriately investigated and resolved.

Competing interests

- Kimura—CARRA (salary support), SOBI (consulting), Novartis (consulting)
- Beukelman—CARRA (salary support), Novartis (consulting), Genentech/Roche (consulting), UCB (consulting)
- Ilowite—CARRA (salary support), Novartis (consulting), SOBI (consulting)
- Prahalad—Novartis (advisory board), Medac Pharma (advisory board)
- Punaro—SOBI (consultant)
- Schanberg – CARRA, SOBI (consulting), UCB (DSMB), Sanofi (DSMB)

Consent for publication

Not applicable.

Author details

[1]Pediatric rheumatology, Joseph M. Sanzari Children's Hospital, Hackensack University Medical Center, 30 Prospect Ave, Hackensack, NJ 07601, USA. [2]Pediatric rheumatology, Seattle Children's Hospital, Seattle, USA. [3]Pediatric rheumatology, University of Alabama at Birmingham, Birmingham, USA. [4]Rheumatology, Cincinnati Children's Hospital Medical Center, Cincinnati, USA. [5]Rheumatology, Immunology and Allergy, Brigham and Women's Hospital, Boston, USA. [6]Childhood Arthritis & Rheumatology Research Alliance, Milwaukee, USA. [7]Pediatric rheumatology, Vanderbilt University, Nashville, USA. [8]Pediatric rheumatology, Children's Mercy Hospital, Kansas

City, USA. [9]Pediatric rheumatology, Children's Hospital at Montefiore, Bronx, NY, USA. [10]Pediatric rheumatology, Ann & Robert H. Lurie Children's Hospital of Chicago, Chicago, USA. [11]Pediatric rheumatology, University of Chicago, Chicago, USA. [12]Pediatric rheumatology, Emory University School of Medicine, Atlanta, USA. [13]Pediatric rheumatology, Texas Scottish Rite Hospital, Dallas, USA. [14]Pediatric rheumatology, St. Christopher's Hospital, Philadelphia, USA. [15]Pediatric rheumatology, Duke University, Durham, NC, USA. [16]Pediatric rheumatology, Children's Hospital of Philadelphia, Philadelphia, USA.

References

1. Prakken B, Albani S, Martini A. Juvenile idiopathic arthritis. Lancet. 2011; 377(9783):2138–49.
2. Quartier P, Allantz F, Cimaz R, Pillet P, Msesiaen C, et al. A multicentre, randomised, double-blind, placebo-controlled trial with the interleukin-1 receptor antagonist anakinra in patients with systemic-onset juvenile idiopathic arthritis (ANAJIS trial). Ann Rheum Dis. 2011;70(5):747–54.
3. Ruperto N, Brunner HI, Quartier P, Constantin T, Wulffraat N, Horneff G, Brik R, McCann L, Kasapcopur O, Rutkowska-Sak L, et al. Two randomized trials of canakinumab in systemic juvenile idiopathic arthritis. N Engl J Med. 2012; 367(25):2396–406.
4. De Benedetti F, Brunner HI, Ruperto N, Kenwright A, Wright S, Calvo I, Cuttica R, Ravelli A, Schneider R, Woo P, et al. Randomized trial of tocilizumab in systemic juvenile idiopathic arthritis. N Engl J Med. 2012; 367(25):2385–95.
5. Yokota S, Imagawa T, Mori M, Miyamae T, Aihara Y, Takei S, Iwata N, Umebayashi H, Murata T, Miyoshi M, et al. Efficacy and safety of tocilizumab in patients with systemic-onset juvenile idiopathic arthritis: a randomised, double-blind, placebo-controlled, withdrawal phase III trial. Lancet. 2008; 371(9617):998–1006.
6. Ringold S, Weiss PF, Beukelman T, DeWitt EM, Ilowite NT, Kimura Y, Laxer RM, Lovell DJ, Nigrovic PA, Robinson AB, et al. 2013 update of the 2011 American College of Rheumatology recommendations for the treatment of juvenile idiopathic arthritis: recommendations for the medical therapy of children with systemic juvenile idiopathic arthritis and tuberculosis screening among children receiving biologic medications. Arthritis Rheum. 2013;65(10):2499–512.
7. Beukelman T, Patkar NM, Saag KG, Tolleson-Rinehart S, Cron RQ, DeWitt EM, Ilowite NT, Kimura Y, Laxer RM, Lovell DJ, et al. 2011 American College of Rheumatology recommendations for the treatment of juvenile idiopathic arthritis: initiation and safety monitoring of therapeutic agents for the treatment of arthritis and systemic features. Arthritis Care Res (Hoboken). 2011;63(4):465–82.
8. Klotsche J, Raab A, Niewerth M, Sengler C, Ganser G, Kallinich T, Niehues T, Hufnagel M, Thon A, Hospach T, et al. Outcome and trends in treatment of systemic juvenile idiopathic arthritis in the German National Pediatric Rheumatological Database from 2000 to 2013. Arthritis Rheum. 2016;68(12): 3023–34.
9. Janow G, Schanberg LE, Setoguchi S, Hasselblad V, Mellins ED, Schneider R, Kimura Y, Investigators CLR. The Systemic Juvenile Idiopathic Arthritis Cohort of the Childhood Arthritis and Rheumatology Research Alliance Registry: 2010–2013. J Rheumatol. 2016;43(9):1755–62.
10. Nigrovic PA, Mannion M, Prince FH, Zeft A, Rabinovich CE, et al. Anakinra as first-line disease-modifying therapy in systemic juvenile idiopathic arthritis: report of forty-six patients from an international multicenter series. Arthritis Rheum. 2011;63(2):545–55.
11. Vastert SJ, de Jager W, Noordman BJ, Holzinger D, Kuis W, Prakken BJ, Wulffraat NM. Effectiveness of first-line treatment with recombinant interleukin-1 receptor antagonist in steroid-naive patients with new-onset systemic juvenile idiopathic arthritis: results of a prospective cohort study. Arthritis Rheum. 2014;66(4):1034–43.
12. Singh-Grewal D, Schenider R, Bayer N, Feldman BM. Predictors of disease course and remission in systemic Juvenile Idiopathic Arthritis. Arthritis Rheum. 2006;54(5):1595–601.
13. Spiegel LR, Schneider R, Lang BA, Silverman ED, Laxer RM, Stephens D. Early predictors of poor functional outcome in systemic-onset juvenile rheumatoid arthritis: a multicenter cohort study. Arthritis Rheum. 2000;43:2402–9.
14. Kimura Y, Weiss JE, Haroldson KL, Lee T, Punaro M, Oliveira S, Rabinovich E, Riebschleger M, Anton J, Blier PR, et al. Pulmonary hypertension and other potentially fatal pulmonary complications in systemic juvenile idiopathic arthritis. Arthritis Care Res (Hoboken). 2013;65(5):745–52.
15. Sox HC, Greenfield S. Comparative effectiveness research: a report from the Institute of Medicine. Ann Intern Med. 2009;151(3):203–5.
16. Yokota S, Itoh Y, Morio T, Origasa H, Sumitomo N, Tomobe M, Tanaka K, Minota S. Tocilizumab in systemic juvenile idiopathic arthritis in a real-world clinical setting: results from 1 year of postmarketing surveillance follow-up of 417 patients in Japan. Ann Rheum Dis. 2016;75(9):1654–60.
17. DeWitt EM, Kimura Y, Beukelman T, Nigrovic PA, Onel K, Prahalad S, Schneider R, Stoll ML, Angeles-Han S, Milojevic D, et al. Consensus treatment plans for new-onset systemic juvenile idiopathic arthritis. Arthritis Care Res (Hoboken). 2012;64(7):1001–10.
18. Kimura Y, DeWitt EM, Beukelman T, Stoll ML, Nigrovic PA, Onel K, Prahalad S, Angeles-Han S, Schneider R, Juvenile Idiopathic Arthritis Disease-Specific Research Committee of the Childhood A, et al. Adding canakinumab to the Childhood Arthritis and Rheumatology Research Alliance consensus treatment plans for systemic juvenile idiopathic arthritis: comment on the article by DeWitt et al. Arthritis Care Res (Hoboken). 2014;66(9):1430–1.
19. Thabane L, Ma J, Chu R, Cheng J, Ismaila A, Rios LP, Robson R, Thabane M, Giangregorio L, Goldsmith CH. A tutorial on pilot studies: the what, why and how. BMC Med Res Methodol. 2010;10:1.
20. Petty RE, Southwood TR, Manners P, Baum J, Glass DN, Goldenberg J, He X, Maldonado-Cocco J, Orozco-Alcala J, Prieur AM, et al. International League of Associations for Rheumatology classification of juvenile idiopathic arthritis: second revision, Edmonton, 2001. J Rheumatol. 2004;31(2):390–2.
21. Wallace CA, Giannini EH, Huang B, Itert L, Ruperto N, Childhood Arthritis Rheumatology Research A, Pediatric Rheumatology Collaborative Study G, Paediatric Rheumatology International Trials O. American College of Rheumatology provisional criteria for defining clinical inactive disease in select categories of juvenile idiopathic arthritis. Arthritis Care Res (Hoboken). 2011;63(7):929–36.
22. Wallace CA, Ruperto N, Giannini E, Childhood Arthritis and Rheumatology Research Alliance; Pediatric Rheumatology International Trials Organization: Pediatric Rheumatology Collaborative Study Group. Preliminary criteria for clinical remission for select categories of juvenile idiopathic arthritis. J Rheumatol. 2004;31:2290–4.
23. Nigrovic PA. Review: is there a window of opportunity for treatment of systemic juvenile idiopathic arthritis? Arthritis Rheum. 2014;66(6):1405–13.
24. Behrens EM, Beukelman T, Gallo L, Spangler J, Rosenkranz M, Arkachaisri T, Ayala R, Groh B, Finkel TH, Cron RQ. Evaluation of the presentation of systemic onset juvenile rheumatoid arthritis: data from the Pennsylvania Systemic Onset Juvenile Arthritis Registry (PASOJAR). J Rheumatol. 2008; 35(2):343–8.
25. Yamaguchi M, Ohta A, Tsunematsu T, Kasukawa R, Mizushima Y, Kashiwagi H, Kashiwazaki S, Tanimoto K, Matsumoto Y, Ota T, et al. Preliminary criteria for classification of adult Still's disease. J Rheumatol. 1992;19(3):424–30.
26. Jiang L, Wang Z, Dai X, Jin X. Evaluation of clinical measures and different criteria for diagnosis of adult-onset Still's disease in a Chinese population. J Rheumatol. 2011;38(4):741–6.
27. Lee J, Kim J, Jung SH. Bayesian analysis of paired survival data using a bivariate exponential distribution. Lifetime Data Anal. 2007;13(1):119–37.

ASAS definition for sacroiliitis on MRI in SpA: applicable to children?

Nele Herregods[1*], Joke Dehoorne[2], Filip Van den Bosch[3], Jacob Lester Jaremko[4], Joke Van Vlaenderen[2], Rik Joos[2], Xenofon Baraliakos[5], Gaëlle Varkas[3], Koenraad Verstraete[1], Dirk Elewaut[3] and Lennart Jans[1]

Abstract

Background: The Assessment of Spondyloarthritis International Society (ASAS) definition for a 'positive' Magnetic Resonance Imaging (MRI) for sacroiliitis is well studied and validated in adults, but studies about the value of this definition in children are lacking. The aim of this study is to evaluate whether the adult ASAS definition of a positive MRI of the sacroiliac joints can be applied to children with a clinical suspicion of Juvenile Spondyloarthritis (JSpA).

Methods: Two pediatric musculoskeletal radiologists blinded to clinical data independently retrospectively reviewed sacroiliac (SI) joint MRI in 109 children suspected of sacroiliitis. They recorded global impression (sacroiliitis yes/no) and whether the adult ASAS definition for sacroiliitis was met at each joint. This was compared to gold-standard clinical diagnosis of JSpA. Additionally, MRI were scored according to'adapted' ASAS definitions including other features of sacroiliitis on MRI.

Results: JSpA was diagnosed clinically in 47/109 (43%) patients. On MRI, sacroiliitis was diagnosed by global assessment in 30/109 patients, of whom 14 also fulfilled ASAS criteria. No patients with negative global assessment for sacroiliitis fulfilled ASAS criteria. Sensitivity (SN) for JSpA was higher for global assessment (SN = 49%) than for ASAS definition (SN = 26%), but the ASAS definition was more specific (SP = 97% vs. 89%). Modifying adult ASAS criteria to allow bone marrow edema (BME) lesions seen on only one slice, synovitis or capsulitis, increased SN to 36%, 32% and 32% respectively, only slightly lowering SP. Including structural lesions increased SN to 28%, but lowered specificity to 95%.

Conclusion: The adult ASAS definition for sacroiliitis has low sensitivity in children. A pediatric-specific definition of MRI-positive sacroiliitis including BME lesions visible on one slice only, synovitis and/or capsulitis may improve diagnostic utility, and increase relevance of MRI in pediatric rheumatology practice.

Keywords: ASAS definition, Sacroiliitis, MRI, Juvenile spondyloarthritis

Background

Juvenile spondyloarthritides (JSpA) have some overlap with adult spondyloarthritis (SpA) but also important differences. JSpA are a group of related inflammatory diseases characterized by enthesitis and arthritis with a strong association to human leukocyte antigen (HLA) B27 [1]. The International League of Associations for Rheumatology (ILAR) classification of juvenile idiopathic arthritis (JIA) includes seven subtypes [2], in which JSpA is represented in enthesitis-related arthritis (ERA), psoriatic arthritis (PsA) and some types of undifferentiated arthritis. In contrast to adult spondyloarthritis (SpA), JSpA generally presents with peripheral arthritis and enthesitis of the lower extremities in the early years of the disease, while involvement of the sacroiliac (SI) and spinal joints typically occurs later [1–3].

In adults, early diagnosis of SpA has become more important to rheumatologists as new therapeutic options have become available to treat inflammation and potentially delay progression of the disease [4–7]. Increasingly, MRI of the sacroiliac (SI) joints is obtained for early detection of inflammatory changes [6], as it shows active

* Correspondence: Nele.Herregods@uzgent.be
[1]Department of Radiology and Medical Imaging, Ghent University Hospital, De Pintelaan 185, 9000 Ghent, Belgium
Full list of author information is available at the end of the article

inflammatory and structural lesions of sacroiliitis, long before radiographic changes become evident [8–11]. The Assessment of Spondyloarthritis International Society (ASAS) criteria are widely used for classification of adult spondyloarthritis [10], with the presence of active sacroiliitis on MRI as a key criterion for disease classification in the imaging arm of the ASAS criteria [10, 12–15]. A clear definition of active sacroiliitis on MRI has been defined and recently updated by the ASAS working group [10, 12].

Unlike in adult spondyloarthritis, classification of the pediatric population remains challenging. In children, many different classification systems have been proposed [2, 6, 10, 16], however none include imaging as a criterion. In adult classification systems, such as the ASAS and New York criteria, imaging plays a key role [3, 10, 14]. Therefore, adult classification criteria have been applied to children as well. An overall classification system that effectively stratifies JSpA into categories of similar clinical and prognostic implications remains elusive. Unlike in adults [12, 13, 17], the value of MRI assessment of sacroiliitis in children is not well studied, although recent studies have postulated the usefulness of MRI in JSpA [11, 18–23]. In daily clinical practice, children are increasingly being referred for MRI of the SI joints. Weiss et al. found active but asymptomatic sacroiliitis on MRI at diagnosis in JSpA, suggesting a potential role for MRI in JSpA [23]. A clear definition for a positive MRI for sacroiliitis in children is needed as much as in adults.

The ASAS definition for a 'positive' MRI for sacroiliitis is well studied and validated in adults [13, 24], but studies about the value of this definition in children are lacking. The aim of this study is to evaluate whether the adult ASAS definition of a positive MRI of the sacroiliac joints can be applied to children with a clinical suspicion of JSpA.

Methods

Patients

A retrospective study of all pediatric MRI of the sacroiliac joint from September 2013 to November 2015 was approved by the institutional ethics committee of the Ghent University Hospital. Informed consent was obtained from all parents and children. All patients were sent from the pediatric rheumatology department in a tertiary care center and were referred for MRI of the SI joints with sacroiliac joint tenderness or clinical (inflammatory) back pain (IBP) suspected for sacroiliitis in the expert opinion of the pediatric rheumatologists. As there is no established definition of IBP symptoms [25] associated with inflammatory spinal disease in children, we defined IBP as a history of back pain for at least three months with either (not and): insidious onset or improvement with exercise or no improvement with rest or pain at night (with improvement upon getting up). Sacroiliac tenderness was defined as tenderness upon palpation of the sacroiliac joint. Patients were only included when age at onset of the disease was < 16 years. The gold standard was the clinical diagnosis of JSpA made by expert opinion of our two pediatric rheumatologists (JD and RJ, respectively 21 and 35 years of experience), who reassessed the clinical files and were blinded to MRI results. They recorded from the clinical files if patients fulfilled the ILAR criteria, and diagnosed JSpA in consensus. Patients with ERA, PsA and IBD-related arthritis were considered positive for JSpA.

Magnetic resonance imaging

MRI was performed on a body flexed array coil in a 1.5 Tesla MRI unit (Avanto, Siemens Medical, Erlangen, Germany). Sequence protocol included: semicoronal (along long axis of the sacral bone perpendicular to the second sacral (S2) vertebral body) T1-weighted (T1) turbo spin echo (TSE) (slice thickness (ST): 3 mm; repetition time/echo time (TR/TE): 368/20 ms; Field of view (FOV): 320; matrix: 512 × 384; Averages: 2; Turbo Factor (TF): 3); semicoronal short tau inversion recovery sequence (STIR) (ST: 3 mm; TR/TE/Inversion Time (TI): 5030/67/150 ms; FOV: 320; matrix: 320 × 320; Averages 2; TF: 7); axial STIR (ST: 5 mm; TR/TE/TI: 7540/67/150 ms; FOV: 400; matrix: 320 × 320; Averages: 1; TF: 7). Contrast-enhanced pulse sequences were also obtained: semicoronal (ST: 3 mm; TR/TE: 558/20 ms; FOV: 320; matrix: 512 × 384; Averages: 2; TF: 3) and axial fat-saturated T1-weighted TSE (ST: 5 mm; TR/TE: 558/9,8 ms; FOV: 350; matrix: 512 × 288; Averages: 2; TF: 3) 120 s after intravenous administration of Gadolinium-DTPA(Gd) contrast (T1/Gd) (Dotarem, 0.1 mmol/kg body weight).

Image review

MR images were reassessed and reviewed separately by two pediatric musculoskeletal radiologists (NH, LJ), with 12 and 13 years of experience, blinded to all clinical information except age and sex.

First, a global diagnostic assessment was made as to whether the MRI was positive for sacroiliitis or not (sacroiliitis yes/no). To make this global assessment, radiologists first considered multiple active and structural features of sacroiliitis on MRI [8, 10, 11, 21].

The MRI features of active disease included bone marrow edema (BME), retro-articular enthesitis, capsulitis and synovitis. Features were scored as positive as follows: BME if periarticular high STIR signal was present in the subchondral bone in ilium or sacrum; retro-articular enthesitis if there was high STIR signal and/or enhancement of the retro-articular entheses representing soft tissue inflammation; capsulitis if high STIR signal and/or enhancement involved the SI joint capsule; synovitis was defined as presence of a hyperintense, linear signal in the joint space on T2-weighted/STIR images (which on T2 images alone is not distinguishable from fluid in the joint space, but post-gadolinium the region of synovitis will enhance, unlike fluid) and/or an enhancing tissue in the synovial part of the joint post-gadolinium administration, with signal intensity similar to vessels [8, 10, 11, 21, 26].

The MRI features implying structural damage from sacroiliitis consisted of sclerosis (lower subchondral signal than normal on all sequences), erosions (irregularities in the osteochondral interface involving both contour and signal on both T1-weighted and STIR images), fat infiltration (higher T1 signal than expected in periarticular bone) and ankylosis (continuous signal bridging all or a portion of an SI joint) [10, 11, 21]. A hazy delineation of the subchondral bone plate was considered to represent normal maturation. Each radiologist then synthesized all the MRI features of active disease and structural damage and formed a global impression as to whether sacroiliitis was present.

Next, each MRI was scored (yes/no) according to the adult ASAS definition of a positive MRI for sacroiliitis [10, 12]: "Bone marrow edema (BME) on T2-weighted sequences or bone marrow enhancement on a T1-weighted fat suppressed sequence is clearly present and located in the typical subchondral or periarticular areas. MRI appearance must be highly suggestive for SpA. If there is only one site of BME, this should be present on at least two consecutive MRI slices. If there is more than one signal present on a single slice, one slice may be enough."[12] Other MRI features representing active inflammation of the SI joint such as enthesitis or capsulitis, or structural lesions alone are not sufficient for a 'positive' MRI for sacroiliitis. If an inflammatory bone marrow lesion appears to be present but it is hard to determine whether the lesion meets the criterion 'highly suggestive for SpA', then the decision may be influenced by the presence of concomitant structural damage and or other signs of inflammation, which in themselves do not suffice to meet the criterion" [12].

We also tested several alternative 'adapted' ASAS definitions for a positive MRI for sacroiliitis, which each used the same definition as above except that: 1. a study is positive even if BME was only seen on one slice or location; or 2. synovitis is present; or 3. capsulitis is present; or 4. retroarticular enthesitis is present; or 5. Any of the structural lesions from sacroiliitis are present; or 6. BME is seen in only one slice or location AND/OR synovitis is present (i.e., a combination of 'adapted' definitions 1 and 2); or 7. BME is seen in only one slice or location AND/OR capsulitis is present (i.e., a combination of 'adapted' definitions 1 and 3); or 8. BME is seen in only one slice or location AND/OR synovitis is present AND/OR capsulitis is present (i.e., a combination of 'adapted' definitions 1,2 and 3).

Statistical analysis

Statistical analysis was performed using SPSS 20.0 software for Windows (SPSS, Chicago, IL, USA). Basic descriptive statistics for categorical data were recorded. The diagnostic utility for clinical diagnosis of JSpA was determined by using decision matrix analysis, generating sensitivity (SN) and specificity (SP) for the global diagnostic impression, ASAS definition and 8 adapted versions of the ASAS definition, each compared to the clinical gold standard diagnosis of JSpA. The likelihood ratio of a positive test (LR+) was calculated as sensitivity/(1-specificity) and the likelihood ratio of a negative test (LR-) value was calculated as (1-sensitivity)/specificity.

Interobserver agreement between the radiologists was calculated using kappa (κ) statistics. The levels of agreement were considered to be slight, fair, moderate, substantial, near-perfect and perfect at κ values of respectively 0–0.20, 0.21–0.40, 0.41–0.60, 0.61–0.80, 0.81–0.99 and 1.00 [27].

Results

Demographics

Of the 109 children, 41 (38%) were boys, 68 (62%) were girls. The mean age of our population was 13.6 years (range 6.8–17.9). HLA-B27 was positive in 31/109 (28%) patients, and negative in 49 (45%). In 29 (27%) patients, HLA-B27 was not obtained by the referring clinician, since this test was not specified to be mandatory in our MRI study design. IBP was reported in 95 patients, SI joint tenderness in 45 patients. In 31 patients, both of these symptoms were present. JSpA was clinically diagnosed in 47 (43%) patients according to the expert opinion of our pediatric rheumatologists, 45 of these children met the ILAR criteria for ERA ($N = 36$) or PsA ($N = 9$). Two patients with inflammatory bowel disease (IBD) and arthritis were also classified as JSpA. Other diagnoses were oligoarticular JIA ($N = 8$), polyarticular JIA ($N = 2$), mechanical pain ($N = 41$), hyperlaxity syndrome ($N = 4$), Behçet disease ($N = 2$), Chronic Recurrent Multifocal Osteomyelitis (CRMO) ($N = 1$), auto-inflammatory syndrome ($N = 1$), reactive arthritis ($N = 1$), psoriasis ($N = 1$) and hyperexcitability ($N = 1$). One patient was diagnosed with lymphoma and was excluded from the study.

Demographics for patients with and without JSpA are summarized in Table 1.

MRI assessment

MRI diagnosis of sacroiliitis according to global assessment and the adult ASAS definition for a positive MRI for sacroiliitis are summarized in Fig. 1. All patients with a positive MRI according to the ASAS definition were positive according to a global assessment for sacroiliitis

Table 1 Demographics of the study population

	Patients with JSpA (N = 47) N (%)		Patients without JSpA (N = 62) N (%)	
	MRI + (N = 23) N (%)	MRI − (N = 24) N (%)	MRI + (N = 7) N(%)	MRI − (N = 55) N (%)
Age (years)	10.8–18 (mean 15.0)	7.7–17.1 (mean 12.6)	12.7–18,8 (mean 15.1)	6.8–18 (mean13.1)
Male	13 (57%)	12 (50%)	1 (14%)	15 (27%)
HLA-B27 +	13 (27%) (0 ND)	8 (33%) (2 ND)	2 (29%) (1 ND)	8 (15%) (25 ND)
Inflammatory back pain	20 (87%)	18 (75%)	7 (100%)	50 (91%)
Sacroiliac joint tenderness	13(57%)	13 (54%)	3 (43%)	16 (29%)
IBP AND sacroiliac joint tenderness	10 (43%)	7 (29%)	3 (43%)	11 (20%)
Arthritis (peripheral)	13 (57%)	16 (67%)	0 (0%)	13 (24%)
Enthesitis (peripheral)	14 (61%)	15 (63%)	1 (14%)	5 (9%)

(*N* Number of patients, *JSpA* Juvenile Spondylarthropathy, *MRI+* sacroiliitis on MRI according to global assessment), *MRI* - normal MRI, *HLA-B27* Human Leukocyte Antigen B27, *ND* Not determined)

(Fig. 2). In 16 of 30 patients considered to have sacroiliitis according to global assessment, the ASAS criteria for a positive MRI for sacroiliitis were not fulfilled (Figs. 3 and 4). The most frequent features which the radiologists considered to indicate sacroiliitis according to global assessment in these 16 patients are BME only seen on one slice or location, synovitis and capsulitis. In 11/16 patients, features of sacroiliitis other than BME (synovitis, capsulitis, retroarticular enthesitis of structural lesions) are seen in the absence of BME (Fig. 3 cd – Fig. 4).

Diagnostic utility of MRI

MRI results according to global diagnostic assessment of sacroiliitis, according to the ASAS definition for a positive MRI for sacroiliitis, and according to the 'adapted' definitions (including small BME lesions visible on one slice only, capsulitis, retro-articular enthesitis, synovitis or structural lesions, and combinations of these features) are correlated with the final clinical diagnosis of JSpA. Sensitivity (SN), specificity (SP), positive (LR+) and negative likelihood ratio's (LR-) for diagnosis of JSpA are shown in Table 2.

When we included BME lesions that are only visible on one slice in the definition, the sensitivity (SN) rose from 26% to 36%, with minimal lowering of specificity (SP) (from 97% to 95%) (Table 2). Including both BME lesions seen on one slice and synovitis in the definition, resulted in a higher SN of 43%, unfortunately lowering SP from 97% to 90%. Including BME lesions seen on one slice and capsulitis in the definition, resulted in a higher SN of 43%, with only minimal lowering of the SP

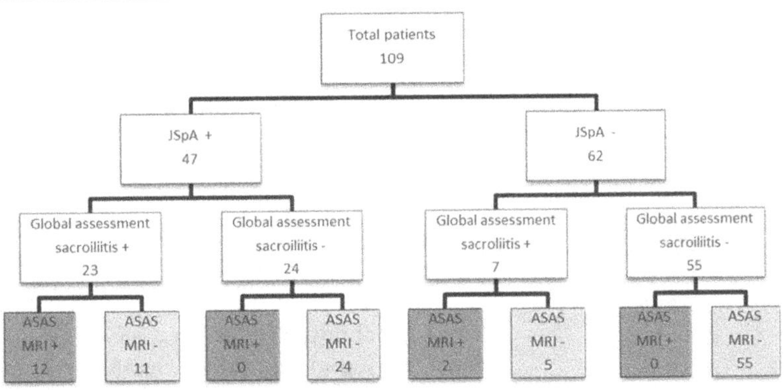

Fig. 1 Flow chart showing the number of patients with and without sacroiliitis according to MRI global diagnostic assessment of sacroiliitis and according to the ASAS definition for a positive MRI for sacroiliitis, both correlated with the final clinical diagnosis of JSpA. (MRI = Magnetic Resonance Imaging; JSpA + = patients with Juvenile Spondyloarthritis; JSpA -: patients without Juvenile Spondyloarthritis; Global assessment sacroiliitis +: one or more features of sacroiliitis present on MRI; global assessment sacroiliitis -: no features of sacroiliitis seen on MRI; ASAS MRI + = sacroiliitis present on MRI as defined by the Assessment of Spondyloarthritis International Society; ASAS MRI -: no sacroiliitis on MRI according to the Assessment of Spondyloarthritis International Society definition)

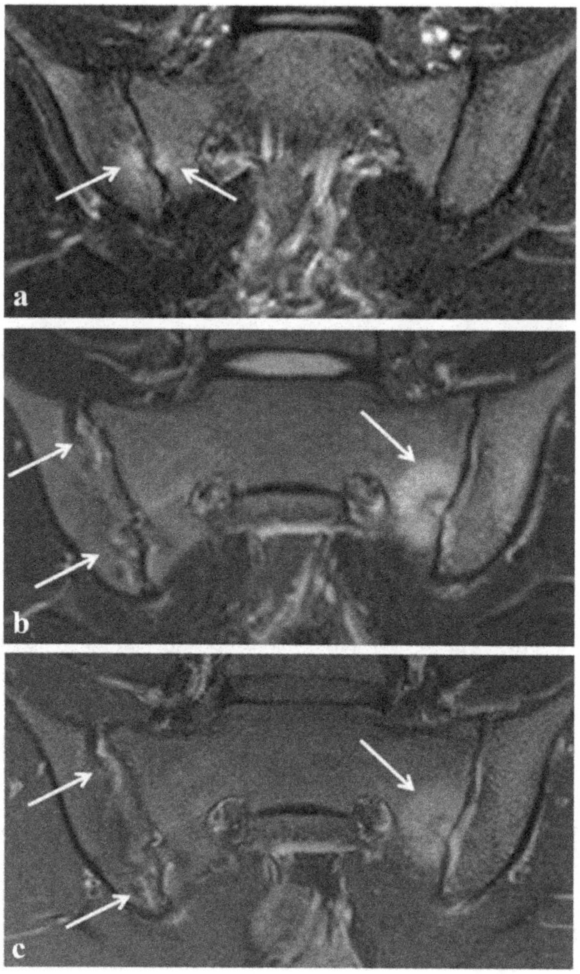

Fig. 2 Active sacroiliitis in a 16-year-old girl with juvenile spondyloarthritis according to global assessment as well as to the ASAS definition of a positive MRI for sacroiliitis. **a** Semicoronal STIR image shows two small, focal spots of BME at the sacral and iliac side of the right sacroiliac joint (arrows). **b** Follow-up MRI 6 months later shows more extensive active sacroiliitis with bilateral high signal in the joint space and an active lesion with surrounding BME at the sacral side of the left sacroiliac joint (arrows). **c** Corresponding semicoronal fat-saturated T1-weighted image of the follow-up MRI shows bilateral enhancement of the synovium (synovitis) and of the active lesion on the left side (arrows)

from 97% to 95%. Including BME lesions seen on one slice, synovitis and capsulitis in the definition, resulted in a higher SN of 47% - almost as high as for global assessment (49%) – at the cost of a lower SP (90%), also comparable to SN for global assessment (89%).

Interobserver agreement

Although the radiologists worked blinded to each other's readings, there was almost perfect inter-observer agreement (κ = 0.98) for the global assessment, and perfect agreement for the ASAS definition (κ = 1). In one case, radiologists were inconclusive for global assessment, and diagnosis of sacroiliitis on MRI in this case was made in consensus.

Discussion

Our study is the first assessing the value of the ASAS definition of a positive MRI for sacroiliitis in children. Currently, there is no clear definition of a 'positive' MRI for sacroiliitis in JSpA.

Recently, Weiss et al. evaluated the prevalence of sacroiliitis and the accuracy of physical examination and back pain to detect sacroiliitis, using pelvic MRI in 40 children with newly diagnosed JSpA [23]. Active sacroiliitis on MRI was defined according to the ASAS definition [10, 12]. They concluded that active sacroiliitis on MRI is common at diagnosis in juvenile SpA and frequently asymptomatic [23]. In 2014, Lin et al. studied 50 children with known or suspected JSpA [20]. In their study, The MRI findings of sacroiliitis were defined as described by Rudwaleit et al. [28] and included the presence of synovial enhancement, bone marrow edema, and/or erosions. However, neither their definition nor the ASAS definition of sacroiliitis on MRI have been validated in children. Furthermore, in adult SpA, it has been controversial whether presence of a structural lesion such as an erosion represents a "positive" MRI when BME is not present [10, 12, 28]. This situation is uncommon in pediatric patients, who generally present with either normal SI joint or signs of active disease, while few established structural lesions are seen until the late teens, and those that are visible are generally still active [21]. Also, Weiss and Lin both only studied children with JSpA, while in our study, all children with a history of inflammatory low back pain (IBP) and/or sacroiliac joint tenderness and were sent for MRI of the SI joints were included.

In our study, we compared the radiologist global assessment of MRI for sacroiliitis with the ASAS definition of a positive MRI in a cohort of children with IBP and/or sacroiliac joint tenderness, regardless of their final diagnosis. MRI global assessment for sacroiliitis had similar diagnostic yield for JSpA as in adult studies, with slightly lower sensitivity (49%) and similar specificity (89%) compared to Aydin et al. and Weber et al. [13, 24]. The ASAS definition for MRI-positive sacroiliitis had a much lower sensitivity for JSpA in children than in adults (26% vs. 67–79%) and was more specific in children (97% vs. 88–89%) (Table 3). Moreover, we found that the sensitivity of the ASAS definition was only half as high as the sensitivity of the global assessment in our pediatric patients (26% vs 49%).

There are several possible explanations for the lower sensitivity in children. First of all, children with JSpA most often present with peripheral arthritis and enthesitis of the lower extremities early in the disease. Axial

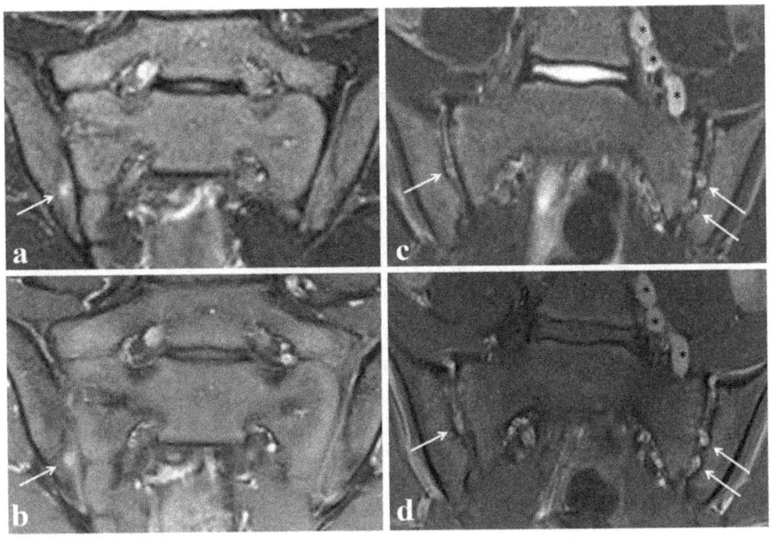

Fig. 3 Active sacroiliitis in a 14-year-old (left) and 13-year-old (right) boy with juvenile spondyloarthritis according to a global assessment of MRI for sacroiliitis, not according to the ASAS definition of a positive MRI for sacroiliitis. Semicoronal STIR (**a** and **c**) and contrast-enhanced fat-saturated T1-weighted (**b** and **d**) images showing on the left side a focal enhancing BME lesion (seen on only one slice) at the iliac side of the right sacroiliac joint (arrows), and on the right side showing bilateral multiple enhancing spots of nodular high signal in the joint space, representing active erosions (arrows). No BME is seen. Note also the enlarged para-iliacal lymph nodes (asterisks)

involvement is often not seen at presentation, but may occur years later [1, 3], and in our experience, may be less extensive at presentation compared to adults [18, 21]. We observed that BME in children, when present, appears not to be as extensive as in adults, frequently insufficient to fulfill the ASAS criteria. In some cases, erosions, capsulitis or synovitis can be seen with little or no surrounding edema, a finding previously reported by Lin et al. [20], thus not fulfilling the ASAS criteria. In 6/30 of the positive MRI for sacroiliitis according to a global assessment, a small focal T2/STIR hyperintense and enhancing lesion was the only finding on MRI. All 6 patients were clinically diagnosed with JSpA by the pediatric rheumatologists, implying that the presence of small lesions in children may therefore be more important than previously suspected. However, caution is needed, as partial volume or other normal features

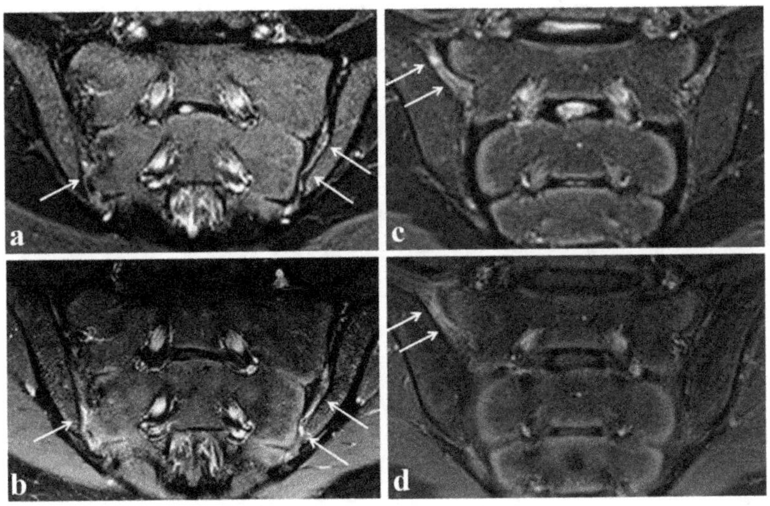

Fig. 4 Active sacroiliitis in a 14-year-old girl (left) and a 14-year-old boy (right) with spondyloarthritis according to a global assessment of MRI for sacroiliitis, not according to the ASAS definition of a positive MRI for sacroiliitis. Semicoronal STIR (**a** and **c**) and contrast-enhanced fat-saturated T1-weighted (**b** and **d**) images on the left side showing synovitis in the caudal part of the left SI joint, also discrete in the caudal part of the right SI joint, seen as high signal in the joint space on STIR with corresponding synovial enhancement. Bone marrow edema is absent. On the right side, synovitis/retro-articular enthesitis is shown at the right sacroiliac joint (arrows). No BME is seen

Table 2 The sensitivity, specificity, positive and negative likelihood ratios for diagnosis of JSpA (clinical gold standard) predicted by MRI global assessment, by the ASAS definition of a positive MRI and for 'adapted' ASAS definitions, including BME lesions only seen on one slice or location, synovitis, capsulitis, retro-articular enthesitis, structural lesions and combinations of these features

	N	Sensitivity % (95% CI)	Specificity % (95% CI)	LR +	LR -
Global assessment	30	49 (34.1–63.9)	89 (78.1–95.3)	4.45	0.57
ASAS definition	14	26 (13.9–40.4)	97 (88.8–99.6)	8.67	0.76
ASAS OR focal lesions	20	36 (22.7–51.5)	95 (86.5–99.0)	7.20	0.67
ASAS OR synovitis	20	32 (19.1–47.1)	92 (82.2–97.3)	4	0.74
ASAS OR capsulitis	17	32 (19.1–47.1)	97 (88.8–99.6)	10.67	0.70
ASAS OR retroarticular enthesitis	18	30 (17.3–44.9)	94 (84.3–98.2)	5	0.74
ASAS OR structural	16	28 (15.6–42.6)	95 (86.5–99.0)	5.60	0.76
ASAS OR focal lesions OR synovitis	26	43 (28.3–57.8)	90 (80.1–96.4)	4.30	0.63
ASAS OR focal lesions OR capsulitis	23	43 (28.3–57.8)	95 (86.5–99.0)	8.60	0.60
ASAS OR focal lesions OR synovitis OR capsulitis	28	47 (32.1–61.9)	90 (80.1–96.4)	4.7	0.59

(*N* Number of sacroiliitis-positive patients, *95% CI* 95% confidence Interval, *LR+* positive likelihood ratio, *LR -* negative likelihood ratio, *ASAS* Assessment of Spondyloarthritis International Society)

such as vessels, cartilage, subchondral defects or osseous clefts may have a high STIR signal and thus mimic active inflammation or erosions [29]. Other potential confounders include features of natural growth including progressive ossification of the segmental and lateral apophyses of the sacral wings and variation of the width of the joint space [30]. Because of the ongoing ossification process, joint margins can look irregular and blurred, especially on T1 weighted images, making it even more difficult to evaluate erosions [21]. Müller et al. reported a high prevalence of bony depressions, signal changes suggestive of bone marrow edema and joint fluid on MRI of the pediatric wrist [31]. However, little is published about the MRI appearance of normal sacroiliac joints in children. Another factor which may contribute to the lower sensitivity for JSpA is the relatively smaller size of the SI joints in younger children, in whom the entire joint is captured in only a few 3-mm slices – BME in a single MRI slice obtained in a small child may represent a similar proportion of the joint as in more than one slice of an adult patient. Thinner slices might be a solution, but this is a technical challenge, especially for the STIR sequence, which already has a low signal to noise ratio.

Table 3 Sensitivity and specificity for diagnosis of JSpA for global assessment of MRI and for the ASAS definition of a positive MRI of children compared to adults according to studies of Ayden et al. [13] and Weber et al. [24]

			Sensitivity	Specificity	LR +	LR -
ADULTS	Aydin et al. [13]	Global	66%	94%	11	0.36
		ASAS	79%	89%	7.18	0.24
	Weber et al. [24]	Global	51%	97%	17	0.51
		ASAS	67%	88%	5.58	0.38
CHILDREN	This study	Global	49%	89%	4.45	0.57
		ASAS	26%	97%	8.67	0.76

(*Global* global assessment of MRI for sacroiliitis, *ASAS* assessment of MRI according to the ASAS definition of a positive MRI for sacroiliitis)

We found the ASAS definition of a positive MRI for sacroiliitis to be more specific (SP = 97%) than global assessment of sacroiliitis in JSpA (SP = 89%), which is an opposite finding compared to adults, where specificity of the ASAS definition is lower compared to global assessment [13, 24]. In adults, BME is also frequently seen in patients presenting with non-rheumatological entities that clinically mimic sacroiliitis such as degenerative disease, lumbosacral transitional anomaly, spondylolysis, fracture, infection and tumor [32, 33]. As these entities, especially degenerative disease, are less frequently seen in children, specificity of BME in children increases. Furthermore, children are frequently physically active, and sacral stress injuries have been described [34]. This suggests that children might also be prone to developing BME secondary to overuse. Grampp et al. described overuse edema in the hand on MRI [35], however, there is a lack of research on this phenomenon in the pelvis. In our pediatric study, global assessment by our two radiologists was about twice as sensitive as the ASAS definition (SN = 49% vs. 26%), implying that the ASAS definition may be too strict in children.

Since specificity of the ASAS definition of a positive MRI for sacroiliitis is very high in children, improving the definition should aim to further increase sensitivity without lowering the specificity, i.e., providing a formal approach to reach at least the level of accuracy achieved by the radiologist's global impression in this study. Simply using the global impression as MRI diagnostic standard would be problematic since this would vary by the level of experience of the MRI reader and also does not provide insight into which features of disease contribute to diagnosis.

We studied several variations of the ASAS definition. We began with the basic adult ASAS definition for sacroiliitis on MRI, and combined it with the other features of active sacroiliitis (synovitis, capsulitis, enthesitis), as well as with structural features (erosions, sclerosis, fat deposition and ankylosis) of sacroiliitis seen in children [21]. As structural lesions such as erosions are not as frequently seen in children compared to adults [9, 21], all structural features were grouped ('+ structural'). Structural lesions are not included in the current ASAS definition, although several recent adult studies indicate that structural lesions, particularly erosions, may contribute substantially to the diagnostic utility of the definition of a positive SI joint MRI [36, 37]. In previous studies, we observed that MRI features of sacroiliitis can be slightly different in the pediatric population compared to adults [9, 18, 21]. As we noticed that BME seen in only one location or slice was the most frequent source of discrepancies, in which sacroiliitis was diagnosed by global impression but not by ASAS definition, we also tested a definition including these small lesions seen on one slice only. Synovitis and capsulitis are also seen in children, but not included in the adult ASAS definition. Finally, we also made combinations of the three most frequent features radiologists consider to indicate sacroiliitis according to global assessment without fulfillment of the ASAS criteria. Assessing all MRI features of sacroiliitis is mandatory to find the best combination of features. However, more and large, prospective, multicentric studies are needed.

Allowing single-slice BME to diagnose sacroiliitis increased SN from 26% to 36%, adding synovitis or capsulitis as individual diagnostic factors each increased SN to 43%, and allowing single-slice BME, synovitis and/or capsulitis to define presence of sacroiliitis achieved SN = 47%, SP 90%, comparable to global impression (SN = 49%, SP = 89%). Structural lesions were less useful; allowing presence of 1 or more structural lesions to diagnose sacroiliitis only slightly increased SN to 28%, also lowering specificity to 95%. The lower specificity when including structural lesions suggests that erosions have been identified by our readers in other than JSpA patients, which partly might be due to misreading. As described, erosions are difficult to assess, especially in smaller children who have irregular delineation of the joint space because of the ongoing ossification process. There still is much debate on the exact definition of sacroiliitis on MRI, and other features than BME are not included currently. According to the most recent revision of the ASAS definition, these other features increase suspicion for sacroiliitis on MRI [12]. Still, this remains difficult, especially in children, as no one knows whether sacroiliitis seen on MRI correlates to a histopathological gold standard. Using other features than just BME is likely to increase the detection rate but will also generate more false positives, which can reduce the specificity. Optimizing this requires more, larger, multicentric studies, assessing different combinations of features as we have done in this study.

Thus, in this study the optimal variation of the ASAS definition to most sensitively detect sacroiliitis with minimum decrease in specificity was to make the ASAS definition for a positive sacroiliac joint MRI less strict by including BME lesions seen on one slice, capsulitis or synovitis. The sensitivity of the 'adapted' definitions was comparable to expert radiologist global impression. Still, as found by others, likely due to the 'limbs-first' pattern of onset of many cases of JSpA, about half of cases of JSpA may be completely imaging-negative at first diagnosis by any criteria [11].

There are some limitations to our study. First, although our study was substantial in size compared to other pediatric studies, we still had a relatively small number of patients (109) compared to adult SpA studies. The patient population represented referrals from a single tertiary center; referral patterns for sacroiliitis may vary elsewhere. However, this reflects clinical practice. As this study is a retrospective study, the patient group that was reassessed partially overlaps with the group of patients of a previous prospective study. However, MRI and clinical files of all patients were reassessed. Secondly, our inclusion criteria might have been not strict enough. The definition used for IBP might have been too sensitive. However, there is no established definition for IBP in children, and in our opinion, applying the adult ASAS definition for IBP in children would be too strict as many children do not meet these adult criteria. MRI was also the only imaging technique, without consistently available radiography or ultrasound. MRI scoring was performed using yes/no decisions and not according to Berlin or Canadian scoring systems [38–40], however, these scoring systems are not validated yet in children. Furthermore, there is little published data on normal appearances of pediatric SI joints. There is a need for studies in healthy children, to determine the range of normal variation in parameters such as joint fluid, enhancement and adjacent marrow signal in normal children. Lacking such studies, there is a risk of misidentifying normal findings as pathology in pediatric SI joints. Since this was a retrospective study, not all clinical criteria were available. In 40/109 patients, HLA-B27 was not obtained by the referring clinician. It may be possible that some patients might have been classified differently if HLA-B27 was obtained. The gold standard for JSpA diagnosis was clinical expert opinion, which although based on well recognized criteria is necessarily subjective. Finally, there was no control group of age- and sex-matched children.

Interpreting the MRI features of pediatric sacroiliac joints remains a challenge, and given the importance of an early diagnosis of JSpA, more experience in this specific topic is needed. There is no clear definition of a 'positive' MRI in JSpA at the moment. More studies are needed to develop and refine pediatric-specific definitions of a 'positive' MRI in juvenile SpA, and to determine the role of MRI in the classification criteria for juvenile JSpA.

Conclusion

In this study, approximately half of pediatric patients with MRI showing some features of sacroiliitis would not have been considered 'positive' according to the current ASAS definition of MRI-positive sacroiliitis in adults. The key feature of the adult ASAS definition limiting sensitivity appears to be the need to show BME on two slices or locations. In children, who have smaller SI joints and less mechanical sources of BME, an adapted definition positive for sacroiliitis if just one BME lesion is seen, or if synovitis or capsulitis are present, appears to maximize sensitivity with little decrease in specificity. With further confirmation in larger / multi-center studies, this could improve clinical diagnostic utility of MRI for sacroiliitis in children.

Abbreviations

ASAS: Assessment of spondyloarthritis international society; BME: Bone marrow edema; CI: Confidence interval; CRMO: Chronic recurrent multifocal osteomyelitis; ERA: Enthesitis-related arthritis; Gd: Gadolinium DTPA; HLA-B27: Human leukocyte antigen B27; IBD: Inflammatory bowel disease; IBP: Inflammatory back pain; ILAR: International league of associations for rheumatology; JIA: Juvenile idiopathic arthritis; JSpA: Juvenile spondyloarthritis; LR-: Negative likelihood ratio; LR+: Positive likelihood ratio; MRI: Magnetic resonance imaging; PsA: Psoriasis arthritis; SI: Sacroiliac; SN: Sensitivity; SP: Specificity; SpA: Spondyloarthritis; ST: Slice thickness; STIR: Short tau inversion recovery sequence; T1/Gd: T1-Weighted post gadolinium sequence; TSE: Turbo spin echo

Acknowledgements

None.

Funding

Research was funded by the ASAS research grant.

Authors' contributions

All authors contributed to the drafting of the manuscript and approved the final version. NH, KV and LJ provided the MRI images. JD, RJ and JVV recorded from the clinical files if patients fulfilled the criteria for JSpA. All authors read and approved the final manuscript.

Competing interests

The authors declare that they have no competing interests.

Author details

[1]Department of Radiology and Medical Imaging, Ghent University Hospital, De Pintelaan 185, 9000 Ghent, Belgium. [2]Department of Pediatric Rheumatology, Ghent University Hospital, De Pintelaan 185, 9000 Ghent, Belgium. [3]Department of Rheumatology and VIB Inflammation Research Center, Unit for Molecular Immunology and Inflammation, Ghent University Hospital, De Pintelaan 185, 9000 Ghent, Belgium. [4]Department of Radiology & Diagnostic Imaging, University of Alberta Hospital, 8440-112 Street, Edmonton T6G 2B7, AB, Canada. [5]Rheumazentrum Ruhrgebiet, Ruhr-University Bochum, Claudiusstr. 45, 44649 Herne, Germany.

References

1. Burgos-Vargas R. The juvenile-onset spondylarthritides. Rheum Dis Clin North Am. 2002;28:531–60.
2. Petty RE, Southwood TR, Manners P, Baum J, Glass DN, Goldenberg J, et al. International League of Association for Rheumatology Classification of juvenile idiopathic arthritis: second revision. Edmonton. 2001. J Rheumatol. 2004;31:390–2.
3. Colbert RA. Classification of juvenile spondyloarthritis: enthesitis-related arthritis and beyond. Nat Rev Rheumatol. 2010;6:477–85.
4. Ravelli A, Martini A. Juvenile Idiopathic Arthritis. Lancet. 2007;369:767–78.
5. Haroon N, Inman RD, Learch TJ, Weisman MH, Lee M, Rahbar MH, et al. The impact of tumor necrosis factor α inhibitors on radiographic progression in ankylosing spondylitis. Arthritis Rheum. 2013;65:2645–54.
6. Tse SML, Laxer RM. New advances in juvenile spondyloarthritis. Nat Rev Rheumatol. 2012;8:269–79.
7. Baraliakos X, Haibel H, Listing J, Sieper J, Braun J. Continuous long-term anti-TNF therapy does not lead to an increase in the rate of new bone formation over 8 years in patients with ankylosing spondylitis. Ann Rheum Dis. 2014;73:710–5.
8. Eshed I, Bollow M, McGonagle DG, Tan AL, Althoff CE, Asbach P, et al. MRI of enthesitis of the appendicular skeleton in spondyloarthritis. Ann Rheum Dis. 2007;66:1553–9.
9. Jans L, Coeman L, Van Praet L, Carron P, Elewaut D, Van den Bosch F, et al. How sensitive and specific are MRI features of sacroiliitis for diagnosis of spondylarthritis in patients with inflammatory back pain? JBR-BTR. 2014;97: 202–5.
10. Sieper J, Rudwaleit M, Baraliakos X, Brandt J, Braun J, Burgos-Vargas R, et al. The Assessment of SpondyloArthritis international Society (ASAS) handbook: a guide to assess spondyloarthritis. Ann Rheum Dis. 2009;68:ii1–ii44.
11. Jaremko JL, Liu L, Winn NJ, Ellsworth JE, Lambert RG. Diagnostic utility of Magnetic Resonance Imaging and Radiography in Juvenile Spondyloarthritis: Evaluation of the Sacroiliac Joints in controls and affected subjects. J Rheumatol. 2014;41:963–70.
12. Lambert RG, Bakker PA, van der Heijde D. Defining active sacroiliitis on MRI for classification of axial spondyloarthritis: update by the ASAS MRI working group. Ann Rheum Dis Published Online First: 14 January 2016. doi: 10. 1136/annrheumdis-2015-2086422016
13. Aydin SZ, Maksymowych WP, Bennett AN, McGonagle D, Emery P, Marzo-Ortega H. Validation of the ASAS criteria and definition of a positive MRI of the sacroiliac joint in an inception cohort of axial spondyloarthritis followed up for 8 years. Ann Rheum Dis. 2012;71:56–60.
14. Rudwaleit M, van der Heijde D, Landewé R, Akkoc N, Brandt J, Chou CT, et al. The Assesment of SpondyloArthritis International Society classification criteria for peripheral spondyloarthritis and for spondyloarthritis in general. Ann Rheum Dis. 2011;70:25–31.
15. Rudwaleit M, van der Heijde D, Landewé R, Listing J, Akkoc N, Brandt J, et al. The development of Assessment of SpondyloArthritis international Society classification criteria for axial spondyloarthritis (part II): validation and final selection. Ann Rheum Dis. 2009;68:777–83.
16. Sezen M, Baru K, Açıkel C, Kasapcopur O. The new proposal classification criteria for juvenile spondyloarthropathies. Pediatr Rheumatol Online J. 2014; 12 Suppl 1:45. doi:10.1186/1546-0096-12-S1-P45. Published online first: 17 September 2014.
17. Maksymowicz H, Kowalewski K, Lubkowska K, Zołud W, Sąsiadek M. Diagnostic value of gadolinium-enhanced MR imaging of active sacroiliitis in seronegative spondyloarthropathy. Pol J Radiol. 2010;75:58–65.

18. Herregods N, Jaremko JL, Baraliakos X, Dehoorne J, Leus A, Verstraete K, et al. Limited role of gadolinium to detect active sacroiliitis on MRI in juvenile spondyloarthritis. Skeletal Radiol. 2015;44:1637–46. doi:10.1007/s00256-015-2211-8. Epub 2015 Jul 24.
19. Bollow M, Biedermann T, Kannenberg J, Paris S, Schauer-Petrowski C, Minden K, et al. Use of dynamic magnetic resonance imaging to detect sacroiliitis in HLA-B27 positive and negative children with juvenile arthritides. J Rheumatol. 1998;25:556–64.
20. Lin C, MacKenzie JD, Courtier JL, Gu JT, Milojevic D. Magnetic resonance imaging findings in juvenile spondyloarthropathy and effects of treatment observed on subsequent imaging. Pediatr Rheumatol. 2014;12:25.
21. Herregods N, Dehoorne J, Joos R, Jaremko JL, Baraliakos X, Leus A, et al. Diagnostic value of MRI features of sacroiliitis in juvenile spondyloarthritis. Clin Radiol. 2015;70:1428–38. doi:10.1016/j.crad.2015.09.003. Published online first: 16 October 2015.
22. Pagnini I, Savelli S, Matucci-Cerinic M, Fonda C, Cimaz R, Simonini G. Early predictors of juvenile sacroiliitis in enthesitis-related arthritis. J Rheumatol. 2010;37:2395–401.
23. Weiss PF, Xiao R, Biko DM, Chauvin NA. Assessment of Sacroiliitis at Diagnosis of Juvenile Spondyloarthritis by Radiography, Magnetic Resonance Imaging, and Clinical Examination. Arthritis Care Res. 2016;68: 187–94.
24. Weber U, Lambert RG, Østergaard M, Hodler J, Pedersen SJ, Maksymowych WP. The diagnostic utility of magnetic resonance imaging in spondylarthritis: an international multicenter evaluation of one hundred eighty-seven subjects. Arthritis Rheum. 2010;62:3048–58.
25. Sieper J, van der Heijde D, Landewé R, Brandt J, Burgos-Vagas R, Collantes-Estevez E, et al. New criteria for inflammatory back pain in patients with chronic back pain: a real patient exercise by experts from the Assessment of SpondyloArthritis international Society (ASAS). Ann Rheum Dis. 2009;68:784–8.
26. Herregods N, Dehoorne J, Pattyn E, Jaremko JL, Baraliakos X, Elewaut D, et al. Diagnositic value of pelvic enthesitis on MRI of the sacroiliac joints in enthesitis related arthritis. Pediatr Rheumatol Online J. 2015;13:46. doi:10. 1186/s12969-015-0045-5. published online first : 10 November 2015.
27. Landis JR, Koch GG. The measurement of observer agreement for categorical data. Biometrics. 1977;33:159–74.
28. Rudwaleit M, Jurik AG, Hermann KA, Landewé R, van der Heijde D, Baraliakos X, et al. Defining active sacroiliitis on magnetic resonance imaging (MRI) for classification of axial spondyloarthritis: a consensual approach by the ASAS/ OMERACT MRI group. Ann Rheum Dis. 2009;68:1520–7.
29. Puhakka KB, Melsen F, Jurik AG, Boel LW, Vesterby A, Egund N. MR imaging of the normal sacroiliac joint with correlation to histology. Skeletal Radiol. 2004;33:15–28. Epub 2003 Nov 12.
30. Bollow M, Braun J, Kannenberg J, Biedermann T, Schauer-Petrowskaja C, Paris S, et al. Normal morphology of sacroiliac joints in children: magnetic resonance studies related to age and sex. Skeletal Radiol. 1997;26(12):697–704.
31. Müller LS, Avenarius D, Damasio B, Eldevik OP, Malattia C, Lambot-Juhan K, et al. The paediatric wrist revisited: redefining MR findings in healthy children. Ann Rheum Dis. 2011;70:605–10. doi:10.1136/ard.2010.135244. Epub 2010 Dec 20.
32. Bereau M, Prati C, Wendling D. Sacroiliac edema by MRI does not always indicate spondylarthritis. Joint Bone Spine. 2011;78:646. doi:10.1016/j.jbspin. 2011.05.011. Published online first: 2 July 2011.
33. Schueller-Weidekamm C, Schueller G. Sacroiliitis oder pseudosacroiliitis? Radiologe. 2012;52:132–40.
34. Grampp S, Henk CB, Mostbeck GH. Overuse edema in the bone marrow ofthe hand: demonstration with MRI. J Comput Assist Tomogr. 1998;22:25.
35. Jaimes C, Jimenez M, Shabshin N, Laor T, Jaramillo D. Taking the stress out of evaluating stress injuries in children. Radiographics. 2012;32(2):537–55.
36. Weber U, Zubler V, Pedersen SJ, Rufibach K, Lambert RG, Chan SM, et al. Development and validation of a magnetic resonance criterion for defining a positive sacroiliac joint magnetic resonance imaging finding in spondyloarthritis. Arthritis Care Res. 2013;65:977–85.
37. Maksymowych WP, Wichuk S, Chiowchanwisawakit P, Lambert RG, Pedersen SJ. Development and preliminary validation of the spondyloarthritis research consortium of Canada magnetic resonance imaging sacroiliac joint structural score. J Rheumatol. 2015;42:79–86.
38. Braun J, Baraliakos X, Golder W, Brandt J, Rudwaleit M, Listing J, et al. Magnetic resonance imaging examinations of the spine in patients with ankylosing spondylitis, before and after successful therapy with infliximab: evaluation of a new scoring system. Arthritis Rheum. 2003;48:1126–36.
39. Haibel H, Rudwaleit M, Brandt HC, Grozdanovic Z, Listing J, Kupper H, et al. Adalimumab reduces spinal symptoms in active ankylosing spondylitis: clinical and magnetic resonance imaging results of a fifty-two-week open-label trial. Arthritis Rheum. 2006;54:678–81.
40. Maksymowych WP, Inman RD, Salonen D, Dhillon SS, Williams M, Stone M, et al. Spondyloarthritis Research Consortium of Canada Magnetic Resonance Imaging index for assessment of sacroiliac joint inflammation in Ankylosing Spondylitis. Arthritis Care Res. 2005;53:703–9.

10

The new Childhood Arthritis and Rheumatology Research Alliance (CARRA) registry: design, rationale, and characteristics of patients enrolled in the first 12 months

Timothy Beukelman[1*], Yukiko Kimura[2], Norman T. Ilowite[3], Kelly Mieszkalski[4], Marc D. Natter[5], Grendel Burrell[4], Brian Best[4], Jason Jones[4], Laura E. Schanberg[6] and For the CARRA Registry Investigators

Abstract

Background: Herein we describe the history, design, and rationale of the new Childhood Arthritis and Rheumatology Research Alliance (CARRA) Registry and present the characteristics of patients with juvenile idiopathic arthritis (JIA) enrolled in the first 12 months of operation.

Methods: The CARRA Registry began prospectively collecting data in the United States and Canada in July 2015 to evaluate the safety of therapeutic agents in persons with childhood-onset rheumatic disease, initially restricted to JIA. Secondary objectives include the evaluation of disease outcomes and their associations with medication use and other factors. Data are collected every 6 months and include clinical assessments, detailed medication use, patient-reported outcomes, and safety events. Follow-up is planned for at least 10 years for each participant and is facilitated by a telephone call center.

Results: As of July 2016, 1192 patients with JIA were enrolled in the CARRA Registry at 49 clinical sites. At enrollment, their median age was 12.4 years old and median disease duration was 2.6 years. Owing to preferential enrollment, patients with systemic JIA (13%) and with a polyarticular course (75%) were over-represented compared to patients in typical clinical practice. Approximately 49% were currently using biologic agents and ever use of oral glucocorticoids was common (47%). The CARRA Registry provides safety surveillance data to pharmaceutical companies to satisfy their regulatory requirements, and several independently-funded sub-studies that use the Registry infrastructure are underway.

Conclusion: The new CARRA Registry successfully enrolled nearly 1200 participants with JIA in the first 12 months of its operation. Sustainable funding has been secured from multiple sources. The CARRA Registry may serve as a model for the study of other uncommon diseases.

* Correspondence: tbeukelman@peds.uab.edu
[1]Division of Pediatric Rheumatology, The University of Alabama at Birmingham, 1600 7th Avenue South, CPP 210, Birmingham, AL 35233-1711, USA
Full list of author information is available at the end of the article

Background

Juvenile idiopathic arthritis (JIA) is a heterogeneous collection of childhood arthritides [1]. Even though JIA is the most common pediatric rheumatologic condition with a prevalence of approximately 1 per 1000 children, the current understanding of its pathogenesis, natural history, and long-term outcomes is limited [2].

Over the last 15 years, the adoption of highly effective biologic therapeutic agents has dramatically changed the treatment and expected outcomes in JIA. Despite the widespread use of biologic agents, important safety questions remain unanswered, particularly regarding potential adverse effects that are rare or have a long latency period. Safety information about more recently approved biologic agents in children remains very limited.

Furthermore, there is little published high-quality evidence to guide pediatric rheumatologists in the management of childhood-onset systemic lupus erythematosus (cSLE), juvenile dermatomyositis (JDM), localized scleroderma, and other less common conditions.

The many current challenges in the treatment of pediatric rheumatic disease were the principal motivation for creation of the Childhood Arthritis and Rheumatology Research Alliance (CARRA) Registry. Herein, we present the history of the CARRA Registry, describe its design and rationale, and present the characteristics of the patients enrolled in the first 12 months of its operation.

Methods

Origins

CARRA was founded in 2002 with the mission to improve the care of children with rheumatic disease by fostering and conducting high-quality clinical and translational research. Since its founding, CARRA has grown to include 460 members in the United States and Canada, including 257 pediatric rheumatologists with sufficient fellowship training to qualify for certification by the American Board of Pediatrics or the Royal College of Physicians and Surgeons of Canada, respectively. In 2014, CARRA became legally recognized in the United States as an incorporated non-profit scientific organization under the name "CARRA Inc." [3].

The initial CARRA Registry (now referred to as the "CARRA Legacy Registry") was established in 2009 through funding from the National Institutes of Health [4]. This funding established the organizational, clinical research, and informatics framework for a 60-site, national registry and enabled development of a multicenter prospective observational study of children with a wide variety of defined rheumatic conditions. During its operation from 2010 through 2014, the CARRA Legacy Registry successfully enrolled the largest number of prospectively followed pediatric rheumatology patients to date: 9,587 participants including 6,607 with JIA, 1,217 with cSLE, and 688 with JDM. Data from the Legacy Registry were analyzed and presented in several peer-reviewed publications [5–16].

To create a scalable registry infrastructure for secure data collection and sharing of research data, the Legacy Registry combined established mechanisms for web-based electronic data collection with new, innovative approaches for data sharing [17]. The Legacy Registry also supported a robust training initiative for site investigators and research coordinators, helping create infrastructure for research at Registry sites and promote an overall culture of universal participation in research.

Despite the obvious success of the CARRA Legacy Registry, there were limitations due to data collection procedures. Legacy Registry participants represented a convenience sample and the generalizability of data was difficult to assess. A parsimonious set of data elements was collected to demonstrate feasibility of the new infrastructure, and detailed medication information was not included. Owing to limited funding, the collection of every 6-month follow-up visit data was not systematic. Therefore, unbiased detailed analyses of medication safety and effectiveness were not possible.

Nevertheless, the Legacy Registry successfully demonstrated the capabilities and infrastructure of the CARRA network to enroll and collect longitudinal data on large numbers of pediatric rheumatic disease participants. This provided the foundation for a suitable platform to conduct United States Food and Drug Administration (FDA) approved, post-marketing pharmacosurveillance, as well as rigorous comparative effectiveness research. In order to fulfill the new missions and accommodate new funding sources, the Legacy Registry closed to enrollment and follow-up in October 2014. Subsequently, in July 2015, the first subjects with JIA were enrolled in the new CARRA Registry.

Objectives

The primary objective of the CARRA Registry is to prospectively collect data essential to evaluate the safety of therapeutic agents in children, adolescents, and young adults with childhood-onset rheumatic diseases. The concept of a disease-based (rather than drug-based) registry for pharmacosurveillance gained important initial traction in May 2009, when the FDA held a public workshop on developing a consolidated pediatric rheumatology observational registry [18]. Over the subsequent years, it was increasingly recognized by all stakeholders that the historical model of drug-based individual prospective registries for each new therapeutic agent was unsustainable and inadequate owing to several challenges [19]. First, competition for enrollment of subjects between individual drug-based registries created difficulties in recruiting an adequate number of comparator patients. Second, dynamic and complex medication histories made the assignment of patients to a single registry implausible. In addition, sample sizes and duration of longitudinal follow up in the existing drug-based registries were generally too small to detect uncommon but important events.

The CARRA Registry has multiple secondary objectives, including documentation of the clinical course and drug treatment patterns of patients over time, evaluation of clinical outcomes (including patient reported outcomes) associated with the use of therapeutic agents, and the evaluation of factors other than drug treatment that are associated with specific disease outcomes. The addition of targeted biospecimen collection to Registry data collection will enable translational studies of disease pathogenesis and response to therapy.

Clinical sites

CARRA Registry sites are comprised of pediatric rheumatology practices that contain at least one active pediatric rheumatologist member of CARRA and are located throughout the United States and Canada.

Enrollment procedures

Potential participants are recruited from activated CARRA Registry clinical sites. The overall inclusion criteria for the CARRA Registry are simple: onset of rheumatic disease prior to age 19 years old (16 years old for JIA) and current age less than 21 years. However, resource constraints initially limited enrollment to children diagnosed with JIA. In addition, to facilitate cohort studies within the Registry database, there was preferential enrollment (produced via per-patient payments to the sites) of children newly diagnosed in the prior 6 months or newly initiated on therapy with methotrexate or a biologic agent. More recently, children with systemic JIA or with a history of arthritis in 5 or more cumulative joints were also preferentially enrolled. The enrollment of children with SLE began in March 2017, and enrollment of children with JDM and localized scleroderma and systemic sclerosis is anticipated later in 2017.

The Registry was approved by Duke University Institutional Review Board (IRB) and each participating site obtained local IRB approval. Fourteen sites use a reliant IRB model in which their local IRB has ceded review to the Duke IRB. Eligible patients are consented for participation by site investigators and research coordinators in the usual manner. The option for electronic informed consent using an interactive tablet device will begin in 2017. Registry participants agree to provide patient/parent reported outcomes at each Registry visit and to be contacted by phone should they discontinue regular medical care at a CARRA Registry site (e.g., transition to an adult rheumatology care provider). Previously collected data from former Registry participants can be linked to data in the new CARRA Registry using the site-provided CARRA Legacy Registry identification number. Participants also agree to potential linkage of their data to external data sources (e.g., cancer registries) with protection of their personal identity. The CARRA Registry maintains two databases for these purposes: one with a limited research data set available to authorized researchers, and a second, separate database containing personal identifiers and contact information, which may only be viewed by a consenting participant's site and the 'honest broker' staff at the central data coordinating call center. This arrangement provides an IRB-approved buffer between data for research versus data for participant contact. Participants also have the option to consent for the future collection of biospecimens.

Data collection

Data are collected in the context of routine clinical care but cannot currently be uploaded directly from an electronic health record. CARRA pays sites for each visit with completed data entry, and most sites employ a research coordinator. Table 1 lists the baseline data collected at the time of enrollment. These same data elements are collected or updated at subsequent follow-up visits occurring approximately every 6 months as part of routine clinical practice. Follow-up data are also collected at initiation of treatment with methotrexate or a biologic agent, irrespective of whether this occurs at a routine 6-month follow-up visit. There is significant overlap between the current Registry data elements and the Legacy Registry data elements; however, the current Registry additionally collects laboratory results, detailed information about medication use, additional clinical assessments, and more patient-reported outcomes. Precise details about data elements may be provided by CARRA to potential collaborators upon request. As shown in Table 1, multiple derived measures, including the American College of Rheumatology (ACR) Pediatric Response [20] and Disease Flare [21], the Juvenile Arthritis Disease Activity Score (JADAS) [22, 23], and the provisional ACR definition of inactive disease [24], can all be determined from data collected at each Registry visit.

In addition to the standard clinical measures and history collected at each follow-up, the CARRA Registry systematically collects data about safety events, specifically serious adverse events (SAEs) and events of special interest (ESIs). SAEs are defined by the standard criteria used by the FDA and others [25]. ESIs are protocol-defined, pre-specified events of particular concern and interest because of a possible association with newer therapeutic agents, but that might not meet the definition of a SAE. Examples of ESIs include optic neuritis and tuberculosis. Data about safety events are reported as soon

Table 1 Data items collected in the CARRA Registry

Data element
Demographics: birthdate, race, sex, household income
Other medical diagnoses
Family medical history
Health insurance provider
Dates of onset of disease symptoms, disease diagnosis, and first pediatric rheumatology evaluation
Current and past rheumatology medications: start date, stop date, dose, frequency, route of administration, reason for discontinuation
Current glucocorticoid dose and presence of any glucocorticoid use since last visit (oral, intravenous, or intra-articular)
JIA ILAR category and associated inclusion criteria
ANA, Anti-CCP, RF, HLA-B27 results
Total number of joints ever affected by arthritis (<5 or ≥5)
Disease manifestations in the past 2 weeks: fever, rash, generalized lymphadenopathy, hepatomegaly, splenomegaly, serositis, psoriasis
Height, weight, blood pressure
Total number of joints with active arthritis
Total number of joints with limited range of motion
Presence and number of tender entheses
Presence of clinically active sacroiliitis
Duration of morning stiffness
Modified Schober test measurement
Radiographic damage
Imaging evidence of sacroiliac joint damage
Imaging evidence of active sacroiliitis
Presence of uveitis (ever)
If uveitis ever present: date of diagnosis, date of most recent eye examination, current best corrected vision, ever/current use of steroid eye drops, ever use of intra-ocular or sub-tenon glucocorticoid injections, presence of anterior chamber cells, uveitis complications, eye surgery
Laboratory results (if obtained): AST, ALT, C-RP, ESR, ferritin, WBC, % neutrophils, hemoglobin, platelet count, total cholesterol, triglycerides
Physician global assessment of disease activity
Study subject contact information
Patient/parent global assessment of overall well-being, patient/parent assessment of disease activity
Childhood Health Assessment Questionnaire (CHAQ)
Pain intensity, PROMIS® pain interference, and pain due to rheumatic condition
PROMIS® upper extremity physical function, PROMIS® mobility
PROMIS® Pediatric Global Health 7

JIA juvenile idiopathic arthritis, *ILAR* International League Against Rheumatism, *ANA* anti-nuclear antibody, *CCP* cyclic citrullinated peptide, *RF* rheumatoid factor, *AST* aspartate aminotransferase, *ALT* alanine aminotransferase, *CR-P* c-reactive peptide, *ESR* erythrocyte sedimentation rate, *WBC* white blood cell count, *PROMIS* Patient Reported Outcomes Measurement Information System

as they are discovered by CARRA Registry site investigators, irrespective of the time elapsed since the last data entry. Data are entered using a standard form that includes detailed information about the event onset, diagnostic studies, event treatment and outcome, and recent medications. MedDRA codes are assigned to all SAE and ESI centrally at the data coordinating center by clinical coding specialists. Additional documentation of safety events, such as hospital discharge summaries or pathology reports, are obtained to increase the specificity and accuracy of any rare safety events identified.

Patient reported outcomes

There is increasing recognition of the importance of patient reported outcomes (PROs) as valuable study endpoints. As shown in Table 1, the CARRA Registry collects patient and/or parent-proxy disease assessments, as well as relevant PROMIS® measures, such as the Pediatric Global Health (PGH-7) Measure. Electronic collection of PROs has been initiated at Registry sites in 2017 using tablet devices, with the option for research participants to also submit PROs electronically between clinical encounters using their own mobile device at home.

As a member organization of the PCORI-funded 'Patients, Advocates and Rheumatology Teams Network for Research and Service' (PARTNERS) Consortium Patient-Powered Research Network [26], the CARRA Registry supports re-contact of Registry participants for collection of new and/or follow-up PROs. PARTNERS also uses the Registry informatics infrastructure to house PRO and associated phenotypic data contributed from other PARTNERS organizations, thereby making this data available for simultaneous, federated querying across all contributed data sources.

Data entry and validation

The Registry data coordinating center is the Duke Clinical Research Institute (DCRI). DCRI personnel have trained all clinical sites on appropriate practices for data collection following standard operating procedures. Data are entered using a web-based interface with programmed validity and consistency checks. If incomplete or inaccurate data are subsequently identified, data clarification requests are sent to the sites until the issues are resolved and all required data are complete. In order to ensure full compliance with FDA regulations for acceptable use of electronic records for clinical trials (i.e., 21 CFR Part 11 compliance), detailed audit trails are maintained for all relevant entries or subsequent revisions of data.

Long-term follow-up

The CARRA Registry intends to collect data for a minimum of 10 years for each enrolled patient. Participants continue to contribute data at a CARRA Registry site as long as they continue to receive care there. If enrolled patients discontinue care from a Registry site (e.g., because of geographic relocation or aging out of pediatric care) their subsequent follow-up is transferred to a centralized Registry call center at the DCRI to maximize the possibility of maintaining long-term contact and longitudinal data collection for each participant. The telephone call center individually contacts each participant and continues to collect patient-reported data about medication use, disease activity, PROs, and safety events. This approach has been successful in other large long-term observational studies performed by the DCRI [27, 28].

Pharmacosurveillance studies

CARRA Inc., as sponsor of the CARRA Registry, has established agreements with pharmaceutical companies to assemble clinical datasets powered to detect pharmacosurveillance safety signals, while also satisfying post-marketing commitments and requirements to regulatory authorities, such as the FDA. Currently, CARRA has active agreements to study the safety of canakinumab (Novartis Pharma AG, Basel, Switzerland) in children with systemic JIA and tocilizumab (Roche Pharmaceuticals, Basel, Switzerland) in children with polyarticular-course JIA. CARRA maintains ownership of all Registry data, as well as full scientific independence and right to publish.

Sub-studies

One of the organizing principals for the CARRA Registry has been the capability to easily add new, modular sub-studies layered upon existing registry infrastructure. With funding from NIAMS/NIH [29], multiple disease-specific Consensus Treatment Plans (CTPs) were developed, standardized, and published contemporaneously with the inception of the CARRA Legacy Registry [30–34]. Following the success of the Arthritis Foundation-funded pilot study of the systemic JIA CTPs [35], funding was obtained from Genentech to conduct a full-scale study entitled "First-line Options for Systemic JIA Treatment (FROST)" and enrollment began in 2016. A similarly designed study of the polyarticular JIA CTPs, entitled "Start Time Optimization in Polyarticular JIA (STOP-JIA)" and funded by PCORI is currently enrolling participants. Companion biospecimen collection for translational studies has been independently funded for both studies: STOP-JIA by the Arthritis Foundation and CARRA; and FROST by the Systemic JIA Foundation. Separate from the CTP-based studies, a modular study to pilot return of research results to patients has completed (NIH/NLM) [36], and a new study to validate PROs among children with JIA and childhood-onset SLE (NIH/NIAMS) [37] is in progress. These studies represent the first of many such modular observational sub-studies anticipated for the CARRA Registry.

Interventional studies

Interventional studies leveraging the CARRA Registry infrastructure and using the CARRA Registry for data collection are under development. Both explanatory/efficacy studies (e.g., placebo-controlled, randomized clinical trial) and pragmatic/effectiveness studies (e.g., large cluster-randomized study of two standards of care) could be incorporated. In addition to the efficiencies provided by the Registry infrastructure, there are other potential benefits of conducting interventional studies of a subset of patients enrolled in the Registry. The disease course and outcomes of patients who meet the interventional study's inclusion criteria but who are not enrolled in the sub-study can be observed in the Registry, thus providing insight into the external validity and generalizability of the interventional study results. Also, interventional study subjects will remain in the Registry following the conclusion of the study, thus greatly aiding the assessment of the long-term effects of the intervention.

Biospecimen collection

Biospecimens initially will be collected from patients enrolled in funded sub-studies to investigate specific translational study aims; plasma, serum, whole blood, and RNA are currently being collected for the STOP-JIA and FROST CTP studies. Future goals include the collection of biospecimens from all Registry participants and the creation of a CARRA biorepository to make the samples available to investigators.

Data sharing

The CARRA Registry utilizes a data infrastructure that provides each participating site with full access to all data its investigators contribute to the network, as well as the ability for each Registry investigator to perform de-identified, aggregate queries of data housed across all network sites [17]. In addition, data access is provided in a tiered fashion, enabling authorized investigators to query for results across multiple CARRA studies and data sources over time, while providing filtering of patient identifiers according to investigator permissions. Specific queries can return comprehensive, longitudinal data on individuals participating in different studies.

CARRA has formulated standardized policies for data and biospecimen sharing (https://carragroup.org/policies_templates) and launched an online platform for investigators to apply for and track the progress of their data and biospecimen sharing requests. Existing data sharing policies are designed for broad access to data while providing formal mechanisms encouraging collaboration rather than competition by investigators, ensuring opportunities and equitable treatment for experienced investigators, junior faculty, and fellows to pursue their research interests, and prioritizing data access to active contributors to the Registry, regardless of site size. Access to data and biosamples is not restricted to CARRA Registry sites.

Financial support

The CARRA Registry is owned and supported by CARRA Inc. The Arthritis Foundation financially supports CARRA Inc., including significant funding for the operation of the CARRA Registry. CARRA Inc. receives funds from pharmaceutical companies in exchange for access to pre-defined sets of post-marketing safety surveillance data. Independent funding for other Registry studies and sub-studies helps to support the general infrastructure costs of the Registry.

Leadership

The CARRA Registry is overseen by an Executive Committee (Chair, Vice-Chair, Scientific Director, CARRA Manager of Research Operations, and DCRI project lead) who receive salary support from CARRA. To develop expertise in the operational and scientific aspects of the Registry and facilitate succession planning, CARRA sponsors year-long Registry research internships for pediatric rheumatologists who have completed clinical training.

Results

As of July 2016, there were 49 active CARRA Registry sites that had enrolled at least one patient. Sites in the United States were broadly representative of the distribution of pediatric rheumatology centers and included at least 1 center from each of the 9 U.S. census divisions.

As of July 2016, 1,192 patients with JIA were enrolled in the CARRA Registry and had completed data entry with less than 1% missing data. The median number of patients with completed data entry at each Registry site was 14, and the largest number at a single site was 178. Thirteen sites had completed data entry for 30 or more participants. The enrollment totals by site location are shown in the Fig. 1.

The participants' characteristics at the time of enrollment are shown in Table 2. Owing to preferential enrollment, patients with a history of polyarthritis (75%) and systemic JIA (13%) were over-represented compared to the general population of children with JIA. Most participants were relatively early in their disease course, with median disease duration of 2.6 years (interquartile range (IQR) 0.5–6.2). Many patients had active disease at the time of enrollment and the median physician global assessment of disease activity was 1.5 out of 10 (IQR 0 – 3.0).

With respect to the creation of analytic cohorts, 295 patients were enrolled within 6 months of their diagnosis of JIA, and 265 patients were enrolled at the time of newly

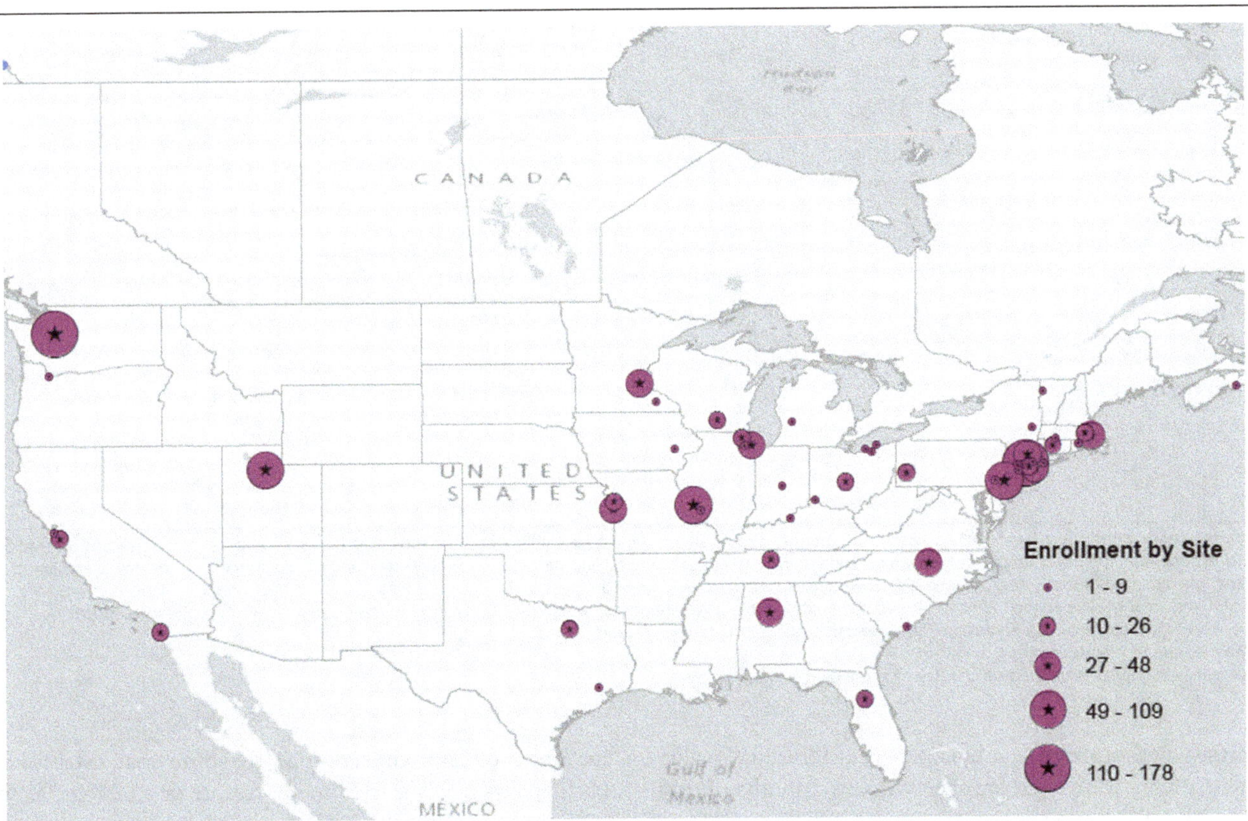

Fig. 1 Location of CARRA Registry participating clinical sites and the number of patients enrolled in the first 12 months. The size of the circle corresponds to the number of patients enrolled, as shown in the figure legend

Table 2 Characteristics of the patients enrolled in the CARRA Registry in the first 12 months of operation. All values are taken from the enrollment visit. Columns 3–5 are not mutually exclusive and patients may appear more than once

Characteristic	Frequency (%) or Median (25–75%)			
	All Participants (*N* = 1,192)	Recent Diagnosis[a] (*N* = 295)	New MTX Use[b] (*N* = 141)	New Biologic Use[b] (*N* = 147)
Age at enrollment (years)	12.4 (7.9–15.7)	10.2 (4.8–14.1)	11.5 (6.8–14.3)	12.7 (7.2–16)
Female	887 (74%)	201 (68%)	109 (77%)	105 (71%)
Race/Ethnicity:				
White	962 (81%)	240 (81%)	112 (79%)	115 (78%)
Black/African-American	58 (5%)	15 (5%)	5 (4%)	8 (5%)
Asian	48 (4%)	15 (5%)	8 (6%)	4 (3%)
Hispanic/Latino	135 (11%)	30 (10%)	14 (10%)	20 (14%)
Middle Eastern/North African	5 (0.4%)	3 (1%)	1 (0.7%)	1 (0.7%)
Native American, American Indian, Alaskan Native	15 (1%)	2 (0.7%)	1 (0.7%)	2 (1%)
Native Hawaiian or Other Pacific Islander	12 (1%)	4 (1%)	2 (1%)	1 (0.7%)
Private health insurance	890 (75%)	217 (74%)	101 (72%)	112 (76%)
Disease duration (years)	2.6 (0.5–6.2)	0.1 (0–0.3)	1.1 (0–4)	2.2 (0.5–6.1)
ILAR category:				
Oligoarthritis, persistent	152 (13%)	90 (31%)	28 (20%)	16 (11%)
Oligoarthritis, extended	102 (9%)	6 (2%)	5 (4%)	11 (7%)
Polyarthritis, RF-	510 (43%)	88 (30%)	66 (47%)	62 (42%)
Polyarthritis, RF+	101 (8%)	18 (6%)	14 (10%)	14 (10%)
Psoriatic arthritis	57 (5%)	20 (7%)	9 (6%)	9 (6%)
Enthesitis related arthritis	104 (9%)	44 (15%)	11 (8%)	20 (14%)
Systemic arthritis	154 (13%)	26 (9%)	6 (4%)	13 (9%)
Undifferentiated arthritis	12 (1%)	3 (1%)	2 (1%)	2 (1%)
ANA+	457/1041 (38%)	107/255 (36%)	64/128 (45%)	64/134 (44%)
RF+	111/907 (9%)	24/213 (8%)	17/107 (12%)	15/118 (10%)
Anti-CCP+	91/585 (8%)	20/129 (7%)	17/74 (12%)	14/73 (10%)
HLA-B27+	98/608 (8%)	32/179 (11%)	15/75 (11%)	16/83 (11%)
Polyarthritis course	895 (75%)	151 (51%)	100 (71%)	107 (73%)
Uveitis, ever	94 (8%)	3 (1%)	8 (6%)	19 (13%)
Number of active joints	1 (0–3)	2 (1–6)	3 (1–6)	3 (1–5.75)
Physician global assessment	1.5 (0–3.0)	3 (1.5–5)	3 (1.75–4.25)	3 (2–5)
CHAQ score	0.125 (0–0.625)	0.375 (0–0.875)	0.25 (0–1)	0.5 (0–1)
ESR	8 (5–17)	9 (5–28)	9 (6–23)	9 (5–27)
CRP	0.6 (0.2–1.7)	0.8 (0.3–1.7)	1.0 (0.5–3.0)	0.8 (0.5–2.6)

Sixty-three participants were recently diagnosed and started methotrexate on the day of enrollment. Thirty-seven participants were recently diagnosed and started a biologic agent on the day of enrollment. Eleven participants were recently diagnosed and started both methotrexate and a biologic agent on the day of enrollment. Twenty-three participants total newly started both methotrexate and a biologic agent on the day of enrollment. Participants could report more than 1 race/ethnicity
ILAR International League Against Rheumatism, *RF* rheumatoid factor, *ANA* antinuclear antibody, *CCP* cyclic citrullinated peptide, *CHAQ* Childhood Health Assessment Questionnaire, *ESR* erythrocyte sedimentation rate, *CRP* C-reactive protein
[a]Within 6 months of diagnosis
[b]New medication was prescribed on the day of enrollment in the Registry

starting methotrexate or a biologic agent (or both). Eighty-nine patients were both enrolled within 6 months of diagnosis and also began methotrexate or a biologic agent at the time of enrollment. The characteristics of these patients are shown in Table 2. In addition, there were 50 instances of data collection at the time that established participants newly started methotrexate or a biologic agent following their enrollment.

Table 3 shows participants' current and ever medication use at the time of enrollment. All medications used

Table 3 Medication use at enrollment by the patients enrolled in the CARRA Registry in the first 12 months of operation

Medication	Number (%) of Current Users	Number (%) of Ever Users
Methotrexate	556 (47%)	868 (73%)
Leflunomide	52 (4%)	71 (6%)
Sulfasalazine	20 (2%)	49 (4%)
Hydroxychloroquine	49 (4%)	69 (6%)
Adalimumab	140 (12%)	235 (20%)
Etanercept	273 (23%)	505 (42%)
Golimumab	7 (1%)	13 (1%)
Infliximab	44 (4%)	95 (8%)
Any TNFi	465 (39%)	664 (56%)
Any TNFi + Methotrexate	255 (21%)	n/a
Abatacept	17 (1%)	55 (5%)
Tocilizumab	59 (5%)	115 (10%)
Tocilizumab + Methotrexate	42 (4%)	n/a
Anakinra	24 (2%)	75 (6%)
Canakinumab	29 (2%)	46 (4%)
Any IL-1 inhibitor + Methotrexate	18 (2%)	n/a
Rituximab	3 (<1%)	16 (1%)
Oral glucocorticoids	124 (10%)	560 (47%)

TNFi tumor necrosis factor inhibitor, *IL-1* interleukin 1, *n/a* not assessed

by at least 1% of participants are shown. As anticipated, participants were enriched for use of biologic agents and there was a broad variety of biologic agents used in addition to the tumor necrosis factor inhibitors. Use of oral glucocorticoids was common.

As of July 2016, 12 safety events had been reported including 8 serious adverse events and 3 episodes of macrophage activation syndrome. There were no deaths or incident malignancies reported.

Discussion

The newly initiated CARRA Registry has built upon the successes of the former CARRA Legacy Registry by leveraging site investigator experience and training as well as coordinating center expertise and innovative technology for integrating and sharing data. Nearly 1,200 patients with JIA were enrolled in the CARRA Registry in the first year since its inception while the number of participating clinical sites was still accumulating. The CARRA Registry has successfully entered collaborations with two pharmaceutical companies to provide data necessary for post-marketing safety surveillance studies. CARRA investigators have successfully secured independent funding to perform observational studies of the published CARRA CTPs. Many additional observational and interventional Registry studies and sub-studies, as well as translational studies using Registry-collected biospecimens linked to Registry clinical data, are anticipated in the near future and will benefit greatly from the growing Registry infrastructure.

Registry data to date demonstrate the ability to rapidly enroll patients with clinical data of the highest utility, namely those newly diagnosed (295; 25% of overall enrollees) and newly starting methotrexate or biologic agents (265; 22% of overall enrollees). Newly diagnosed patients provide prospective data about the natural history of disease and its treatment course that are less prone to bias; nevertheless, the CARRA Registry is not truly population-based and data may not be generalizable to all children diagnosed with JIA. Patients newly starting medications establish retrospective and prospective analytic cohorts within the Registry, enabling the unbiased evaluation of the safety and effectiveness of therapeutic agents. This "new user" analytic design greatly improves the validity of study results [38, 39].

One of the keys to the sustained success of the CARRA Registry will be providing investigators as well as participants with added value for their engagement in the Registry. The most obvious added value will result from published studies and improved knowledge of the safety and effectiveness of therapeutic agents. For research investigators, the ability to freely access and analyze data collected on their own patients, in combination with straightforward policies and rapid processes for previewing and then accessing data sourced across the entire network, will foster additional opportunities to conduct research of interest to them in a timely fashion. For clinicians, providing personalized, up-to-date benchmarks of their own site's practices and therapeutic decisions in context to many other pediatric rheumatologists is likely to be of considerable interest and benefit, and should catalyze meaningful follow-up discussions and analyses, supporting "learning health system" cycles [40]. For patients and their families, providing feedback of results of self-identified importance, and incorporating patient preferences across the spectrum of research into long-term outcomes, is likely to be of high value.

Conclusion

Single product registries in the United States have disappointed both patient and provider communities due to their limited enrollment and inability to address many important questions. The disease-specific CARRA Registry offers an alternative approach designed to directly address these concerns and provide broader opportunities to streamline clinical research in understudied populations. We hope the CARRA Registry will serve as a valuable paradigm for the study of uncommon diseases.

Abbreviations

ACR: American College of Rheumatology; CARRA: Childhood arthritis and rheumatology research alliance; cSLE: Childhood-onset systemic lupus erythematosus; CTPs: Consensus treatment plans; DCRI: Duke Clinical Research Institute; ESI: Event of special interest; FDA: United States Food and Drug Administration; FROST: First-line options for systemic JIA treatment; IRB: Institutional review board; JADAS: Juvenile arthritis disease activity score; JDM: Juvenile dermatomyositis; JIA: Juvenile idiopathic arthritis; PARTNERS: Patients, Advocates, and Rheumatology Teams Network for Research and Service; PGH-7: Pediatric Global Health 7; PROs: Patient reported outcomes; SAE: Serious adverse event; STOP-JIA: Start time optimization in polyarticular JIA

Acknowledgements
We thank Anne Dennos for assistance with data analysis.
We acknowledge the following CARRA Registry investigators and research coordinators: Leslie Abramson, Shoghik Akoghlanian, Edwin Anderson, Margaret Andrew, Kevin Baszis, Mara Becker, Heather Bell-Brunson, Heather Benham, James Birmingham, Peter Blier, Hermine Brunner, Elizabeth Chalom, Johanna Chang, Paula Charpentier, Nazma Chowdhury, Joni Dean, Fatma Dedeoglu, Marija Dionizovik-Dimanovski, Brian Feldman, Polly Ferguson, Marie Fox, Kimberly Francis, Lourdes Franco, Mary Gervasini, Ingrid Goh, Donald Goldsmith, T. Brent Graham, Thomas Griffin, Dawn Helfrich, Kristin Hickey, Mark Hoeltzel, Sarah Holtschlag, Joyce Hsu, Adam Huber, Anna Huttenlocher, Lisa Imundo, Christi Inman, Jane Jaquith, Rita Jerath, Suzy Jones, Philip Kahn, Daniel Kingsbury, Kristin Klein, Marisa Klein-Gitelman, Sara Kramer, Ann Kunkel, Sivia Lapidus, Deborah Latham, Thomas Lehman, Carol Lindsley, Sean Linehan, Jennifer Lorenzo, Bipin Malla, Alexandra Martyniuk, Thomas Mason, Karen McConnell, Deborah McCurdy, Kieran McKibben, Chivon McMullen-Jackson, Diana Milojevic, Katie Mims, Christine Moniz, Sheri Morgan, Elizabeth Murray, Karen Nicely, Kathleen O'Neil, Karen Onel, Jordan Orange, Lori Ponder, Sampath Prahalad, Marilynn Punaro, C. Egla Rabinovich, Amy Rakestraw, Susan Rauch, Luke Reichley, Ariel Rhea, Sarah Ringold, Mary Ellen Riordan, Staci Roberson, Angela Robinson, Margalit Rosenkranz, Krista Ross, Deborah Rothman, Yonit Ruas, Natasha Ruth, Rosemary Sanders, Kenneth Schikler, Nora Singer, Chelsey Smith, Heidi Stapp, Shameka Swann, Reema Syed, Ashlee Tangarone, Akaluck Thatayatikom, Danielle Trejo, Jenna Tress, Richard Vehe, Emily von Scheven, Allen Watts, Jennifer Weiss, Pamela Weiss, Jennifer Woo, Ali Yalcindag, Andrew Zeft, Lawrence Zemel, Aihua Zhu.

Funding
The CARRA Registry is financially supported by CARRA Inc., the Arthritis Foundation, Novartis, and Roche. The Arthritis Foundation, Novartis, and Roche played no role in design of the study; the collection, analysis, or interpretation of data; or the writing of the manuscript.
Drs. Beukelman, Kimura, Ilowite, Natter, and Schanberg, and Ms. Miezkalski, Ms. Burrell, and Mr Best receive salary support from CARRA Inc. Mr. Jones was an employee of CARRA Inc.

Authors' contributions
All authors made substantial contributions to the conception of the CARRA Registry and the acquisition of data. TB, YK, and LES analyzed and interpreted the data. TB, YK, MDN, and LES drafted the manuscript. All authors critically revised the manuscript and approved of the final version.

Competing interests
JJ was an employee of CARRA Inc. TB, YK, NI, MN, LES, KM, GB, and BB receive salary support from CARRA Inc. TB has received consulting fees from Novartis, Genentech/Roche, and UCB.

Consent for publication
Not applicable.

Author details
[1]Division of Pediatric Rheumatology, The University of Alabama at Birmingham, 1600 7th Avenue South, CPP 210, Birmingham, AL 35233-1711, USA. [2]Hackensack University Medical Center, Hackensack, USA. [3]Children's Hospital at Montefiore, Bronx, USA. [4]Childhood Arthritis and Rheumatology Research Alliance, Durham, USA. [5]Children's Hospital Boston, Boston, USA. [6]Duke University, Durham, USA.

References

1. Petty RE, Southwood TR, Manners P, Baum J, Glass DN, Goldenberg J, et al. International League of Associations for Rheumatology classification of juvenile idiopathic arthritis: second revision, Edmonton, 2001. J Rheumatol. 2004;31:390–2.
2. Gowdie PJ, Tse SM. Juvenile idiopathic arthritis. Pediatr Clin North Am. 2012;59:301–27.
3. CARRA Website https://carragroup.org/.
4. Schanberg LE, Ilowite NT, Sandborg CI, Wallace CA. CARRA: Accelerating Toward an Evidence Based Culture in Pediatric Rheumatology (1RC2AR058934-01) https://projectreporter.nih.gov/project_info_description.cfm?aid=7855553. Accessed 11 Apr 2017.
5. Beukelman T, Ringold S, Davis TE, DeWitt EM, Pelajo CF, Weiss PF, et al. Disease-modifying antirheumatic drug use in the treatment of juvenile idiopathic arthritis: a cross-sectional analysis of the CARRA Registry. J Rheumatol. 2012;39:1867–74.
6. Weiss PF, Beukelman T, Schanberg LE, Kimura Y, Colbert RA, Investigators CR. Enthesitis-related arthritis is associated with higher pain intensity and poorer health status in comparison with other categories of juvenile idiopathic arthritis: the Childhood Arthritis and Rheumatology Research Alliance Registry. J Rheumatol. 2012;39:2341–51.
7. Angeles-Han ST, Pelajo CF, Vogler LB, Rouster-Stevens K, Kennedy C, Ponder L, et al. Risk markers of juvenile idiopathic arthritis-associated uveitis in the Childhood Arthritis and Rheumatology Research Alliance (CARRA) Registry. J Rheumatol. 2013;40:2088–96.
8. Kimura Y, Weiss JE, Haroldson KL, Lee T, Punaro M, Oliveira S, et al. Pulmonary hypertension and other potentially fatal pulmonary complications in systemic juvenile idiopathic arthritis. Arthritis Care Res (Hoboken). 2013;65:745–52.
9. Ringold S, Beukelman T, Nigrovic PA, Kimura Y, CRSP Investigators. Race, ethnicity, and disease outcomes in juvenile idiopathic arthritis: a cross-sectional analysis of the Childhood Arthritis and Rheumatology Research Alliance (CARRA) registry. J Rheumatol. 2013;40:936–42.
10. Boneparth A, Ilowite NT, CR Investigators. Comparison of renal response parameters for juvenile membranous plus proliferative lupus nephritis versus isolated proliferative lupus nephritis: a cross-sectional analysis of the CARRA registry. Lupus. 2014;23:898–904.
11. Robinson AB, Hoeltzel MF, Wahezi DM, Becker ML, Kessler EA, Schmeling H, et al. Clinical characteristics of children with juvenile dermatomyositis: the Childhood Arthritis and Rheumatology Research Alliance Registry. Arthritis Care Res (Hoboken). 2014;66:404–10.
12. Driest KD, Sturm MS, O'Brien SH, Spencer CH, Stanek JR, Ardoin SP, et al. Factors associated with thrombosis in pediatric patients with systemic lupus erythematosus. Lupus. 2016;25(7):749–53.
13. Fitzpatrick L, Broadaway KA, Ponder L, Angeles-Han ST, Jenkins K, Rouster-Stevens K, et al. Phenotypic characterization of juvenile idiopathic arthritis in African American children. J Rheumatol. 2016;43:799–803.
14. Henderson LA, Zurakowski D, Angeles-Han ST, Lasky A, Rabinovich CE, Lo MS, et al. Medication use in juvenile uveitis patients enrolled in the Childhood Arthritis and Rheumatology Research Alliance Registry. Pediatr Rheumatol Online J. 2016;14:9.
15. Prahalad S, McCracken CE, Ponder LA, Angeles-Han ST, Rouster Stevens KA, Vogler LB, et al. Familial autoimmunity in the Childhood Arthritis and Rheumatology Research Alliance Registry. Pediatr Rheumatol Online J. 2016;14:14.
16. Janow G, Schanberg LE, Setoguchi S, Hasselblad V, Mellins ED, Schneider R, et al. The systemic juvenile idiopathic arthritis cohort of the Childhood

Arthritis and Rheumatology Research Alliance Registry: 2010–2013. J Rheumatol. 2016;43:1755–62.
17. Natter MD, Quan J, Ortiz DM, Bousvaros A, Ilowite NT, Inman CJ, et al. An i2b2-based, generalizable, open source, self-scaling chronic disease registry. J Am Med Inform Assoc. 2013;20:172–9.
18. Public Workshop on Developing a Consolidated Pediatric Rheumatology Observational Registry - Executive Summary. http://www.regulations.gov/#!documentDetail;D=FDA-2009-N-0145-0055. Accessed 11 Apr 2017.
19. Lionetti G, Kimura Y, Schanberg LE, Beukelman T, Wallace CA, Ilowite NT, et al. Using registries to identify adverse events in rheumatic diseases. Pediatrics. 2013;132:e1384–94.
20. Giannini EH, Ruperto N, Ravelli A, Lovell DJ, Felson DT, Martini A. Preliminary definition of improvement in juvenile arthritis. Arthritis Rheum. 1997;40:1202–9.
21. Brunner HI, Lovell DJ, Finck BK, Giannini EH. Preliminary definition of disease flare in juvenile rheumatoid arthritis. J Rheumatol. 2002;29:1058–64.
22. Consolaro A, Ruperto N, Bazso A, Pistorio A, Magni-Manzoni S, Filocamo G, et al. Development and validation of a composite disease activity score for juvenile idiopathic arthritis. Arthritis Rheum. 2009;61:658–66.
23. McErlane F, Beresford MW, Baildam EM, Chieng SE, Davidson JE, Foster HE, et al. Validity of a three-variable juvenile arthritis disease activity score in children with new-onset juvenile idiopathic arthritis. Ann Rheum Dis. 2013;72:1983–8.
24. Wallace CA, Giannini EH, Huang B, Itert L, Ruperto N, Childhood Arthritis Rheumatology Research A, et al. American College of Rheumatology provisional criteria for defining clinical inactive disease in select categories of juvenile idiopathic arthritis. Arthritis Care Res (Hoboken). 2011;63:929–36.
25. United States Food and Drug Administration Code of Federal Regulations Title 21. [cited 2016 Novermber 28]. Available from: https://www.accessdata.fda.gov/scripts/cdrh/cfdocs/cfCFR/CFRSearch.cfm?fr=312.32.
26. PARTNERS Website http://www.arthritis.org/partners/.
27. Chin CT, Wang TY, Anstrom KJ, Zhu B, Maa JF, Messenger JC, et al. Treatment with adenosine diphosphate receptor inhibitors-longitudinal assessment of treatment patterns and events after acute coronary syndrome (TRANSLATE-ACS) study design: expanding the paradigm of longitudinal observational research. Am Heart J. 2011;162:844–51.
28. Hess CN, McCoy LA, Duggirala HJ, Tavris DR, O'Callaghan K, Douglas PS, et al. Sex-based differences in outcomes after percutaneous coronary intervention for acute myocardial infarction: a report from TRANSLATE-ACS. J Am Heart Assoc. 2014;3:e000523.
29. Wallace CA, Ilowite NT. Comparative effectiveness research in pediatric rheumatic diseases: leveraging CARRA (1RC1AR058605-01) https://projectreporter.nih.gov/project_info_description.cfm?aid=7832335. Accessed 11 Apr 2017.
30. Mina R, von Scheven E, Ardoin SP, Eberhard BA, Punaro M, Ilowite N, et al. Consensus treatment plans for induction therapy of newly diagnosed proliferative lupus nephritis in juvenile systemic lupus erythematosus. Arthritis Care Res (Hoboken). 2012;64:375–83.
31. Huber AM, Robinson AB, Reed AM, Abramson L, Bout-Tabaku S, Carrasco R, et al. Consensus treatments for moderate juvenile dermatomyositis: beyond the first two months. Results of the second Childhood Arthritis and Rheumatology Research Alliance consensus conference. Arthritis Care Res (Hoboken). 2012;64:546–53.
32. DeWitt EM, Kimura Y, Beukelman T, Nigrovic PA, Onel K, Prahalad S, et al. Consensus treatment plans for new-onset systemic juvenile idiopathic arthritis. Arthritis Care Res (Hoboken). 2012;64:1001–10.
33. Li SC, Torok KS, Pope E, Dedeoglu F, Hong S, Jacobe HT, et al. Development of consensus treatment plans for juvenile localized scleroderma: a roadmap toward comparative effectiveness studies in juvenile localized scleroderma. Arthritis Care Res (Hoboken). 2012;64:1175–85.
34. Ringold S, Weiss PF, Colbert RA, DeWitt EM, Lee T, Onel K, et al. Childhood Arthritis and Rheumatology Research Alliance consensus treatment plans for new-onset polyarticular juvenile idiopathic arthritis. Arthritis Care Res (Hoboken). 2014;66:1063–72.
35. Kimura Y, Grevich S, Beukelman T, Morgan E, Mieszkalski K, Graham TB, et al. Pilot study results comparing the Childhood Arthritis and Rheumatology Research Alliance (CARRA) Consensus Treatment Plans for new-onset systemic juvenile idiopathic arthritis.
36. Mandl KD, Weitzman ER. Active patient participation in a disease registry for comparative effectiveness (1R01LM011185-01) https://projectreporter.nih.gov/project_info_description.cfm?aid=8226504. Accessed 11 Apr 2017.
37. Reeve BB, Schanberg LE. Enhancing clinical meaningfulness and usefulness of PROMIS pediatric measures via validation in children and adolescents with rheumatic disease, cancer, or inflammatory bowel disease (1U19AR069522-01) https://projectreporter.nih.gov/project_info_description.cfm?aid=9077742&icde=30170784. Accessed 11 Apr 2017.
38. Ray WA. Evaluating medication effects outside of clinical trials: new-user designs. Am J Epidemiol. 2003;158:915–20.
39. Solomon DH, Lunt M, Schneeweiss S. The risk of infection associated with tumor necrosis factor alpha antagonists: making sense of epidemiologic evidence. Arthritis Rheum. 2008;58:919–28.
40. IOM (Institute of Medicine). In: Smith M, Saunders R, Stuckhardt L, McGinnis JM, Committee on the Learning Health Care System in America, editors. Best care at lower cost: the path to continuously learning health care in America. Washington, DC: The National Academic Press; 2013.

A survey of national and multi-national registries and cohort studies in juvenile idiopathic arthritis: challenges and opportunities

Timothy Beukelman[1,19*], Janneke Anink[2], Lillemor Berntson[3], Ciaran Duffy[4], Justine A. Ellis[5], Mia Glerup[6], Jaime Guzman[7], Gerd Horneff[8], Lianne Kearsley-Fleet[9], Ariane Klein[8], Jens Klotsche[10], Bo Magnusson[11], Kirsten Minden[10], Jane E. Munro[12], Martina Niewerth[10], Ellen Nordal[13], Nicolino Ruperto[14], Maria Jose Santos[15], Laura E. Schanberg[16], Wendy Thomson[9], Lisette van Suijlekom-Smit[2], Nico Wulffraat[17] and Kimme Hyrich[18]

Abstract

Background: To characterize the existing national and multi-national registries and cohort studies in juvenile idiopathic arthritis (JIA) and identify differences as well as areas of potential future collaboration.

Methods: We surveyed investigators from North America, Europe, and Australia about existing JIA cohort studies and registries. We excluded cross-sectional studies. We captured information about study design, duration, location, inclusion criteria, data elements and collection methods.

Results: We received survey results from 18 studies, including 11 national and 7 multi-national studies representing 37 countries in total. Study designs included inception cohorts, prevalent disease cohorts, and new treatment cohorts (several of which contribute to pharmacosurveillance activities). Despite numerous differences, the data elements collected across the studies was quite similar, with most studies collecting at least 5 of the 6 American College of Rheumatology core set variables and the data needed to calculate the 3-variable clinical juvenile disease activity score. Most studies were collecting medication initiation and discontinuation dates and were attempting to capture serious adverse events.

Conclusion: There is a wide-range of large, ongoing JIA registries and cohort studies around the world. Our survey results indicate significant potential for future collaborative work using data from different studies and both combined and comparative analyses.

Keywords: Juvenile idiopathic arthritis, Registry, Observational study, Pharmacosurveillance, Pediatric rheumatology

Background

Juvenile idiopathic arthritis (JIA), a heterogeneous collection of inflammatory arthritides, is the most common rheumatic condition of childhood [1]. Despite this, our understanding of the long-term outcomes for many children with this condition, in terms of disease status, functional limitation, need for long-term immunosuppression as well as the development of comorbidities, remains relatively limited. Similarly, we have an incomplete understanding of the potential adverse effects of new therapeutic agents, especially effects that are rare or have a long latency period.

The epidemiological study of JIA is challenging. Compared to the 1% prevalence of rheumatoid arthritis (RA) in adults, JIA is rare. The approximate worldwide yearly incidence is 8 per 100,000 children and most prevalence estimates range from 15 to 150 per 100,000 depending on geographic region and

* Correspondence: tbeukelman@peds.uab.edu
[1]University of Alabama at Birmingham, Birmingham, USA
[19]Division of Pediatric Rheumatology, The University of Alabama at Birmingham, 1600 7th Avenue South, CPP 210, Birmingham, AL 35233-1711, USA
Full list of author information is available at the end of the article

study methodology [2]. In contrast to the categorization of the arthritis counterparts in adulthood, JIA encompasses a wide range of inflammatory arthritides, from self-limited oligoarthritis to severe, persistent polyarthritis, and it also includes psoriatic arthritis, spondyloarthritis, and systemic arthritis (an autoinflammatory condition). Results from long-term follow-up studies of JIA may not be broadly generalizable; they may exclude children with milder forms of disease who are discharged from rheumatology care, and they may include too few children to adequately study the less common disease phenotypes. The long-term study of childhood-onset diseases is complicated when patients transition to the adult healthcare setting, making the capture of health outcome data challenging. However, patients and parents identify long-term outcomes, such as physical ability in adulthood, successful schooling and employment, and the consequences of long-term exposure to immunosuppression in childhood, as some of their key priorities for research [3, 4].

With the advent of biological therapies and their increasing use, reliable outcome data in JIA has become even more crucial. Little is known about the background rates of serious outcomes, such as infections and malignancies, making it difficult to interpret the safety of new medications. Extrapolation from studies of these drugs in adults with RA has limited accuracy because most children with JIA do not have RA (only approximately 5% have rheumatoid factor positive polyarthritis) and children have far fewer serious comorbid conditions compared to adults. Exposure to immune modulating drugs in developing immune systems may also result in different longer-term adverse health outcomes compared to more mature immune systems.

Given the rarity of JIA and the now frequent use of potentially high risk treatments in the absence of robust, large, long-term safety studies, the capture of data in longitudinal cohorts is essential. Appropriately combining data from various cohorts enables detection of rare adverse events and more accurate assessment of disease outcomes. Comparing data from different countries may provide information about genotypic variations in disease and geographic variation in environmental risk factors. It may also allow for comparisons of treatment differences that result largely from local availability of therapeutic agents rather than differences in disease characteristics.

The purpose of this study was to survey the international landscape of prospective longitudinal registries and cohort studies in JIA to assess the breadth and depth of data being collected. This information will inform future international collaborative work in JIA, including data harmonization for future studies.

Methods

A list of existing JIA registries and cohort studies was compiled through known contacts of the authors, ongoing collaborations, and a review of the recent literature. This included studies conducted in the United States of America (USA), Canada, United Kingdom (UK), Germany, the Netherlands, Sweden, Norway, Portugal, and Australia, as well as some multi-national studies. A survey developed in Microsoft Excel (2010) was emailed to the principal investigators of each registry or cohort. The survey also asked for additional registries or cohorts known to the respondent. Surveys were completed between October and December 2014. Owing to delays in manuscript preparation and in an effort to provide the most recent information possible, all respondents were given the opportunity to revise their responses in March 2016.

The survey captured details about each registry or cohort study, including study design, study duration, location, inclusion criteria and number of participants, and data elements and collection method. Cross-sectional studies, defined as those with less than 12 months of planned follow-up per participant, were excluded.

Results

In total, 20 investigators were contacted, and the replies described 20 studies. Two identified studies were not included (CLARITY from Australia [5] and EPOCA from PRINTO [6]) due to cross-sectional design. The remaining 18 studies contain more than 60,000 patients with JIA (Table 1). These studies include 11 national and 7 multi-national cohorts (covering more than 37 countries in total), with data spanning from 1993 until 2016 onwards. These included 5 JIA inception cohorts (recruiting exclusively from disease onset), 6 prevalent disease cohorts (without strict requirements about disease duration or treatment), and 7 treatment cohorts (restricted to children starting certain anti-rheumatic therapies, such as biologics). Data from treatment cohorts were often part of pharmacosurveillance regulatory requirements. A majority of studies had been established within the past 15 years. Despite the long duration of some studies, the number of total subjects recruited to each study remained relatively low, with few national studies exceeding 1500 children.

Most studies are still recruiting and continuing to follow-up children previously recruited. The planned length of follow-up varied across studies and was generally dependent on the amount or nature of funding available (data not shown). A majority of studies were based in a single country or a small number of countries within a geographic area. One noted exception is the large multi-national Pharmacovigilance in Juvenile Idiopathic Arthritis Patients (Pharmachild) collaboration,which was initiated with a European Union grant from the Framework

Table 1 Summary of JIA registries and cohort studies

Study Name and Published Reference	Country	Start Year	Approx. number of patients	Children/adults enrolled	Minimum Follow-up (Years)	Active Follow-up after Transition of Care	Active Recruitment	Active Follow-up
Inception Cohorts								
CAPS [Childhood Arthritis Prospective Study] [19]	UK	2001	1500	Children	10 years or transition	No (patient questionnaire at age 18 and 21 years)	Yes	Yes
ICON [Inception Cohort of Newly Diagnosed Children with JIA] [35]	Germany	2010	950	Children	10	Yes	No	Yes
JACS [Juvenile Arthritis Cohort Study]	Australia	2012	25	Children	To transition	No	Yes	Yes
Nordic JIA Cohort [24]	Sweden, Finland, Denmark, Norway, Iceland	1997	1200	Children	15	Yes	Yes	Yes
ReACCh Out [Research in Arthritis in Canadian Children Emphasizing Outcomes] [36]	Canada	2005	1500	Children	5	No	No	Yes
Prevalent Disease Cohorts								
CARRA Legacy [Childhood Arthritis and Rheumatology Research Alliance] [37]	USA, Canada	2010	6600	Children	Until 2013	No	No	No
CARRA (current)[a] [Childhood Arthritis and Rheumatology Research Alliance] [14]	USA, Canada	2015	994	Children	10	Yes, via Call centre	Yes	Yes
NPRD [National Pediatric Rheumatology Database] [38]	Germany	1997	~29,000	Children	Unlimited	No	Yes	Yes
PHARMACHILD (Retrospective) [Pharmacovigilance in Juvenile Idiopathic Arthritis Patients]	Multi-national	2011	7000	Children	Retrospective data collection only	No	Yes	Yes
Reuma.pt [9]	Portugal/Brazil	2009	1188/310	Both	Unlimited	Yes	Yes	Yes
Swedish JIA Register	Sweden	2009	1800	Children	To transition	No	Yes	Yes
Treatment Cohorts								
ABC [Arthritis and Biologicals in Children] [39]	Netherlands	1999	425	Children	To transition	No	No	No
BiKeR [Biologics in Pediatric Rheumatology] [10, 11]	Germany, Austria	2001	3743	Children	To transition	No	Yes	Yes
JuMBO [Juvenile Arthritis Methotrexate Biologics Long-Term Observation] [8]	Germany	2007	1100	Adults	10	Follow-up to BIKER study	Yes	Yes
BCRD[b]	UK	2010	850	Children	10	Yes	Yes	Yes

Table 1 Summary of JIA registries and cohort studies *(Continued)*

[Biologics for Children with Rheumatic Diseases] [13]								
BSPAR-ETN[b] [British Society for Pediatric and Adolescent Rheumatolgy-Etanercept] [12]	UK	2003	1400	Children	Unlimited	Yes	Yes	Yes
BSRBR[c] [British Society for Rheumatology Biologics Register] [7]	UK	2001	550	Adults	Unlimited	N/A	Yes	Yes
PHARMACHILD (Prospective) [Pharmacovigilance in Juvenile Idiopathic Arthritis Patients]	28 countries	2011	1450	Children	10	Yes, via JAMAR questionnaire	Yes	Yes

[a]The CARRA Registry preferentially enrols children with systemic arthritis, polyarticular JIA, new diagnosis of JIA, or initiation of treatment with methotrexate or biologic agents
[b]BCRD and BSPAR-ETN preferentially recruit children at point of starting MTX or a biologic drug
[c]BSRBR recruits adults starting a biologic drug. The primary focus is RA but includes adults with JIA

Table 2 Data Capture Across JIA Registries and Cohort Studies

Study	ILAR Category	AJC	LJC	MD global	Parent global	CHAQ/ HAQ	ESR	CRP	Full ACR Core Set	JADAS	cJADAS	Pain	Uveitis data	JIA Medication Start/Stop dates	Serious Adverse Events	Stored Bio-samples	Imaging results	Link to external data sources	Industry pharmaco-surveillance studies
Inception Cohorts																			
CAPS	Y	Y	Y	Y	Y	Y	Y	Y	Y	Y	Y	Y	Y	Y	Y	Y	Y	Y	N
ICON	Y	Y	Y	Y	Y	Y	Y	Y	Y	Y	Y	Y	Y	Y	Y	Y	Limited	N	N
JACS	Y	Y	Y	Y	Y	Y	Y	Y	Y	Y	Y	Y	Y	Y	Y	Y	N	Y	N
Nordic JIA Cohort	Y	Y	Y	Y	Y	Y	Y	Y	Y	Y	Y	Y	Y	N	N	Y	N	N	N
ReACCh Out	Y	Y	Y	Y	Y	Y	Y	Y	Y	Y	Y	Y	Y	Y	N	Y	N	N	N
Prevalent Cohorts																			
CARRA Legacy	Y	Y	N	Y	Y	Y	N	N	N	N	Y	Y	Y	N	Limited	N	Y	N	N
CARRA (current)	Y	Y	Y	Y	Y	Y	Y	Y	Y	Y	Y	Y	Y	Y	Y	Limited	Y	Potential	Y
NPRD	Y	Y	Y	Y	Y	Y	Y	Y	Y	Y	Y	Y	Y	Start only	Y	Limited	N	N	N
PHARMACHILD (retrospective)	Y	N	N	N	N	N	N	N	N	N	N	N	Y	Y	Y	N	N	N	N
Reuma.pt	Y	Y	Y	Y	Y	Y	Y	Y	Y	Y	Y	Y	Y	Y	Y	Limited	Limited	N	N
Swedish JIA Register	Y	Y	N	Y	Y	Y	Y	Y	N	Y	Y	Y	Y	Y	N	Limited	N	N	Y
Treatment Cohorts																			
ABC	Y	Y	Y	Y	Y	Y	Y	N	Y	Y	Y	Y	Y	Y	Y	Y	Limited	N	N
BCRD	Y	Y	Y	Y	Y	Y	Y	Y	Y	Y	Y	Y	Y	Y	Y	Y	N	Y	N
BIKER	Y	Y	Y	Y	Y	Y	Y	Y	Y	Y	Y	Y	Y	Y	Y	Y	N	N	Y
BSPAR-ETN	Y	Y	Y	Y	Y	Y	Y	Y	Y	Y	Y	Y	Y	Y	Y	Y	N	Y	Y
PHARMACHILD (prospective)	Y	Y	Y	Y	Y	N	Y	Y	N	Y	Y	Y	Y	Y	Y	Limited	Y	N	Y
BSRBR	N	N[a]	N	N	Y	Y	Y	Y	N	N	N	N	N	Y	Y	Limited	N	Y	Y
JuMBO	Y	Y	Y	Y	Y	Y	Y	Y	Y	Y	Y	Y	Y	Y	Y	Limited	N	N	Y

ILAR International League of Associations for Rheumatology, *AJC* active joint count, *LJC* limited joint count, *MD* physician, *(C)HAQ* (Childhood) Health Assessment Questionnaire, *ESR* erythrocyte sedimentation rate, *CRP* C-reactive protein, *ACR* American College of Rheumatology, *JADAS* Juvenile Arthritis Disease Activity Score, *cJADAS* clinical (3-variable) Juvenile Arthritis Disease Activity Score, *Y* yes, *N*-no

[a]Captures 28-swollen and tender joint count only

Programme 7, managed by the Pediatric Rheumatology International Trials Organization (PRINTO), and has recruited children from 28 countries.

The vast majority of studies recruited children, although 2 studies (The British Society for Rheumatology Biologics Register (BSRBR) [7] and The German Juvenile Arthritis - Methotrexate/Biologics Long-term Observation Study (JUMBO) [8], specifically recruit adult patients with JIA receiving biologic therapies. Most studies stop follow-up after children leave paediatric care; however, there are several exceptions. The Portuguese register, Reuma.pt, is built into routine care and continues to capture data from patients into adulthood [9]. JUMBO is a follow-on study that links adults who were followed in the German BiKeR registry [10, 11] as children. Similarly, the UK BSPAR [12] and BCRD registers [13] continue to capture outcome data about young adults from their adult care providers. The CARRA Registry follows young adults after transition of care via a structured survey conducted by a telephone call center [14]. Pharmachild has the option for adult rheumatology centers to submit data and plans to collect data directly from young adults after transition of care by use of the JAMAR questionnaire [15].

Despite differences in geographic location, time since study inception, and study designs, the data elements collected across studies appears to be quite similar (Table 2). All studies but one capture the International League of Associations for Rheumatology (ILAR) category of JIA [1]. More than two-thirds of studies capture the full American College of Rheumatology JIA core outcome set (count of joints with active arthritis, count of joints with limited range of motion, physician global assessment of overall disease activity, patient/parent global assessment of overall well-being, functional ability (Childhood Health Assessment Questionnaire (CHAQ) score), inflammatory markers) [16]. Nearly all of the remaining studies capture 5 of the ACR core outcome variables. Fifteen studies (83%) collect the data needed to calculate the 10 or 71-joint Juvenile Arthritis Disease Activity Score (JADAS-10 or JADAS-71) [17], and 16 can calculate the 3-variable clinical JADAS (cJADAS) which omits inflammatory markers [18]. All studies enrolling children captured data on the presence or absence of uveitis. Most studies (83%) captured medication start and stop dates. Fourteen studies (78%) captured the occurrence of serious adverse events (e.g., requiring hospitalisation), but only 28% had the ability to capture these data additionally through external data sources (the majority based in the UK). Seven registries were working with industry to perform pharmacosurveillance studies and included monitoring of data and adjudication of adverse event reports.

Biosample collection was performed in most of the registries. Nine registries had relatively systematic collection, and 7 had more limited collection on a subset of patients. Serum, plasma, and whole blood/DNA were the most commonly collected samples. Synovial fluid was collected less frequently.

Discussion

This is the first report to bring together information about the numerous existing JIA registries and longitudinal cohort studies, highlighting a wealth of JIA outcome data being collected around the world. Many important questions surround the etiology, pathogenesis, optimal management, and long-term outcomes of JIA. No single registry can answer all questions. Registries must have a clearly defined purpose that determines the process of data collection and the specific data items collected.

Three primary patient enrolment strategies are being used: diagnosis inception cohorts, prevalence or convenience cohorts, and treatment initiation cohorts. Although all studies aim to assess disease outcomes over time, inception cohorts better identify predictors of short and long-term outcomes (e.g. social, clinical, psychological, laboratory and genetic) [19], whereas treatment initiation cohorts are superior to evaluate treatment effectiveness and safety. Of course, with sufficient patient enrolment and procedures to collect data at times when medications are newly started, treatment cohort studies can be performed within a subset of patients from any registry.

Whilst one study started collecting data as early as 1993, most initiated recruitment following the introduction of biologic therapies for JIA around 2000. This was likely a direct result of increased monitoring and safety concerns among investigators, sponsors, and patients with JIA. The relatively recent increase of JIA cohort studies coincided with a movement in the late 1990's to classify children with chronic arthritis into homogenous groups to facilitate research using the ILAR classification [1], and this is reflected by all paediatric studies classifying children according to this system. Most studies continue to actively recruit and follow previously recruited patients.

Unfortunately, many studies cease to follow patients after they transition into adult care. The transition of care period presents many challenges. Patients not only change clinicians and often their place of residence, but also may change medical systems and third-party payers. The most relevant outcome measures may also change, such as a change from active and limited joint counts in paediatric clinics to counts of tender and swollen joints in adult clinics, or change from JADAS to RA disease activity measures (e.g., DAS28).

With the majority of JIA studies initiating in the 2000's only preliminary results on adult-aged patients are currently available. Two studies specifically assess effectiveness and safety of biologics in adult patients with JIA. The German JuMBO study has published outcome data of 346 children (median age 21 years) who had received the biologic etanercept in childhood [8]. The UK BSRBR study has published data on outcomes of 225 adults with JIA who started a biological therapy in childhood [7]. In previous studies, outcomes of adults with JIA have been assessed cross-sectionally [20–22], retrospectively [23], or by identifying adult patients diagnosed as children from medical records [24–27]. These studies reported approximately 40 to 60% of children with JIA continue to have some level of active disease in adulthood [22, 24, 25, 27–29]. Given the relative rarity of JIA and that not all children continue to have active disease in adulthood, it will be important for registries to share their experiences to develop robust methods to track children through adulthood. Because few patients enrolled in the current studies have reached adulthood, this may be an opportunity now to align the data to be collected in the future across studies.

The studies included in our survey do not reflect the entirety of long-term outcomes studies in JIA. Several recent studies have used administrative data to investigate the risk of rare outcomes in JIA, such as malignancy or serious infection [30–32]. Administrative data sources provide readily available data and often very large sample sizes, but provide scant clinical data compared to clinical cohorts. Accordingly, administrative data are typically most useful for studies of adverse effects of medications, but are less useful for studies of medication effectiveness or long-term outcomes in JIA.

Although there were many differences among the studies, there was significant overlap in the data being collected. This may allow for the determination of a minimal data set that all existing and future prospective observational studies could collect, enabling nearly identical analysis plans to be conducted across all data sources.

Our survey was able to summarize the extent of data items captured, but did not collect estimates of the amount of missing data for each variable. Missing data are a common problem in observational research due to clinic non-attendance by patients, variable clinical need for investigation (e.g. inflammatory marker and other blood testing), and failure to report adverse events in busy outpatient clinics, among others. This can result in biases that require careful consideration of how to handle missing data and missing patients. This issue is compounded further in JIA due to the heterogeneity of disease, with many children who are well being discharged from secondary care and therefore no longer contributing to longer term outcome studies. Also, our survey did not enquire in detail about the timing of data capture, particularly in relation to disease onset or start of therapies.

In order to understand the risk of rare outcomes, large sample sizes and long term follow up are needed. Combining data from multiple studies increases statistical power, but must be done carefully. It is reassuring that there is significant commonality on the data items captured across studies, which may permit the creation of a common data model to pool data. However, differing methods of outcome ascertainment (e.g., assessing adverse events by patient report, physician report, or through an external data source) may produce important differences in results. It will also be important to ensure that no patients are double-counted if they have been simultaneously enrolled in more than one registry effort; this is likely currently best addressed at the individual clinical site level, but assignment of a universal identification number allowing patients to contribute to various different registries over time (e.g., in response to changes in age or geographic location) would have potential additional benefits.

This survey did not account for the differences in health care systems, clinical expertise in JIA, or funding for arthritis medications around the world. Because patients are enrolled from pediatric rheumatology centers, differences in health care systems may influence enrolment into JIA registries through physician referral bias. Differential access to biologics likely results in substantial differences in disease duration and severity at the time of starting treatment. Given the differences in patient enrolment and data collection techniques, as well as geographical differences in treatment approaches, genetic background of the patients, and varying incidences of comorbid conditions and endemic pathogens (such as tuberculosis), simple pooling of data may not be the most appropriate approach to evaluate drug safety or effectiveness. In addition, there may be restrictions on the sharing of data, depending on the ethical approval and patient consent obtained in each study. Overcoming these hurdles to facilitate collaborative research in JIA will be challenging and will require an international effort involving multiple stakeholders. Within the JIA research community, initial steps have been taken to begin to address these obstacles [33].

Sophisticated methods for combining data should be explored, such as nested case-control studies or meta-analyses of individual register data analysis. These approaches were adopted by the EULAR Registers and Observational Drug Studies (RODS) Working Group to explore the risk of malignant melanoma associated with TNFi therapies in patients with RA across Europe [34]. Methodological approaches that consider the individual data source will likely provide more accurate results and new insights about confounders and effect modifiers of outcome. Despite the significant resources required, these analyses would be a unique opportunity to answer critical questions about JIA and should be undertaken.

Conclusions

This study identified a wide range of ongoing JIA cohort studies and registries around the world. Many of the challenges in the long-term study of childhood-onset diseases were highlighted. Nevertheless, the results indicate significant potential for future collaborative work using both combined and comparative analyses of data from different studies. New approaches to maximise data capture beyond childhood will be crucial to answer important questions about long-term outcomes.

Abbreviations

ABC: Arthritis and biologicals in children; ACR: American college of rheumatology; AJC: Active joint count; BCRD: Biologics for children with rheumatic diseases; BiKeR: Biologics in pediatric rheumatology; BSPAR-ETN: British society for pediatric and adolescent rheumatolgy-etanercept; BSRBRc: British society for rheumatology biologics register; CAPS: Childhood arthritis prospective study; CARRA: Childhood arthritis and rheumatology research alliance; CHAQ: Childhood health assessment questionnaire; CRP: C-reactive protein; ESR: Erythrocyte sedimentation rate; HAQ: Health assessment questionnaire; ICON: Inception cohort of newly diagnosed children with jia; ILAR: International league of associations for rheumatology; JACS: Juvenile arthritis cohort study; JADAS: Juvenile arthritis disease activity score; JAMAR: Juvenile arthritis multidimensional assessment report; JIA: Juvenile idiopathic arthritis; JuMBO: Juvenile arthritis methotrexate biologics long-term observation; LJC: Limited joint count; MD: Physician; N: No; NPRD: National pediatric rheumatology database; Pharmachild: Pharmacovigilance in juvenile idiopathic arthritis patients; PRINTO: Pediatric rheumatology international trials organization; RA: Rheumatoid arthritis; ReACCh Out: Research in arthritis in canadian children emphasizing outcomes; RODS: Registers and observational drug studies; UK: United Kingdom; USA: United States of America; Y: Yes

Acknowledgements

The authors thank all children with JIA and their families who have contributed to these studies.
ICON: coordinator Angela Zink; consortium partners Dirk Foell and Arnd Heiligenhaus; funded by a research grant of the Federal Ministry of Education and Research (FKZ 01ER0812); made possible by the support and participation of more than 300 German paediatric and adult rheumatologists whom we thank.
NPRD: funded by the German child arthritis foundation; made possible by the support and participation of more than 300 German paediatric and adult rheumatologists whom we thank.
JuMBO: Co-PI Angela Zink; funded by an unconditional grant from Pfizer and Abbvie; made possible by the support and participation of more than 300 German paediatric and adult rheumatologists whom we thank.
CAPS: funded by Arthritis Research UK (Grant # 20542)
BCRD: funded by Arthritis Research UK (Grant # 20747)
BSRBR: funded by British Society for Paediatric and Adolescent Rheumatology and the British Society for Rheumatology
BSPAR-ETN: funded by British Society for Paediatric and Adolescent Rheumatology and the British Society for Rheumatology
CARRA Legacy Registry: funded by United States National Institutes of Health/National Institute of Arthritis and Musculoskeletal and Skin Diseases (1RC2AR058934), Friends of CARRA, Arthritis Foundation
CARRA Registry: funded by Arthritis Foundation, Novartis, Roche; Executive Committee members Laura Schanberg, Yukiko Kimura, Timothy Beukelman, Jason Jones, and Helen Bristow
JACS: Justine Ellis was supported by an Australian Research Council Future Fellowship, FT120100253
Pharmachild: funded by European Union Framework Programme 7 grant (260353); Chiara Pallotti (PRINTO coordination center)
BiKeR: made possible by the collaboration of numerous German and Austrian pediatric rheumatologists, patients and their parents and by non-restricted grants from Abbvie, Chugai, Novartis, Pfizer, and Roche.
Swedish JIA Register: Board of the Registry
Reuma.pt: made possible by the collaboration of pediatric and adult rheumatologists, rheumatology nurses, patients, and by unrestricted grants from AbbVie, Celegene, Hospira, MSD, Pfizer, Roche, and UCB.
Nordic JIA Study: conducted by the Nordic Study Group of Pediatric Rheumatology (NoSPeR)

Funding

This work was supported in part by the Arthritis Research UK Centre for Epidemiology (Grant #20380). The funding body had no role in the design of the study or the collection, analysis, or interpretation of the data, or the writing of the manuscript.

Authors' contributions

The study was conceived by TB, LES, and KH. All authors contributed to the acquisition and interpretation of data. The manuscript was drafted by TB, LKF, and KH. All authors revised the manuscript critically and gave approval of the final version.

Competing interests

The authors declare that they have no competing interests.

Consent for publication

Not applicable

Author details

[1]University of Alabama at Birmingham, Birmingham, USA. [2]Erasmus Medical Center, Rotterdam, The Netherlands. [3]Uppsala University Hospital, Uppsala, Sweden. [4]Children's Hospital of Eastern Ontario, Ottawa, Canada. [5]Murdoch Children's Research Institute, Genes, Environment & Complex Disease, Parkville, Australia. [6]Aarhus University Hospital, Aarhus, Denmark. [7]University of British Columbia, Vancouver, Canada. [8]Asklepios Klinik Sankt Augsutin, Sankt Augustin, Germany. [9]University of Manchester, Manchester, UK. [10]German Rheumatism Research Center, Berlin, Germany. [11]Karolinska University Hospital, Stockholm, Sweden. [12]Royal Children's Hospital, Melbourne, Australia. [13]University Hospital of North Norway, Tromso, Norway. [14]Istituto Giannina Gaslini, Genoa, Italy. [15]Hospital Garcia de Orta, Almada, Portugal. [16]Duke University, Durham, USA. [17]University Medical Center Utrecht, Utrecht, The Netherlands. [18]University of Manchester and Central Manchester Foundation Trust, Manchester, UK. [19]Division of Pediatric Rheumatology, The University of Alabama at Birmingham, 1600 7th Avenue South, CPP 210, Birmingham, AL 35233-1711, USA.

References

1. Petty RE, Southwood TR, Manners P, Baum J, Glass DN, Goldenberg J, et al. International league of associations for rheumatology classification of juvenile idiopathic arthritis: second revision, Edmonton, 2001. J Rheumatol. 2004;31:390–2.
2. Thierry S, Fautrel B, Lemelle I, Guillemin F. Prevalence and incidence of juvenile idiopathic arthritis: a systematic review. Joint Bone Spine. 2014;81:112–7.

3. Guzman J, Gomez-Ramirez O, Jurencak R, Shiff NJ, Berard RA, Duffy CM, et al. What matters most for patients, parents, and clinicians in the course of juvenile idiopathic arthritis? a qualitative study. J Rheumatol. 2014;41: 2260–9.
4. van Pelt P, Wulffraat NM. Transition of care in rheumatology: managing the rheumatic patient from childhood to adulthood. In: Harrison A, editor. Insights and perspectives in rheumatology: InTech. 2012. p. 255–74.
5. Ellis JA, Ponsonby AL, Pezic A, Chavez RA, Allen RC, Akikusa JD, et al. CLARITY - ChiLdhood arthritis risk factor identification sTudY. Pediatr Rheumatol Online J. 2012;10:37.
6. Consolaro A, Ruperto N, Filocamo G, Lanni S, Bracciolini G, Garrone M, et al. Seeking insights into the EPidemiology, treatment and outcome of childhood arthritis through a multinational collaborative effort: introduction of the EPOCA study. Pediatr Rheumatol Online J. 2012;10:39.
7. McErlane F, Foster HE, Davies R, Lunt M, Watson KD, Symmons DP, et al. Biologic treatment response among adults with juvenile idiopathic arthritis: results from the British society for rheumatology biologics register. Rheumatology (Oxford). 2013;52:1905–13.
8. Minden K, Niewerth M, Zink A, Seipelt E, Foeldvari I, Girschick H, et al. Long-term outcome of patients with JIA treated with etanercept, results of the biologic register JuMBO. Rheumatology (Oxford). 2012;51:1407–15.
9. Canhao H, Faustino A, Martins F, Fonseca JE. Rheumatic diseases Portuguese register board coordination PSoR. Reuma.pt - the rheumatic diseases Portuguese register. Acta Reumatol Port. 2011;36:45–56.
10. Horneff G, De Bock F, Foeldvari I, Girschick HJ, Michels H, Moebius D, et al. Safety and efficacy of combination of etanercept and methotrexate compared to treatment with etanercept only in patients with juvenile idiopathic arthritis (JIA): preliminary data from the German JIA registry. Ann Rheum Dis. 2009;68:519–25.
11. Schmeling H, Minden K, Foeldvari I, Ganser G, Hospach T, Horneff G. Efficacy and safety of adalimumab as the first and second biologic agent in juvenile idiopathic arthritis: the German biologics JIA registry. Arthritis Rheumatol. 2014;66:2580–9.
12. Davies R, Southwood TR, Kearsley-Fleet L, Lunt M, Hyrich KL, British Society for P, et al. Medically significant infections Are increased in patients with juvenile idiopathic arthritis treated with etanercept: results from the British society for paediatric and adolescent rheumatology etanercept cohort study. Arthritis Rheumatol. 2015;67:2487–94.
13. Kearsley-Fleet L, Davies R, Baildam E, Beresford MW, Foster HE, Southwood TR, et al. Factors associated with choice of biologic among children with juvenile idiopathic arthritis: results from two UK paediatric biologic registers. Rheumatology (Oxford). 2016;55:1556–65.
14. Beukelman T, Kimura Y, Ilowite NI, Mieszkalski K, Natter MD, Burrell G, et al. The new Childhood Arthritis and Rheumatology Research Alliance (CARRA) Registry: design, rationale, and characteristics of patients enrolled in the first 12 months. (in press).
15. Filocamo G, Consolaro A, Schiappapietra B, Dalpra S, Lattanzi B, Magni-Manzoni S, et al. A new approach to clinical care of juvenile idiopathic arthritis: the juvenile arthritis multidimensional assessment report. J Rheumatol. 2011;38:938–53.
16. Giannini EH, Ruperto N, Ravelli A, Lovell DJ, Felson DT, Martini A. Preliminary definition of improvement in juvenile arthritis. Arthritis Rheum. 1997;40:1202–9.
17. Consolaro A, Ruperto N, Bazso A, Pistorio A, Magni-Manzoni S, Filocamo G, et al. Development and validation of a composite disease activity score for juvenile idiopathic arthritis. Arthritis Rheum. 2009;61:658–66.
18. McErlane F, Beresford MW, Baildam EM, Chieng SE, Davidson JE, Foster HE, et al. Validity of a three-variable juvenile arthritis disease activity score in children with new-onset juvenile idiopathic arthritis. Ann Rheum Dis. 2013;72:1983–8.
19. Adib N, Hyrich K, Thornton J, Lunt M, Davidson J, Gardner-Medwin J, et al. Association between duration of symptoms and severity of disease at first presentation to paediatric rheumatology: results from the childhood arthritis prospective study. Rheumatology (Oxford). 2008;47:991–5.
20. Packham JC, Hall MA. Long-term follow-up of 246 adults with juvenile idiopathic arthritis: functional outcome. Rheumatology (Oxford). 2002;41:1428–35.
21. Bruinooge LN, El Moussaoui R, Taal E, Dijkmans BA, Van Soesbergen RM. Outcome in adults with juvenile idiopathic arthritis. Comparison of the DUTCH-AIMS2 between JIA and RA. Scand J Rheumatol. 2003;32:89–94.
22. Foster HE, Marshall N, Myers A, Dunkley P, Griffiths ID. Outcome in adults with juvenile idiopathic arthritis: a quality of life study. Arthritis Rheum. 2003;48:767–75.
23. Peterson LS, Mason T, Nelson AM, O'Fallon WM, Gabriel SE. Psychosocial outcomes and health status of adults who have had juvenile rheumatoid arthritis: a controlled, population-based study. Arthritis Rheum. 1997;40:2235–40.
24. Nordal E, Zak M, Aalto K, Berntson L, Fasth A, Herlin T, et al. Ongoing disease activity and changing categories in a long-term nordic cohort study of juvenile idiopathic arthritis. Arthritis Rheum. 2011;63:2809–18.
25. Zak M, Pedersen FK. Juvenile chronic arthritis into adulthood: a long-term follow-up study. Rheumatology (Oxford). 2000;39:198–204.
26. French AR, Mason T, Nelson AM, O'Fallon WM, Gabriel SE. Increased mortality in adults with a history of juvenile rheumatoid arthritis: a population-based study. Arthritis Rheum. 2001;44:523–7.
27. Arkela-Kautiainen M, Haapasaari J, Kautiainen H, Leppanen L, Vilkkumaa I, Malkia E, et al. Functioning and preferences for improvement of health among patients with juvenile idiopathic arthritis in early adulthood using the WHO ICF model. J Rheumatol. 2006;33:1369–76.
28. Fantini F, Gerloni V, Gattinara M, Cimaz R, Arnoldi C, Lupi E. Remission in juvenile chronic arthritis: a cohort study of 683 consecutive cases with a mean 10 year followup. J Rheumatol. 2003;30:579–84.
29. Selvaag AM, Aulie HA, Lilleby V, Flato B. Disease progression into adulthood and predictors of long-term active disease in juvenile idiopathic arthritis. Ann Rheum Dis. 2016;75:190–5.
30. Beukelman T, Xie F, Chen L, Baddley JW, Delzell E, Grijalva CG, et al. Rates of hospitalized bacterial infection associated with juvenile idiopathic arthritis and its treatment. Arthritis Rheum. 2012;64:2773–80.
31. Beukelman T, Haynes K, Curtis JR, Xie F, Chen L, Bemrich-Stolz CJ, et al. Rates of malignancy associated with juvenile idiopathic arthritis and its treatment. Arthritis Rheum. 2012;64:1263–71.
32. Nordstrom BL, Mines D, Gu Y, Mercaldi C, Aquino P, Harrison MJ. Risk of malignancy in children with juvenile idiopathic arthritis not treated with biologic agents. Arthritis Care Res (Hoboken). 2012;64:1357–64.
33. Robinson E, Albani S, Beresford MW, de Jager W, de Roock S, Duong T, et al. Towards stratified medicine in juvenile idiopathic arthritis [abstract]. 2016 Pediatric Rheumatology European Society (PReS) Congress.
34. Mercer LK, Askling J, Raaschou P, Dixon WG, Dreyer L, Hetland ML, et al. Risk of invasive melanoma in patients with rheumatoid arthritis treated with biologics: results from a collaborative project of 11 European biologic registers. Ann Rheum Dis. 2017;76(2):386–91.
35. Sengler C, Klotsche J, Niewerth M, Liedmann I, Foll D, Heiligenhaus A, et al. The majority of newly diagnosed patients with juvenile idiopathic arthritis reach an inactive disease state within the first year of specialised care: data from a German inception cohort. RMD open. 2015;1:e000074.
36. Oen K, Tucker L, Huber AM, Miettunen P, Scuccimarri R, Campillo S, et al. Predictors of early inactive disease in a juvenile idiopathic arthritis cohort: results of a Canadian multicenter, prospective inception cohort study. Arthritis Rheum. 2009;61:1077–86.
37. Beukelman T, Ringold S, Davis TE, DeWitt EM, Pelajo CF, Weiss PF, et al. Disease-modifying antirheumatic drug use in the treatment of juvenile idiopathic arthritis: a cross-sectional analysis of the CARRA Registry. J Rheumatol. 2012;39:1867–74.
38. Minden K, Niewerth M, Listing J, Zink A. German study group of pediatric R. Health care provision in pediatric rheumatology in Germany–national rheumatologic database. J Rheumatol. 2002;29:622–8.
39. Prince FH, Twilt M, ten Cate R, van Rossum MA, Armbrust W, Hoppenreijs EP, et al. Long-term follow-up on effectiveness and safety of etanercept in juvenile idiopathic arthritis: the Dutch national register. Ann Rheum Dis. 2009;68:635–41.

12

When a patient suspected with juvenile idiopathic arthritis turns out to be diagnosed with an infectious disease

Krzysztof Orczyk, Joanna Świdrowska-Jaros and Elżbieta Smolewska*

Abstract

The Lyme arthritis is a common manifestation of infection with *Borrelia burgdorferi* spirochete. Despite its infectious background, the inflammation clinically and histopatologically resembles juvenile idiopathic arthritis. As it affects a considerable number of Lyme disease patients, it should be routinely considered in differential diagnosis. Development of arthritis is partially dependent on spirochetal factors, including the ribosomal spacer type and the sequence of outer surface protein C. Immunological background involves Th1-related response, but IL-17 provides an additional route of developing arthritis. Autoimmune mechanisms may lead to antibiotic-refractory arthritis. The current diagnostic standard is based on a 2-step testing: ELISA screening and immunoblot confirmation. Other suggested methods contain modified two-tier test with C6 ELISA instead of immunoblot. An initial 28-day course of oral antibiotics (doxycycline, cefuroxime axetil or amoxicillin) is a recommended treatment. Severe cases require further anti-inflammatory management. Precise investigation of new diagnostic and therapeutic approaches is advisable.

Keywords: Lyme arthritis, Lyme disease, Pathogenesis, Symptoms, Treatment

Background

Lyme arthritis (LA) is a feature of late stage infection with the tick-borne spirochete, *Borrelia burgdorferi (B. burgdorferi)*. It usually occurs weeks to months after the initial tick bite and may be preceded by erythema migrans (EM) [1]. This erythematous patch with a characteristic central clearing forming a typical "bull's eye lesion" is considered to be a pathognomonic manifestation of Lyme disease (LD) [2]. However, there is a growing body of evidence that the earlier stage of the infection frequently tends to remain asymptomatic and arthritis is becoming the presenting manifestation of the disease [3].

Steere et al. were the first to describe LD in Lyme, Connecticut, the United States, in patients initially suspected of juvenile idiopathic arthritis (JIA) [4]. Thorough diagnostic process in the aforementioned group revealed that reported episodes of arthritis were provoked by a novel infectious trigger [5]. To date, there are 20 identified genospecies of *B. burgdorferi sensu lato* [6]. Nine of them infect humans: *B. burgdorferi sensu stricto, B. garinii, B. afzelii, B. bavariensis, B. bissetii, B. kurtenbachii, B. lusitaniae, B. spielmanii, B. valaesiana* [7]. The highest arthrogenic potential is presented by *B. burgdorferi sensu stricto* [8]. It induced arthritis in 46% of infected patients in the United States observed by Cerar et al. [9]. Its immunogenicity plays a crucial role in differences in clinical course of spirochetal infection between the United States, where *B. burgdorferi sensu stricto* is the main etiological factor of LD [10], and Europe, which is dominated by two other genospecies: *B. garinii* and *B. afzelii* [11]. As reported by Cerar et al. who assessed clinical images of LD in Slovenia, patients infected with *B. garinii* and *B. afzelii* developed arthritis in 18 and 15%, respectively [9]. According to Kocbach et al., *B. garinii* infection frequently produces neurological symptoms and patients infected with *B. afzelii* regularly present with fatigue and myalgia [8].

* Correspondence: e.smolewska@wp.pl
Department of Pediatric Rheumatology, Medical University of Lodz, Sporna 36/50, 91-738 Lodz, Poland

Epidemiology

LD usually affects people in northern hemisphere [12]. The highest incidence in Europe was reported in southern Sweden (464/100,000) [13]. Sykes et al. calculated average incidence rate in Western Europe as 22,05/100,000, what results in approximately 230,000 of cases in Western Europe per year [14]. In the United States, The Centers for Disease Control and Prevention (CDC) reported nearly 30,000 of cases of LD in 2008 [15], whereas a survey regarding LD testing performed by large commercial laboratories gave a result of estimated 300,000 of cases per year [16].

There is a tendency towards an upswing in incidence of LD in the last few years [17]. Incidence rate reported in Poland in 2014 was 36/100,000 and it was 52,9% higher than median from years 2008–2012 [18]. It is caused not only by better awareness of the disease and changes in human recreational behavior, but also by dispersion of reservoir hosts [19]. Colonization of urban areas in Poland by blackbirds [6] may provide a potential explanation, as one of the genospecies which dominate in Europe, *B. garinii*, most commonly affects birds [20].

There are two peaks of age in incidence of spirochetal infection. Most cases of LD are reported in age groups which spend more time outdoors near the natural reservoirs of ticks, specifically children between 5 and 9 years of age and adults >50 years [21]. Period between tick bite and its removal is considered to be a pivotal risk factor for infection [22], which is more likely to occur if a tick remains attached to the skin for more than first 24 h after bite [23]. Owning dogs has been also considered as a potential risk factor for LD, but Aenishaenslin et al. did not find significantly higher risk of tick bites in dog owners [24].

LA affects 3–15% of LD patients in Europe [25]. As for the United States, CDC reported LA in 33% of LD patients diagnosed in 2001 and 2002 [26]. LD caused 51% of pediatric knee arthritis (341 out of 673 patients) observed by Deanehan et al. [27] and 5,2% of pediatric hip arthritis (20 out of 385 patients) reported by Bachur et al. [28]. Therefore it is frequent enough to be included in differential diagnosis, which should consider other inflammatory arthritides, such as reactive arthritis and JIA (including psoriatic arthritis). Autoinflammatory arthritis may also develop within months after LD, presumably triggered by the spirochetal infection [3].

Clinical features

EM (Fig. 1), a characteristic sign mentioned above as a common initial manifestation of *B. burgdorferi* infection, is frequently accompanied, or sometimes preceded, by systemic symptoms, in particular fatigue, fever, headache, stiff neck, myalgias, arthralgias, nausea and dysesthesia [29]. However, according to Glaude et al.,

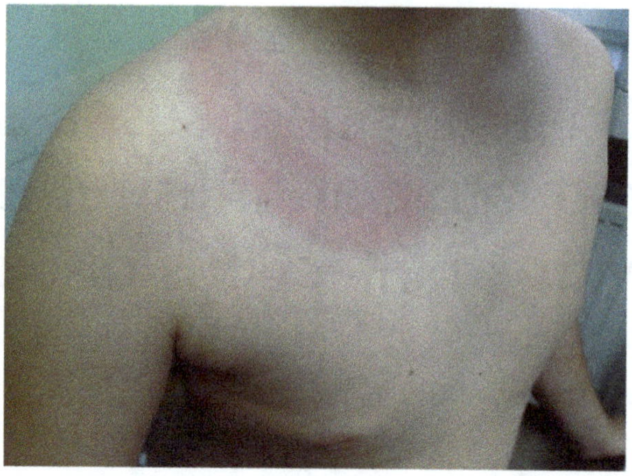

Fig. 1 Erythema migrans in a 9-year-old boy after tick bite

the majority (72%) of patients observed in Canada had arthritis as their first symptom of LD. 76% of patients did not recall a tick bite, and only 18% of patients had previous EM [30].

In patients who developed EM, arthralgias appeared 1 day to 8 weeks after onset of rash in a study of 55 patients performed by Steere et al. [31]. When EM is absent, symptoms of LA may occur months or even years after initial tick bite [32]. Therefore, it can be manifested in every month of the year, not only within time of increased outdoor activity [33]. In accordance with aforementioned diversity of genospecies, LA observed in Europe (caused mainly by *B. garinii* and *B. afzelii)* tends to occur in shorter period after initial tick bite comparing to *B. burgdorferi sensu stricto* infections [9].

On clinical presentation, LA usually affects large synovial joints asymmetrically [34]. Recurrent swelling of the affected joint with a presence of moderate inflammatory effusion is a common clinical finding in children suspected of LA [35]. Although more acute presentation may mimic septic arthritis, pain of the affected joints reported in patients with LA is usually less severe [27]. All patients reported by Huppertz et al. experienced joint swelling or limitation of range of motion, but no pain [36]. Additionally, 38% of patients assessed by Thompson et al. were incapable of bearing weight on the affected limb [37].

The knee is affected (Fig. 2) in over 90% of cases [38]. The ankle is found to be the second most commonly involved joint [38]. Correspondingly, the clinical image can resemble a mono- or oligoarticular JIA. Still, polyarticular involvement should not automatically exclude LA. Sá et al. reported a case of a 6-year-old girl with serological confirmation of spirochetal infection who developed swelling of the proximal inter-phalangeal joints of hands and wrist and both tibiotarsal joints within several months after initial tick bite and was finally diagnosed with polyarticular JIA [39].

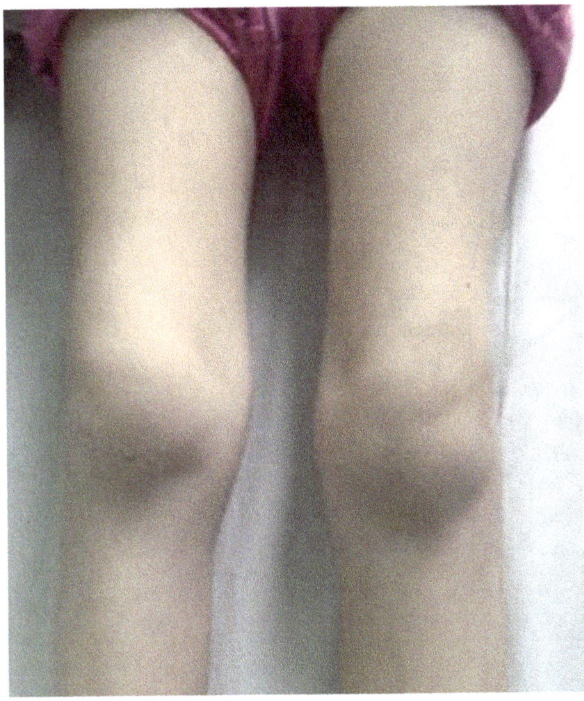

Fig. 2 Bilateral knee arthritis in a serological-positive (*Borrelia burgdorferi*) 6-year-old girl

LA that does not recover during first 3 months after initiation of recommended treatment regimens (described below) has been referred to as antibiotic-refractory LA [36, 40]. In a study published by Tory et al. 23% of pediatric patients had persistent synovitis after 8 weeks of oral antibiotic therapy or 4 weeks of intravenous therapy or both [41]. LA eventually resolves spontaneously, but this may take even 8 years in extreme cases [42].

Spirochetal factors of inflammation

The *B. burgdorferi* genome has a unique structure. More than 40% of genetic material is located in linear and circular plasmids therefore spirochetes are able to rapidly adapt to new environmental conditions [43]. *B. burgdorferi* genotypes are classified on the basis of the 16S-23S ribosomal spacer type (RST) and the sequence of outer surface protein C (OspC) [9]. RST1 strains are more likely to cause disseminated *B. burgdorferi* infection, whereas RST2 and RST3 strains are less frequently detected peripherally. Moreover, RST1 isolates induce significantly greater interferon (IFN)-γ production by peripheral blood mononuclear cells comparing to RST3 strains [44]. Infection of C3H/HeJ mice with RST1 strains resulted in more severe arthritis and carditis than did infection with RST3 isolates in a study performed by Wang et al. [45].

Spirochetal antigen OspC is a factor crucial for the invasion of a host [46]. OspC facilitates bacterial transmission with tick saliva during a bite by forming a complex with a tick salivary protein, Salp15 [47]. OspC is highly immunogenic and is one of the primary inductors of host immune response [48]. Moreover, it interacts with plasminogen which is likely to enable spirochetal dissemination to peripheral tissues [46].

Through its surface molecules, *B. burgdorferi* is able to bind host proteins and, in that way, hide from the host immune system. As reviewed by Nardelli et al., it can bind to fibronectin, type I collagen, glycosaminoglycans, proteoglycans and integrins [49].

B. burgdorferi has also been shown to rapidly inhibit human complement by binding host complement regulators (such as FH, FHR-1, C4Bp, C1r, C7, C8, C9, TCC) through a family of surface-exposed molecules (CspA, CspZ, ErpP, ErpC, ErpA, p43, BBK32, BGA66, BGA71 and CD59-like protein) [50].

Additionally, *B. burgdorferi* produces protease with aggrecanase activity, which is postulated by Russell et al. to be involved in direct mechanism of tissue damage in LA [51].

There is also evidence of roles for several constituents of tick saliva. Prostaglandin E2 inhibits the production of the T helper (Th)1-associated cytokines interleukin (IL)-12 and tumor necrosis factor (TNF)-α by dendritic cells in an infection site [52]. B-cell inhibitory protein and sialostatin L are also involved in local suppression of immune response [53, 54].

Immunological background

Presence of spirochetes at synovial sites triggers development of joint inflammation (Fig. 3) characterized by effusion dominated with neutrophils. As they bind spirochetal lipoprotein to Toll-like receptor 2 [55], neutrophils produce proinflammatory cytokines: IL-1, TNF-α, IL-8 and IL-15 [49]. They can also eliminate spirochetes through phagocytosis [56].

Additionally, spirochetal stimulation of macrophages results in release of proinflammatory mediators typical for M1 macrophages, namely: TNF-α, IL-1β, IL-12, IL-18 and nitric oxide [57].

Subsequently, development of joint inflammation involves Th1 lymphocytes. Activated T lymphocytes from LD patients produce IFN-γ following *ex vivo* stimulation with *B. burgdorferi* constituents [58]. In addition, IFN-γ and IFN-responsive genes are expressed in the joints of *B. burgdorferi*-infected mice [59, 60]. Surprisingly, the levels of IFN-γ did not correlate with the severity of other symptoms in a study performed by Callister et al. [61].

Zeidner et al. found that treating mice with the Th1-associated cytokines TNF-α and IFN-γ during tick feeding provided a 95 and 55% protection rate against transmission, respectively [62].

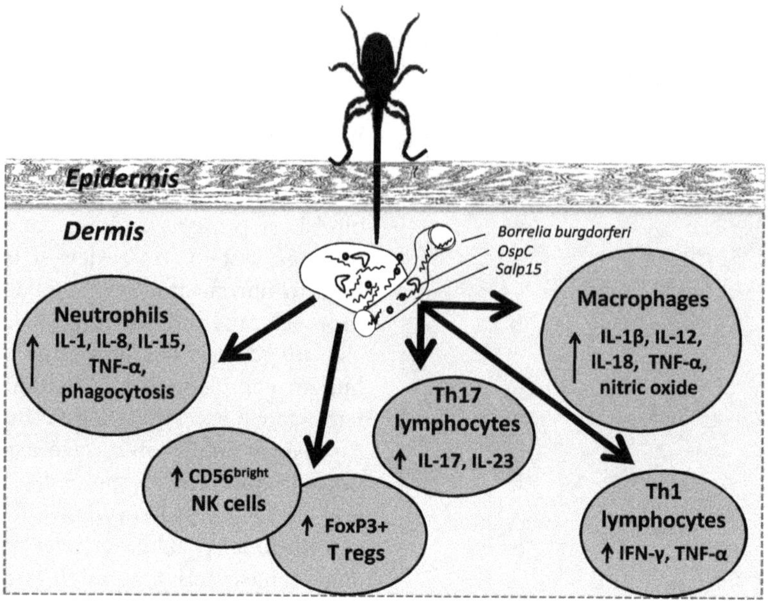

Fig. 3 Set of changes in cytokine profile and concentrations of cells in the pathogenesis of LA; abbreviations explained in the text

Th1-related inflammation is not the only possible immunological route of developing LA. *B. burgdorferi* has been shown to be a strong inducer of IL-10 which inhibits Th1 activity and may contribute to the immune tolerance of the microbe [63].

Several studies reviewed by Kuo et al. showed that arthritis observed in IFN-γ-deficient mice was dependent on IL-17 [64]. Infante-Duarte et al. reported compatible results in humans [65]. However, Bachmann et al. did not observe production of IL-17 by *B. burgdorferi*-stimulated human peripheral blood mononuclear cells [66].

Production of IL-17, as well as another Th17-supporting cytokine, IL-23, is induced by borrelial neutrophil activating protein A (NapA) [67]. There is mounting evidence that levels of these cytokines tend to be elevated in patients with severe, persisting symptoms, namely in antibiotic-refractory LA [67, 68].

Patients with LA have also high frequencies of CD56bright natural killer (NK) cells in synovial fluid [69]. It has been suggested that CD56bright NK cells may either exacerbate or regulate immune responses [70]. Presence of CD56bright NK cells producing IFN-γ in synovial fluid suggests that these cells contribute to elimination of spirochetes [52]. Barthold et al. reported less severe LA in mice genetically deficient in granulocytes and NK cells [71].

FoxP3+ regulatory T cells in synovial fluid also play a role in LA [72]. Low frequencies of FoxP3+ regulatory T cells in synovial fluid lead to slower arthritis resolution [73, 74].

The progression into antibiotic-refractory LA is presumably independent of persistent spirochetal infection. Underlying autoimmune background has been postulated by Steere et al. [75]. There are seven human leukocyte antigen-D-related (HLA-DR) alleles identified, including the DRB1*0101, 0401 and 1501 alleles, that are predominant in patients with antibiotic-refractory patients [76]. Moreover, Arvikar et al. listed 4 Lyme-associated autoantigens that are more frequent in the aforementioned group [77]. They include: endothelial cell growth factor (ECGF), apolipoprotein B-100 (apoB-100), matrix metalloproteinase-10 (MMP-10) and annexin-A2. Of these, only the response to annexin-A2 is not LA-specific, as it is elevated in both LA and RA [78].

Diagnostics

The current diagnostic standard of LA requires both clinical and laboratory criteria [79]. Laboratory testing relies predominantly on serology. Overall, a two-step approach is recommended: initial screening with an enzyme-linked immunosorbent assay (ELISA) followed by a supplemental Western immunoblot test (WB) in case the first step is positive [80]. In the United States, current criteria for a positive WB established by CDC require the presence of 2 (of 3) specified bands on the IgM WB or 5 (of 10) specified bands on the IgG WB [81]. There are also several other types of immunoblotting assays (including the EUROIMMUN Anti-Borrelia EUROLINE-WB which is frequently utilized in Europe) with variation in antigen composition and modified interpretation criteria which are provided by the producers [82].

Patients with signs and symptoms ≤30 days may be considered positive based on either IgM or IgG, whereas those with signs and symptoms >30 days, that is the majority of patients with LA, require IgG positivity [83]. Serology results may be falsely positive due to cross-reactivity, especially in patients with infectious mononucleosis [84] or in the presence of rheumatoid factor (RF) [7].

The diagnostic value of testing LA patients for IgM is questionable. A positive IgM WB may be falsely positive, particularly if a patient has manifested symptoms for more than 1 month [85]. Sensitivity of IgM testing in LA patients assessed by Leeflang et al. was insufficient (0.392) to be considered reliable, whereas IgG testing was sensitive enough (0.941) to be informative [86]. Specificity of IgM and IgG was comparable: 0.951 and 0.969, respectively.

Serology results are inadequate to monitor the treatment of LA [7]. It may be expected that some individuals with LA will be found to have positive IgM WB months to years later, due to the persistence of OspC-specific antibody response [87]. Polymerase chain reaction (PCR) on synovial fluid performed no sooner than 2 months after treatment is postulated to serve as a marker of eradication of spirochetes [87]. However, it is not yet properly standardized to use routinely in the diagnostic process [88].

There are several limitations of WB which affect the results of the standard two-tier test. As reviewed by Branda et al., it is insensitive in early phase of LD due to slow development of the humoral immune response [89]. Moreover, it is a complex procedure with a potential risk of false results influenced by subjective visual scoring. Therefore it frequently needs to be performed at reference laboratories and, for that reason, it consumes more time and expenses [90].

A newer, first-step ELISA, the C6 antibody test, uses a peptide from the constant region of a *B. burgdorferi* protein called Vmp-like sequence lipoprotein E (VlsE) [91]. Anti-VlsE antibodies develop early therefore C6 test provides comparable to higher sensitivity than a standard two-tier test [84, 92]. As it is less time-consuming than a standard two-tier test, it may be helpful in early decision whether to consider treatment [92]. Nevertheless, C6 seroprevalence in healthy blood donors tends to be high in endemic areas [93].

Branda et al. postulated an alternative diagnostic algorithm, in which WB is replaced by C6 ELISA as the second step in modified two-tier test (MTTT) [94]. As evaluated by Molins et al., it offered a simplified procedure as it was free of WB limitations. MTTT had enhanced sensitivity in diagnosing LD and was equivalent or significantly better than the standard algorithm [84]. Therefore this approach should be further investigated.

Treatment

According to current recommendations (B/III level) from the Infectious Diseases Society of America (IDSA), children with LA should be treated initially with a 28-day course of oral antibiotics: doxycycline 4 mg/kg per day in 2 divided doses (maximum of 100 mg per dose), cefuroxime axetil 30 mg/kg per day in 2 divided doses (maximum of 500 mg per dose) or amoxicillin 50 mg/kg per day in 3 divided doses (maximum of 500 mg per dose) [35]. Doxycycline is typically preferred because of its activity against *B. burgdorferi sensu lato*. However, doxycycline is not recommended for children <8 years of age due to its contribution to discoloration of teeth [95].

In patients who are still symptomatic after the recommended treatment, another 4-week course of oral antibiotics or a 2–4-week course of intravenous ceftriaxone should be administered [35]. Nevertheless, there is no benefit in further prolongation of antibiotic therapy. In a study performed by Berende et al. there was no significant difference of health-related quality of life between groups of patients who received 2 weeks of intravenous ceftriaxone and then continued treatment with a 12-week course of oral doxycycline, clarithromycin plus hydroxychloroquine or placebo [96].

As even antibiotic-refractory cases of LA were shown by Steere et al. to eventually improve [31], further treatment is questionable. In persistent cases, symptomatic therapies with non-steroidal anti-inflammatory drugs (NSAIDs), disease-modifying antirheumatic drugs (DMARDs), or intra-articular corticosteroids are recommended in the United States according to the IDSA [35]. Oral or intra-articular corticosteroids are contraindicated until antibiotic treatment is completed since these drugs permit greater growth of spirochetes [97], and because intra-articular steroid injections were reported to prolong duration of LA [3]. DMARDs are typically prescribed for only 6–12 months rather than indefinitely as in the treatment of patients with JIA. Arthroscopic synovectomy may be an option when pharmacotherapy is eventually ineffective [98].

Spirochetal infection provides plethora of potential therapeutic targets for new designer drugs [99]. These include, among others: ClpP protease which is upregulated by spirochetal persister cells [100] and HtrA protease which plays a role in pathogenicity of *B. burgdorferi* [101].

Conclusions

The clinical picture of LA resembles a classic autoimmune arthritis, similar to other rheumatoid disease, with immunomodulation and tissue damage. The active infection requiring antibiotic treatment is a factor that constitutes the essential difference. As a single-centre experience, the authors recommend ELISA screening in all patients suspected with JIA in regions endemic for

LD. As WB confirmation may be time-consuming, simultaneous two-tier testing is advisable when patient's history suggests a possibility of potential tick bite.

New diagnostic approaches should be elaborated on to evaluate their relevance. The assessment of the C6 antibody test in children is particularly essential for the future progress in diagnostic process and therapy.

Development of consistent worldwide guidelines would simplify diagnostic process in everyday pediatric practice.

Abbreviations

apoB-100: apolipoprotein B-100; *B. burgdorferi*: *Borrelia burgdorferi*; CDC: The centers for disease control and prevention; DMARDs: Disease modifying antirheumatic drugs; ECGF: Endothelial cell growth factor; ELISA: Enzyme-linked immunosorbent assay; EM: Erythema migrans; HLA-DR: Human leukocyte antigen-D-related; IDSA: Infectious diseases society of America; IFN-γ: Interferon gamma; IL: Interleukin; JIA: Juvenile idiopathic arthritis; LA: Lyme arthritis; LD: Lyme disease; MMP-10: metalloproteinase 10; MTTT: Modified two-tier test; NapA: Neutrophil activating protein A; NK: Natural killer; NSAIDs: Non-steroidal anti-inflammatory drugs; OspC: Outer surface protein C; PCR: Polymerase chain reaction; RF: Rheumatoid factor; RST: Ribosomal spacer type; Th: T helper; TNF-α: Tumor necrosis factor alpha; VlsE: Vmp-like sequence lipoprotein E; WB: Western immunoblot test

Acknowledgements
Not applicable

Funding
This work was partially the grant from Medical University of Lodz, Poland No. 502-03/8-000/01/502-64-094.

Authors' contributions

KO and JSJ collected literature and prepared manuscript with equal contribution. ES supervised the content of the manuscript and provided images. All authors read and approved the final manuscript.

Competing interests

The authors declare that they have no competing interests.

References

1. Steere AC, Broderick TF, Malawista SE. Erythema chronicum migrans and Lyme arthritis: epidemiologic evidence for a tick vector. Am J Epidemiol. 1978;108:312–21.
2. Torbahn G, Hofmann H, Allert R, et al. Efficacy and safety of pharmacological agents in the treatment of erythema migrans in early Lyme borreliosis-systematic review protocol. Syst Rev. 2016;5:73.
3. Arvikar SL, Steere AC. Diagnosis and treatment of Lyme arthritis. Infect Dis Clin North Am. 2015;29:269–80.
4. Steere AC, Malawista SE, Snydman DR, et al. Lyme arthritis: an epidemic of oligoarticular arthritis in children and adults in three connecticut communities. Arthritis Rheum. 1977;20:7–17.
5. Steere AC, Bartenhagen NH, Craft JE, et al. The early clinical manifestations of Lyme disease. Ann Intern Med. 1983;99:76–82.
6. Gryczynska A, Welc-Faleciak R. Long-term study of the prevalence of Borrelia burgdorferi s.l. infection in ticks (Ixodes ricinus) feeding on blackbirds (Turdus merula) in NE Poland. Exp Appl Acarol. 2016;70:381–94.
7. Kmieciak W, Ciszewski M, Szewczyk EM. Tick-borne diseases in Poland: Prevalence and difficulties in diagnostics [in Polish]. Med Pr. 2016;67:73–87.
8. Kocbach PP, Kocbach BP. Prevalence of Lyme disease among forestry workers [in Polish]. Med Pr. 2014;65:335–41.
9. Cerar T, Strle F, Stupica D, et al. Differences in genotype, clinical features, and inflammatory potential of borrelia burgdorferi sensu stricto strains from Europe and the United States. Emerging Infect Dis. 2016;22:818–27.
10. van Dam AP, Kuiper H, Vos K, et al. Different genospecies of Borrelia burgdorferi are associated with distinct clinical manifestations of Lyme borreliosis. Clin Infect Dis. 1993;17:708–17.
11. Stanek G, Reiter M. The expanding Lyme Borrelia complex–clinical significance of genomic species? Clin Microbiol Infect. 2011;17:487–93.
12. Jaenson TG, Jaenson DG, Eisen L, Petersson E, Lindgren E. Changes in the geographical distribution and abundance of the tick Ixodes ricinus during the past 30 years in Sweden. Parasit Vectors. 2012;5:8.
13. Lindgren E, Jaenson TGT. Lyme borreliosis in Europe: influences of climate and climate change, epidemiology, ecology and adaptation measures. WHO Europe. 2006. http://www.euro.who.int/__data/assets/pdf_file/0006/96819/E89522.pdf. Accessed 22 Dec 2016.
14. Sykes RA, Makiello P. An estimate of Lyme borreliosis incidence in Western Europe. J Public Health (Oxf). 2016. doi:10.1093/pubmed/fdw017.
15. Centers for Disease Control and Prevention (CDC). Summary of notifiable diseases, United States, 2008. MMWR Morb Mortal Wkly Rep. 2010;57:19.
16. Hinckley AF, Connally NP, Meek JI, et al. Lyme disease testing by large commercial laboratories in the United States. Clin Infect Dis. 2014;59:676–81.
17. Czupryna P, Moniuszko-Malinowska A, Pancewicz S, et al. Lyme disease in Poland - A serious problem? Adv Med Sci. 2016;61:96–100.
18. Sadkowska-Todys M, Zielinski A, Czarkowski MP. Infectious diseases in Poland in 2014 [in Polish]. Przegl Epidemiol. 2016;70:167–81.
19. Zeman P, Benes C. Spatial distribution of a population at risk: an important factor for understanding the recent rise in tick-borne diseases (Lyme borreliosis and tick-borne encephalitis in the Czech Republic). Ticks Tick Borne Dis. 2013;4:522–30.
20. Richter D, Schlee DB, Matuschka FR. Reservoir competence of various rodents for the lyme disease Spirochete Borrelia spielmanii. Appl Environ Microbiol. 2011;77(11):3565–70.
21. Borchers AT, Keen CL, Huntley AC, Gershwin ME. Lyme disease: a rigorous review of diagnostic criteria and treatment. J Autoimmun. 2015;57:82–115.
22. Sood SK, Salzman MB, Johnson BJ, et al. Duration of tick attachment as a predictor of the risk of Lyme disease in an area in which Lyme disease is endemic. J Infect Dis. 1997;175:996–9.
23. Hodzic E, Feng S, Freet KJ, Borjesson DL, Barthold SW. Borrelia burgdorferi population kinetics and selected gene expression at the host-vector interface. Infect Immun. 2002;70:3382–8.
24. Aenishaenslin C, Bouchard C, Koffi JK, Ogden NH. Exposure and preventive behaviours toward ticks and Lyme disease in Canada: Results from a first national survey. Ticks Tick Borne Dis. 2016. doi:10.1016/j.ttbdis.2016.10.006.
25. Pancewicz SA, Rutkowski R, Rutkowski K, Zajkowska J, Kondrusik M. Immunopathology of Lyme Arthrites [in Polish]. Pol Merk Lek. 2007;134:141–4.
26. Centers for Disease Control and Prevention (CDC). Lyme disease–United States, 2001–2002. MMWR Morb Mortal Wkly Rep. 2004;53:365–9.
27. Deanehan JK, Kimia AA, Tan tanny SP, et al. Distinguishing Lyme from septic knee monoarthritis in Lyme disease-endemic areas. Pediatrics. 2013;131:e695–701.
28. Bachur RG, Adams CM, Monuteaux MC. Evaluating the child with acute hip pain ("irritable hip") in a Lyme endemic region. J Pediatr. 2015;166:407–11.e1.
29. Devauchelle-Pensec V, Thepaut M, Pecquery R, Houx L. Managing monoarthritis in children. Joint Bone Spine. 2016;83:25–30.
30. Glaude PD, Huber AM, Mailman T, Ramsey S, Lang B, Stringer E. Clinical characteristics, treatment and outcome of children with Lyme arthritis in Nova Scotia. Paediatr Child Health. 2015;20:377–80.
31. Steere AC, Schoen RT, Taylor E. The clinical evolution of Lyme arthritis. Ann Intern Med. 1987;107(5):725–31.
32. Szer IS, Taylor E, Steere AC. The long-term course of Lyme arthritis in children. N Engl J Med. 1991;325:159–63.
33. Daikh BE, Emerson FE, Smith RP, Lucas FL, McCarthy CA. Lyme arthritis: a comparison of presentation, synovial fluid analysis, and treatment course in children and adults. Arthritis Care Res (Hoboken). 2013;65:1986–90.
34. Miller JR, Dunn KW, Braccia D, et al. Lyme disease manifestations in the foot and ankle: a retrospective case series. J Foot Ankle Surg. 2016;55:1241–4.

35. Wormser GP, Dattwyler RJ, Shapiro ED, et al. The clinical assessment, treatment, and prevention of lyme disease, human granulocytic anaplasmosis, and babesiosis: clinical practice guidelines by the Infectious Diseases Society of America. Clin Infect Dis. 2006;43:1089–134.
36. Huppertz HI, Karch H, Suschke HJ, et al. Lyme arthritis in European children and adolescents. The pediatric rheumatology collaborative group. Arthritis Rheum. 1995;38:361–8.
37. Thompson A, Mannix R, Bachur R. Acute pediatric monoarticular arthritis: distinguishing lyme arthritis from other etiologies. Pediatrics. 2009;123:959–65.
38. Aiyer A, Hennrikus W, Walrath J, Groh B, Ostrov B. Lyme arthritis of the pediatric lower extremity in the setting of polyarticular disease. J Child Orthop. 2014;8:359–65.
39. Sá MC, Moreira C, Melo C, Sousa Á, Carvalho S. Lyme disease and juvenile idiopathic arthritis - A pediatric case report. Rev Bras Reumatol. 2015. doi:10.1016/j.rbr.2015.08.003.
40. Steere AC, Levin RE, Molloy PJ, et al. Treatment of Lyme arthritis. Arthritis Rheum. 1994;37:878–88.
41. Tory HO, Zurakowski D, Sundel RP. Outcomes of children treated for Lyme arthritis: results of a large pediatric cohort. J Rheumatol. 2010;37:1049–55.
42. Bennet L, Berglund J. Reinfection with Lyme borreliosis: a retrospective follow-up study in southern Sweden. Scand J Infect Dis. 2002;34:183–6.
43. Schnarr S, Franz JK, Krause A, Zeidler H. Infection and musculoskeletal conditions: Lyme borreliosis. Best Pract Res Clin Rheumatol. 2006;20:1099–118.
44. Strle K, Jones KL, Drouin EE, Li X, Steere AC. Borrelia burgdorferi RST1 (OspC type A) genotype is associated with greater inflammation and more severe Lyme disease. Am J Pathol. 2011;178:2726–39.
45. Wang G, Ojaimi C, Wu H, et al. Disease severity in a murine model of lyme borreliosis is associated with the genotype of the infecting Borrelia burgdorferi sensu stricto strain. J Infect Dis. 2002;186:782–91.
46. Edmondson DG, Prabhakaran S, Norris SJ, et al. Enhanced protective immunogenicity of homodimeric Borrelia burgdorferi Outer Surface Protein C. Clin Vaccine Immunol. 2016. doi:10.1128/CVI.00306-16.
47. Ramamoorthi N, Narasimhan S, Pal U, et al. The Lyme disease agent exploits a tick protein to infect the mammalian host. Nature. 2005;436:573–7.
48. Fung BP, Mchugh GL, Leong JM, Steere AC. Humoral immune response to outer surface protein C of Borrelia burgdorferi in Lyme disease: role of the immunoglobulin M response in the serodiagnosis of early infection. Infect Immun. 1994;62:3213–21.
49. Nardelli DT, Callister SM, Schell RF. Lyme arthritis: current concepts and a change in paradigm. Clin Vaccine Immunol. 2008;15:21–34.
50. Kraiczy P. Hide and seek: how Lyme disease spirochetes overcome complement attack. Front Immunol. 2016;7:385.
51. Russell TM, Johnson BJ. Lyme disease spirochaetes possess an aggrecan-binding protease with aggrecanase activity. Mol Microbiol. 2013;90:228–40.
52. Sjöwall J, Fryland L, Nordberg M, et al. Decreased Th1-type inflammatory cytokine expression in the skin is associated with persisting symptoms after treatment of erythema migrans. PLoS ONE. 2011;6:e18220.
53. Hannier S, Liversidge J, Sternberg JM, Bowman AS. Characterization of the B-cell inhibitory protein factor in Ixodes ricinus tick saliva: a potential role in enhanced Borrelia burgdoferi transmission. Immunology. 2004;113:401–8.
54. Kotsyfakis M, Sá-Nunes A, Francischetti IM, Mather TN, Andersen JF, Ribeiro JM. Antiinflammatory and immunosuppressive activity of sialostatin L, a salivary cystatin from the tick Ixodes scapularis. J Biol Chem. 2006;281:26298–307.
55. Parker LC, Whyte MK, Dower SK, Sabroe I. The expression and roles of Toll-like receptors in the biology of the human neutrophil. J Leukoc Biol. 2005;77:886–92.
56. Szczepanski A, Fleit HB. Interaction between Borrelia burgdorferi and Polymorphonuclear Leukocytes. Ann NY Acad Sci. 1988;539:425–8.
57. Swidrowska-Jaros J, Orczyk K, Smolewska E. Macrophages - silent enemies in juvenile idiopathic arthritis. Postepy Hig Med Dosw (Online). 2016;70:743–50.
58. Jin C, Roen DR, Lehmann PV, Kellermann GH. An enhanced ELISPOT assay for sensitive detection of antigen-specific T cell responses to borrelia burgdorferi. Cells. 2013;2:607–20.
59. Crandall H, Dunn DM, Ma Y, et al. Gene expression profiling reveals unique pathways associated with differential severity of lyme arthritis. J Immunol. 2006;177:7930–42.
60. Miller JC, Ma Y, Bian J, et al. A critical role for type I IFN in arthritis development following Borrelia burgdorferi infection of mice. J Immunol. 2008;181:8492–503.
61. Callister SM, Jobe DA, Stuparic-Stancic A, et al. Detection of IFN-γ secretion by T cells collected before and after successful treatment of early Lyme disease. Clin Infect Dis. 2016;62:1235–41.
62. Zeidner N, Dreitz M, Belasco D, Fish D. Suppression of acute Ixodes scapularis-induced Borrelia burgdorferi infection using tumor necrosis factor-alpha, interleukin-2, and interferon-gamma. J Infect Dis. 1996;173:187–95.
63. Sonderegger FL, Ma Y, Maylor-hagan H, et al. Localized production of IL-10 suppresses early inflammatory cell infiltration and subsequent development of IFN-γ-mediated Lyme arthritis. J Immunol. 2012;188:1381–93.
64. Kuo J, Warner TF, Munson EL, Nardelli DT, Schell RF. Arthritis is developed in Borrelia-primed and -infected mice deficient of interleukin-17. Pathog Dis. 2016. doi:10.1093/femspd/ftw077.
65. Infante-Duarte C, Horton HF, Byrne MC, Kamradt T. Microbial lipopeptides induce the production of IL-17 in Th cells. J Immunol. 2000;165:6107–15.
66. Bachmann M, Horn K, Rudloff I, et al. Early production of IL-22 but not IL-17 by peripheral blood mononuclear cells exposed to live Borrelia burgdorferi: the role of monocytes and interleukin-1. PLoS Pathog. 2010;6:e1001144.
67. Codolo G, Amedei A, Steere AC, et al. Borrelia burgdorferi NapA-driven Th17 cell inflammation in lyme arthritis. Arthritis Rheum. 2008;58:3609–17.
68. Strle K, Stupica D, Drouin EE, Steere AC, Strle F. Elevated levels of IL-23 in a subset of patients with post-lyme disease symptoms following erythema migrans. Clin Infect Dis. 2014;58:372–80.
69. Katchar K, Drouin EE, Steere AC. Natural killer cells and natural killer T cells in Lyme arthritis. Arthritis Res Ther. 2013;15:R183.
70. Pausa M, Pellis V, Cinco M, et al. Serum-resistant strains of Borrelia burgdorferi evade complement-mediated killing by expressing a CD59-like complement inhibitory molecule. J Immunol. 2003;170:3214–22.
71. Barthold SW, De Souza M. Exacerbation of Lyme arthritis in beige mice. J Infect Dis. 1995;172:778–84.
72. Hori S, Nomura T, Sakaguchi S. Control of regulatory T cell development by the transcription factor Foxp3. Science. 2003;299:1057–61.
73. Vudattu NK, Strle K, Steere AC, Drouin EE. Dysregulation of CD4 + CD25(high) T cells in the synovial fluid of patients with antibiotic-refractory Lyme arthritis. Arthritis Rheum. 2013;65:1643–53.
74. Shen S, Shin JJ, Strle K, et al. Treg cell numbers and function in patients with antibiotic-refractory or antibiotic-responsive Lyme arthritis. Arthritis Rheum. 2010;62:2127–37.
75. Steere AC, Glickstein L. Elucidation of Lyme arthritis. Nat Rev Immunol. 2004;4:143–52.
76. Steere AC, Klitz W, Drouin EE, et al. Antibiotic-refractory Lyme arthritis is associated with HLA-DR molecules that bind a Borrelia burgdorferi peptide. J Exp Med. 2006;203:961–71.
77. Arvikar SL, Crowley JT, Sulka KB, Steere AC. Autoimmune arthritides, rheumatoid arthritis, psoriatic arthritis, or peripheral spondyloarthropathy, following lyme disease. Arthritis Rheumatol. 2016. doi:10.1002/art.39866.
78. Pianta A, Drouin EE, Crowley JT, et al. Annexin A2 is a target of autoimmune T and B cell responses associated with synovial fibroblast proliferation in patients with antibiotic-refractory Lyme arthritis. Clin Immunol. 2015;160:336–41.
79. Lipsett SC, Nigrovic LE. Diagnosis of Lyme disease in the pediatric acute care setting. Curr Opin Pediatr. 2016;28:287–93.
80. Hu LT. Lyme disease. Ann Intern Med. 2016;165:677.
81. Fallon BA, Pavlicova M, Coffino SW, Brenner C. A comparison of lyme disease serologic test results from 4 laboratories in patients with persistent symptoms after antibiotic treatment. Clin Infect Dis. 2014;59:1705–10.
82. Ang CW, Notermans DW, Hommes M, Simoons-smit AM, Herremans T. Large differences between test strategies for the detection of anti-Borrelia antibodies are revealed by comparing eight ELISAs and five immunoblots. Eur J Clin Microbiol Infect Dis. 2011;30(8):1027–32.
83. Centers for Disease Control and Prevention (CDC). Recommendations for test performance and interpretation from the Second National Conference on Serologic Diagnosis of Lyme Disease. MMWR Morb Mortal Wkly Rep. 1995;44:590–1.
84. Molins CR, Delorey MJ, Sexton C, Schriefer ME. Lyme borreliosis serology: performance with several commonly used laboratory diagnostic tests and a large resource panel of well-characterized patient samples. J Clin Microbiol. 2016. doi:10.1128/JCM.00874-16.
85. Seriburi V, Ndukwe N, Chang Z, Cox ME, Wormser GP. High frequency of false positive IgM immunoblots for Borrelia burgdorferi in clinical practice. Clin Microbiol Infect. 2012;18:1236–40.
86. Leeflang MM, Ang CW, Berkhout J, et al. The diagnostic accuracy of serological tests for Lyme borreliosis in Europe: a systematic review and meta-analysis. BMC Infect Dis. 2016;16:140.
87. Pawinska A. Lyme borreliosis – microbiological diagnostics and treatment [in Polish]. Stand Med Pediatr. 2009;6:757–66.

88. Flisiak R, Pancewicz S. Diagnostics and treatment of Lyme borreliosis. Recommendations of Polish Society of Epidemiology and Infectious Diseases [in Polish]. Department of Infectious Diseases and Hepatology – Medical University of Bialystok. 2011. http://www.choroby-zakazne.pl/uploads/pdf/borelioza.pdf. Accessed 22 Dec 2016.
89. Branda JA, Strle K, Nigrovic LE, et al. Evaluation of modified 2-tiered serodiagnostic testing algorithms for early Lyme disease. Clin Infect Dis. 2017;64(8):1074–80.
90. Wormser GP, Levin A, Soman S, Adenikinju O, Longo MV, Branda JA. Comparative cost-effectiveness of two-tiered testing strategies for serodiagnosis of lyme disease with noncutaneous manifestations. J Clin Microbiol. 2013;51(12):4045–9.
91. Bacon RM, Biggerstaff BJ, Schriefer ME, et al. Serodiagnosis of Lyme disease by kinetic enzyme-linked immunosorbent assay using recombinant VlsE1 or peptide antigens of Borrelia burgdorferi compared with 2-tiered testing using whole-cell lysates. J Infect Dis. 2003;187:1187–99.
92. Lipsett SC, Branda JA, Mcadam AJ, et al. Evaluation of the C6 Lyme enzyme immunoassay for the diagnosis of Lyme disease in children and adolescents. Clin Infect Dis. 2016;63(7):922–8.
93. Johansson M, Manfredsson L, Wistedt A, Serrander L, Tjernberg I. Significant variations in the seroprevalence of C6 ELISA antibodies in a highly endemic area for Lyme borreliosis: evaluation of age, sex and seasonal differences. APMIS. 2017. doi:10.1111/apm.12664.
94. Branda JA, Linskey K, Kim YA, Steere AC, Ferraro MJ. Two-tiered antibody testing for Lyme disease with use of 2 enzyme immunoassays, a whole-cell sonicate enzyme immunoassay followed by a VlsE C6 peptide enzyme immunoassay. Clin Infect Dis. 2011;53:541–7.
95. Barton-forbes M, Leonard E, Lindsay LR, Langley JM, Koffi JK, Ogden NH. Tick bites in the Lyme light. Paediatr Child Health. 2015;20:237–8.
96. Berende A, Ter Hofstede HJ, Vos FJ, et al. Randomized trial of longer-term therapy for symptoms attributed to Lyme disease. N Engl J Med. 2016;374:1209–20.
97. Pachner AR, Delaney E, O'neill T. Neuroborreliosis in the nonhuman primate: Borrelia burgdorferi persists in the central nervous system. Ann Neurol. 1995;38:667–9.
98. Schoen RT, Aversa JM, Rahn DW, Steere AC. Treatment of refractory chronic Lyme arthritis with arthroscopic synovectomy. Arthritis Rheum. 1991;34:1056–60.
99. Stricker RB, Johnson L. Lyme disease: the promise of Big Data, companion diagnostics and precision medicine. Infect Drug Resist. 2016;9:215–9.
100. Feng J, Shi W, Zhang S, Zhang Y. Persister mechanisms in Borrelia burgdorferi: implications for improved intervention. Emerg Microbes Infect. 2015;4:e51.
101. Gherardini FC. Borrelia burgdorferi HtrA may promote dissemination and irritation. Mol Microbiol. 2013;90:209–13.

13

Juvenile idiopathic arthritis in relation to perinatal and maternal characteristics

Samantha W. Bell[1,4,5*], Susan Shenoi[2], J. Lee Nelson[3], Parveen Bhatti[1,3] and Beth A. Mueller[1,3]

Abstract

Background: Existing data on associations between maternal and early childhood exposures and juvenile idiopathic arthritis (JIA) risk is scant and inconsistent with previous studies showing potential role for prematurity, number of siblings and infections. We explored JIA and International League of Associations for Rheumatology (ILAR) JIA categories in relation to selected infant (birthweight, size-for-gestational-age, gestational age), and maternal (parity, delivery type, prior fetal loss) characteristics that may be markers for exposures related to two pathways (hygiene hypothesis, microchimerism) potentially associated with autoimmune disorder occurrence.

Methods: A case–control analysis with 1,234 JIA cases and 5,993 birth year-matched controls was conducted. Exposure information was obtained from WA state birth certificates. Multivariable logistic regression was used to estimate adjusted odds ratios (OR) and 95% confidence intervals (CI) for associations with maternal and early life exposures for JIA and JIA categories.

Results: Greater maternal parity was associated with a decreased OR for JIA (most marked for persistent oligoarticular JIA, OR 0.32, 95% CI 0.15; 0.71, p for trend = 0.0001). Prior fetal loss (except for oligoarticular JIA) was associated with an increased OR for JIA. Prematurity was associated with increased risk of enthesitis related arthritis (OR 1.9, 95% CI: 1.3–2.9) and rheumatoid factor positive polyarticular JIA (OR 2.2, 95% CI: 1.0–4.8).

Conclusions: We observed associations of selected maternal factors with JIA, some of which varied across JIA categories. The findings of decreased ORs for JIA in relation to greater maternal parity may be consistent with the hygiene and microchimerism hypotheses. Future studies with biomarkers relevant to these hypotheses will help elucidate any associations.

Keywords: Juvenile arthritis, Maternal reproductive history, Case-control study, Perinatal factors, Birth certificate

Background

Juvenile Idiopathic Arthritis (JIA) is a heterogeneous group of seven categories of chronic inflammatory arthritides in children with onset before 16 years of age [1]. JIA likely has a complex etiology, with multiple genetic and environmental factors contributing to its development [2]. Concordance rates of JIA among monozygotic twins are estimated at 25–40%; suggesting that environmental factors may influence JIA risk [3]. Evidence suggests that adult rheumatoid arthritis (RA) [4], JIA [5, 6], and other autoimmune diseases such as multiple sclerosis [7, 8] may be associated with maternal or early childhood exposures such as maternal parity, birthweight, or gestational age.

Two hypotheses have been suggested relating perinatal and maternal reproductive characteristics to JIA. The "Hygiene hypothesis" suggests that early exposure to infection results in decreased risk of childhood autoimmune disease [9] due to modulation of the developing immune system. Proxy measures often used to assess this include maternal parity (a greater number of prior births being consistent with a greater number of older daycare- or school-aged siblings at home and greater

* Correspondence: Samantha.Bell@ucsf.edu
[1]Department of Epidemiology, School of Public Health, University of Washington, Seattle, WA, USA
[4]School of Medicine, University of California, San Francisco, San Francisco, CA, USA
Full list of author information is available at the end of the article

possibility of early infection); infant birthweight, small size-for-gestational age, or gestational age (small, or preterm infants may be less resistant to infection), and mode of delivery (vaginal deliveries may more likely elicit a normal immune response due to early exposure to vaginal flora). The microchimerism hypothesis relates to maternal and/or sibling origin microchimerism (harboring of cells or DNA from another genetically distinct individual) from exchange of cells/DNA *in utero* from the mother or older siblings during gestation [10]. Microchimerism may potentially increase or decrease disease risk based on the specificity of the acquired genetic material from another individual [11], and some studies suggest that its presence may alter rheumatoid arthritis (RA) risk in women [12–17] although we could locate no studies of this in JIA. It has been suggested that the decreased RA risk in parous women may be due to microchimerism among women with prior births [12]. Proxy measures potentially associated with increased microchimerism may include greater maternal parity (greater likelihood that infant has acquired genetic material from older sibling(s)); plurality (twins and higher-order multiples may have acquired genetic material from their sibling *in utero*); and a maternal history of prior fetal loss (maternally-retained genetic material from a fetus may be passed to subsequent offspring).

Lacking direct indicators of early prior infection relevant to the hygiene hypothesis, or of the presence of microchimerism, we explored associations of JIA and its individual categories in relation to selected maternal reproductive and infant characteristics as proxies for these, as assessed by birth certificate data among children with, and without JIA. Elucidation of these relationships will enhance understanding of possible JIA risk factors.

Methods

Study design

This case-control study identified JIA cases at a regional children's hospital in the Seattle-Puget Sound region of Washington State using methods described previously [18]. Appropriate Institutional Review Board approvals were obtained. Potential JIA cases were identified though International Classification of Diseases (ICD-9), Ninth Revision diagnosis codes (720.0, 696.0, 714.32, 714.31, 714.30, 720.89, 714.33, 714.3) from 1997–2010 ($N = 2{,}274$) and linked to WA State birth records to identify children born in-state ($N = 1{,}518$). Controls were randomly selected in a 4:1 control: case ratio from remaining birth records, matched on year of birth ($N = 6{,}072$).

Chart review further refined JIA identification and categorized cases into ILAR categories including: polyarticular rheumatoid factor (RF) positive, polyarticular RF negative, oligoarticular arthritis (persistent and extended), psoriatic JIA, enthesitis related arthritis, systemic JIA, and undifferentiated JIA. We excluded 228 cases who did not meet ILAR criteria [1], and 38 cases with disease onset at > 16 years, resulting in 1,252 cases for analyses. After examining the OR for JIA in relation to plurality status, all remaining analyses were restricted to singleton infants only (1,234 cases; 5,993 controls) because characteristics (for example, birthweight and gestational age) of infants and pregnancies differ for singleton and multiple gestation pregnancies.

Exposure information from birth records included: birthweight (<2500, 2500- < 4000, 4000+ grams); size-for-gestational-age (SGA; small, AGA; appropriate, or LGA; large, based on above/below the 10th percentile for size/gestational age in Washington birth record standards); and gestational age (<37, 37- < 42, 42+ weeks). Maternal and infant factors relevant to the hygiene hypothesis included: number of prior births; delivery method (vaginal, cesarean (C) section), infant birthweight, gestational age and size for gestational age. To examine the microchimerism hypothesis, we examined birth order (as measured by maternal parity), plurality (singleton, twin/multiple gestation), and number of prior fetal losses (any; and by <20, 20+ weeks gestation).

Statistical analysis

Multivariable logistic regression was used to estimate odds ratios (OR) and 95% confidence intervals (CIs) for associations, adjusted for maternal age, and the matching variable birth year. Other factors evaluated for possible effects on the relationships of interest included paternal age; maternal race/ethnicity, educational level, prenatal smoking, and marital status; medical insurance at birth (Medicaid vs. other); sex; and trimester prenatal care began. We adjusted for factors that altered the OR by greater than 10% in univariate analyses. Potential effect modifiers were evaluated by inspection of stratum-specific ORs and the Breslow-Day test for homogeneity. Trends were evaluated using Wilcoxon rank sum test. Analyses were initially conducted to examine JIA overall, and repeated for JIA categories (restricted to factors with at least 5 subjects in a cell). Analyses were conducted using Stata (version 11; StataCorp, College Station, Texas).

Results

The majority of cases (67%) were female. Mothers of cases' were more likely to be white (81%), married (80% v), college graduates (34%), have first trimester prenatal care (86%) and less likely to have Medicaid insurance (26%) (Table 1). Maternal gravidity was similar among cases and controls, with about 30% of mothers being nulliparous. Distribution of JIA categories included:

Table 1 Infant and Maternal Characteristics of JIA Cases and non-JIA Controls born in Washington State 1997–2010

Characteristics	Cases (N = 1,252)[a]		Controls (N = 6,072)[a]	
	n	%	n	%
Infant Factors				
Female	843	67.3	2,903	47.8
Twin/multiple gestation[b]	18	1.4	79	1.3
Race/Ethnicity				
White	984	81.3	4,425	74.8
Black	37	3.1	316	5.3
Asian/Pacific Islander	60	4.9	426	7.2
Native American	38	3.1	150	2.5
Hispanic	91	7.5	598	10.1
Other	1	0.1	3	0.1
Maternal Factors				
Age (years)				
< 20	106	8.5	694	11.4
20–24	233	18.6	1,536	25.3
25–29	385	30.8	1,774	29.2
30–34	341	27.2	1,326	21.9
35+	187	14.9	739	12.2
Education (years)				
< 12	100	12.9	639	18.0
12	227	29.3	1,092	30.8
12–16	188	24.2	927	26.1
16+	261	33.6	888	25.0
Unmarried	250	20.0	1,577	26.1
Trimester of inception of prenatal care				
First	987	85.9	4,591	81.1
Second	133	11.6	897	15.8
Third	29	2.5	175	3.1
Medicaid insurance	282	26.3	1,789	37.0

[a]Numbers may not add up to totals due to missing data
[b]OR for association with JIA = 1.04, 95% CI: 0.62–1.74

oligoarticular; persistent (31.5%) and extended (5.9%), enthesitis related arthritis (21.2%), RF negative polyarticular (20.7%), systemic arthritis (5.8%), psoriatic arthritis (5.0%), RF positive polyarticular arthritis (4.9%), and undifferentiated arthritis (3.2%). The remaining 1.8% was polyarticular arthritis with unknown RF status.

Infant and maternal characteristics in relation to JIA

Multiple gestation pregnancy was not associated with JIA (Table 1); OR 1.04, 95% CI: 0.62–1.74). Among singletons, birthweight >4000 g was associated with a decreased OR for JIA (OR 0.81, 95% CI: 0.67–0.98) (Table 2). The OR for JIA decreased with increasing number of prior maternal deliveries, with the lowest OR observed for children of women with two prior deliveries (0.68, 95% CI: 0.56–0.83 for 2 deliveries, p for trend =0.0007). No associations of JIA were observed with gestational age, size-for-gestational age, C-section delivery or maternal history of prior fetal losses.

Infant and maternal characteristics in relation to individual JIA categories

We observed an increased ORs for prematurity and RF+ polyarthritis (OR 2.23, 95% CI: 1.04–4.80) and enthesitis-related arthritis (OR 1.90, 95% CI: 1.27–2.86) (Table 3). SGA was associated with increased risk of undifferentiated JIA (OR 2.64, 95% CI: 1.18–5.94). Birthweight <2500 grams was associated with RF+ polyarthritis (OR 2.29, 95% CI: 1.03–5.13).

The pattern we observed for overall JIA of decreasing ORs in relation to increasing number of maternal prior deliveries was marked for persistent oligoarthritis, with a monotonically decreasing trend ranging from 0.88 (95% CI: 0.69–1.12) for one prior birth, to 0.32 (95% CI: 0.15–0.71) for 4+ prior deliveries (p for trend =0.0001), and a suggestion of trend for extended oligoarthritis. Non-statistically significant decreased ORs were observed for greater numbers of prior deliveries for most other JIA categories, except for RF- (OR 1.24, 95% CI: 0.70–2.18 for 4+ prior deliveries) and RF+ (OR 1.77, 95% CI: 0.75–4.14 for 3+ prior deliveries) polyarthritis.

ORs were increased in relation to maternal fetal loss for psoriatic JIA (OR 2.85, 95% CI: 1.57–5.17); RF- polyarthritis (OR 2.20, 95% CI: 1.55–3.12); RF+ polyarthritis (OR 2.00, 95% CI: 1.00–4.00); systemic JIA (OR 1.90, 95% CI: 1.00–3.64) and enthesitis-related arthritis (OR 1.59, 95% CI: 1.16–2.17). Increased ORs were noted with maternal history of early fetal loss (<20 weeks) for enthesitis-related arthritis (OR 1.56, 95% CI: 1.13–2.14), RF- polyarthritis (OR 2.08, 95% CI: 1.46–2.96), and psoriatic (OR 2.62, 95% CI: 1.44–4.79).

Discussion

We observed a decreased risk of JIA overall in relation to greater maternal parity, with a significant monotonic trend for persistent oligoarthritis, and suggestion of decreased ORs in relation to increasing maternal parity for most other JIA categories. This finding may be consistent with the hygiene hypotheses as children with older siblings likely have greater opportunity for infection exposure, both *in utero* and during post-natal life. Additionally a modest, non-statistically significant increased risk of JIA with Cesarean delivery similar to a Swedish registry report [5] provides weak support for the hygiene hypothesis, although this has not been supported in all studies [4].

Table 2 Infant and maternal characteristics among singleton Juvenile Idiopathic Arthritis (JIA) cases and controls born in WA State, 1997–2010

Characteristics	Cases ($N = 1,234$)		Controls ($N = 5,993$)			
	n	%	N	%	OR[a]	95% CI
Infant factors						
Gestational age (weeks)						
< 37	72	6.0	352	6.0	0.99	0.76, 1.29
37–42	1,030	85.5	4,903	83.9	1.00	reference
42+	102	8.5	587	10.1	0.88	0.70, 1.10
Size for gestational age						
SGA	102	9.4	496	9.6	1.01	0.81, 1.27
AGA	878	80.5	4,181	80.8	1.00	reference
LGA	110	10.1	500	9.6	1.01	0.81, 1.26
Birth weight (grams)						
< 2500	64	5.2	292	4.9	1.05	0.79, 1.39
2500–3999	1,026	83.3	4,880	81.7	1.00	reference
≥ 4000	142	11.5	803	13.4	0.81	0.67, 0.98
Maternal factors						
Cesarean Section						
Yes	256	20.7	1,110	18.5	1.08	0.93, 1.26
No	978	79.3	4,878	81.5	1.00	reference
Number of prior births[b]						
0	525	43.6	2,488	42.5	1.00	reference
1	418	34.7	1,893	32.3	0.95	0.82, 1.10
2	157	13.0	931	15.9	0.68	0.56, 0.83
3	60	5.0	325	5.6	0.71	0.53, 0.96
4+	44	3.7	216	3.7	0.72	0.51, 1.02
Any fetal loss (early or late)						
None	482	67.0	2,388	67.4	1.00	reference
1+	237	33.0	1,154	32.6	0.99	0.84, 1.18
Number of prior fetal losses (<20 weeks)[c]						
None	500	69.5	2,472	69.8	1.00	reference
1+	219	30.5	1,069	30.2	0.99	0.83, 1.18
Number of prior fetal losses (≥20 weeks)[c,d]						
None	698	97.1	3,429	97.1	1.00	reference
1+	21	2.9	104	2.9	1.09	0.67, 1.77

[a]Adjusted for maternal age and birth year
[b]p for trend ****P0.0007
[c]Restricted to 839 cases and 4,015 control whose mothers had a prior pregnancy
[d]Adjusted for maternal age, birth year, and paternal age

Consistent with our data, a previous Australian clinic-based study showed that having any siblings (vs. none) was protective for JIA in (OR 0.46, 95% CI 0.28; 0.74, using clinic-based controls); a result slightly attenuated (OR 0.50, 95% CI 0.24; 1.02) when community controls were used [10]. An OR of 1.6 for JIA was observed in relation to being an only child in a Danish registry-based study [19]. In contrast, no risk reduction was observed in relation to having increased numbers of older siblings in a Swedish registry-based study [5]. Birth order was not found to be associated with JIA in two previous studies [6, 20].

The presence of microchimerism might increase or decrease JIA risk based on the nature of the acquired genetic material. An inverse association of JIA with greater maternal parity may be related to the presence of

Table 3 Infant and maternal characteristics among singleton Juvenile Idiopathic Arthritis (JIA) case categories and controls born in WA State, 1997–2010

	Persistent Oligoarthritis		Extended Oligoarthritis		RF+ Polyarthritis		RF- Polyarthritis		Systemic JIA		Enthesitis Related Arthritis		Psoriatic Arthritis		Undifferentiated JIA	
N[a] (%)	389	31.50%	73	5.90%	60	4.90%	256	20.70%	71	5.80%	262	21.20%	62	5.00%	39	3.20%
	OR[b]	95% CI	OR[b]	95% CI	OR[b]	95% CI	OR[b]	95% CI	OR[b]	95% CI	OR[b]	95% CI	OR[b]	95% CI	OR[b]	95% CI
Infant factors																
Gest. age (wks)																
< 37	0.71	0.43, 1.18	-	-	*2.23*	*1.04, 4.80*	0.64	0.33,1.21	1.67	0.76, 3.69	*1.9*	*1.27, 2.86*	-	-	-	-
37–42	1	reference	1	reference	1	reference	1	reference	1	reference	1	reference	1	reference	1	reference
42+	0.88	0.60, 1.29	1.31	0.62, 2.75	0.74	0.29, 1.89	0.83	0.52, 1.33	1.07	0.48, 2.35	0.81	0.51, 1.29	0.79	0.31, 2.00	-	-
Size for gest age																
SGA	0.95	0.64, 1.40	0.79	0.31, 1.99	-	-	0.97	0.60, 1.55	1.03	0.44, 2.41	1.03	0.65, 1.62	1.31	0.55, 3.13	*2.64*	*1.18, 5.94*
AGA	1	reference	1	reference	1	reference	1	reference	1	reference	1	reference	1	reference	1	reference
LGA	1.16	0.82, 1.63	0.99	0.45, 2.18	1.42	0.60, 3.40	1.07	0.69, 1.65	0.8	0.32, 2.01	0.93	0.59, 1.47	-	-	-	-
Birth weight (g)																
< 2500	0.84	0.51, 1.40	0.24	0.03, 1.77	*2.29*	*1.03, 5.13*	1.1	0.63, 1.92	1.88	0.85, 4.15	1.18	0.69, 2.02	-	-	-	-
2500–3999	1	reference	1	reference	1	reference	1	reference	1	reference	1	reference	1	reference	1	reference
≥ 4000	0.85	0.62, 1.17	0.55	0.24, 1.28	0.66	0.26, 1.67	0.89	0.61, 1.31	-	-	0.96	0.67, 1.38	0.79	0.35, 1.74	-	-
Maternal Factors																
Cesarean Section																
Yes	1.17	0.92,1.66	0.93	0.52, 1.66	*1.8*	*1.00, 3.20*	1.07	0.78, 1.46	0.9	0.49, 1.65	1.14	0.84, 1.55	1.15	0.62, 2.13	0.84	0.35, 2.01
No	1	Reference	1	reference	1	reference	1	reference	1	reference	1	reference	1	reference	1	reference
No. prior birth[c,e]																
0	1	Reference	1	reference	1	reference	1	reference	1	reference	1	reference	1	reference	1	reference
1	0.88	0.69, 1.12	1.02	0.60, 1.74	0.72	0.38, 1.37	0.78	0.58, 1.06	0.92	0.53, 1.59	*1.36*	*1.02, 1.82*	1.15	0.65, 2.04	0.66	0.31, 1.41
2	*0.71*	*0.52, 0.98*	0.53	0.27, 1.04	0.67	0.27,1.67	*0.63*	*0.42, 0.95*	0.94	0.47, 1.86	0.83	0.56, 1.24	0.53	0.21, 1.33	0.6	0.25, 1.44
3	*0.55*	*0.32, 0.94*	-	-	1.77	0.75, 4.14	0.89	0.51, 1.53	0.64	0.24, 1.70	0.96	0.54, 1.69	0.71	0.26, 1.94	-	-
4+	*0.32*	*0.15, 0.71*	-	-	-	-	1.24	0.70, 2.18	-	-	0.65	0.31, 1.39	-	-	-	-
Any fetal loss																
None	1	reference	1	reference	1	reference	1	reference	1	reference	1	reference	1	reference	1	reference
1+	1.06	0.76, 1.47	0.77	0.35, 1.70	*2*	*1.00, 4.00*	*2.2*	*1.55, 3.12*	*1.9*	*1.00, 3.64*	*1.59*	*1.16, 2.17*	*2.85*	*1.57, 5.17*	1.42	0.61, 3.30
No. prior fetal losses (<20 w)[c]																
None	1	reference	1	reference	1	reference	1	reference	1	reference	1	reference	1	reference	1	reference
1+	1.11	0.80, 1.54	0.84	0.38, 1.88	1.71	0.83, 3.51	*2.08*	*1.46, 2.97*	1.68	0.86, 3.28	*1.56*	*1.13, 2.14*	*2.62*	*1.44, 4.78*	1.57	0.68, 3.65
No. prior fetal losses ((≥20 w)[c, d]																
None	1	reference	1	reference	1	reference	1	reference	1	reference	1	reference	1	reference	1	reference
1+	-	-	-	-	-	-	2.25	0.96, 5.25	-	-	1.9	0.86, 4.20	-	-	-	-

[a]Estimates do not include polyarthritis with unknown RF status
[b]All estimates are adjusted for maternal age and birth year
[c]Estimates are restricted to 839 case mothers and 4,015 control mothers with prior pregnancy
[d]In addition to maternal age and birth year, also adjusted for paternal age
[e]P for trends: persistent oligo: ****P0.0001; extended oligo, ***P0.0075. All others are > 0.05
Estimates in italics are statistically significant

acquired genetic material carrying JIA-protective Human Leukocyte Antigen (HLA) alleles from an older sibling. In our study, most JIA category-specific risk estimates for maternal fetal loss were increased; a finding that could be consistent with the microchimerism hypothesis only if presence of increased levels of acquired microchimerism from a mother's prior pregnancy carried JIA-associated risk HLA alleles [11]. However, it has been demonstrated that mothers of children with JIA have impaired reproductive capacity [21], so history of maternal fetal loss may also simply be an indicator of this observed association. Ultimately, we had no information about specific gene traits of children or their families, and this is speculation.

In contrast with previous studies from Sweden and United States [5, 6], high birthweight in our study was associated with a significantly decreased risk of JIA overall. Reasons for this difference are not clear.

Previous studies related to a gestational age effect vary. Although Swedish registry data suggest a borderline decreased OR in relation to preterm delivery [5], Shenoi et al [6] noted a significantly increased risk of JIA in relation to prematurity. While our results suggest no association with gestational age overall, enthesitis-related arthritis and RF+ polyarticular JIA had significantly increased ORs in relation to preterm gestation. Mothers of children with JIA have higher rates of preterm delivery [21] and the association of prematurity with JIA needs to be further explored in future studies.

The use of outpatient and inpatient medical records maintained by board-certified pediatric rheumatologists at a large regional children's medical center, with data linkage to state birth records, are major strengths of this study enabling identification of a relatively large number of cases. Exposure information was assessed from birth records prior to onset and diagnosis of JIA, and was not subject to recall bias. Because of the known polygenic genetic predispositions and heterogeneity of the pathogenesis of differing JIA categories, it is important to examine these relationships separately for each category; to our knowledge, this is the first study to do so. Medical chart review allowed us to confirm and ascertain JIA categories, thereby reducing misclassification.

Some limitations of our study include possible inaccuracies in reporting of mother's reproductive history; in particular, inaccurate reporting of fetal loss on the birth certificates may have lead to non-differential misclassification, biasing the OR estimates towards the null. Birthweight and number of prior live births, however, have been assessed as reliable in comparison to medical records [22]. There is potential for unmeasured confounding due to unrecognized pregnancy loss, psychosocial support factors, and lack of information on fertility, or residual confounding due to the necessity of reliance on birth records for exposure information. The inability to measure these could lead to residual confounding in our risk estimates and could bias the estimates either way. Although we attempted to identify all children with JIA at the sole facility with board-certified pediatric rheumatologists in Washington State during the study period, and free care is available for families without resources, it is possible that our JIA cases may not be representative of all children with JIA in Washington State. Some cases may have been treated by adult rheumatologists or other practitioners outside this facility, or they may differ from the underlying population in ways that we could not measure. We attempted to evaluate any related bias due to this, although adjustment for socio-economic and other factors potentially related to care access had no effect on the results. Our inability to examine the presence of younger siblings is also a limitation.

Conclusions

We observed decreased JIA risk with increasing parity, which potentially supports the hygiene or microchimerism hypotheses, with consistent results demonstrated in many JIA categories. Of note, our results indicate the need to consider JIA categories as separate entities; indeed our results were often inconsistent across categories, suggesting potentially different etiologies. Given the current lack of preventative or curative treatments for JIA, further studies, particularly those capable of examining category-specific JIA associations, are warranted. A better understanding of these associations will help inform prevention programs and hopefully reduce the burden of this debilitating disease.

Abbreviations

CI: Confidence interval; ICD-9: International classification of diseases; JIA: Juvenile idiopathic arthritis; OR: odds ratio; RF: Rheumatoid factor

Acknowledgements

We would like to thank the Washington State Department of Health for data access, and Mr. Bill O'Brien for programming assistance.

Funding

This project was supported in part by the Health Resources and Services Administration's Maternal and Child Health Bureau (Title V, Social Security Act), grant # T76MC00011-21-00. Dr Shenoi's work was supported by an NIH T32AR007108 grant.

Authors' contributions

All authors were involved in drafting the article or revising it critically for important intellectual content, and all authors approved the final version to be submitted for publication. Ms. SWB had full access to all of the data in the study and takes responsibility for the integrity of the data and the accuracy of the data analysis. Study conception and design. SWB, BAM, SS, PB. Acquisition of data. SS, SWB, BAM. Analysis and interpretation of data. SS, SWB, BAM, JLN.

Competing interests

The authors declare that they have no competing interests.

Consent for publication

Not applicable.

Author details

[1]Department of Epidemiology, School of Public Health, University of Washington, Seattle, WA, USA. [2]Department of Pediatrics, Division of Rheumatology, Seattle Children's Hospital, University of Washington School of Medicine, Seattle, WA, USA. [3]Public Health Sciences Division, Fred Hutchison Cancer Research Center, Seattle, WA, USA. [4]School of Medicine, University of California, San Francisco, San Francisco, CA, USA. [5]University of California, San Francisco, 513 Parnassus Ave., Room S245, San Francisco, CA 94143, USA.

References

1. Petty RE, Southwood TR, Manners P, et al. International league of associations for rheumatology classification of juvenile idiopathic arthritis: Second revision, edmonton, 2001. J Rheumatol. 2004;31(2):390–2.
2. Cassidy J, Petty R, Laxer R, Lindsley C. Textbook of pediatric rheumatology: Expert consult. Vol 6th ed. 2011.
3. Ellis JA, Munro JE, Ponsonby AL. Possible environmental determinants of juvenile idiopathic arthritis. Rheumatology (Oxford). 2010;49(3):411–25.
4. Colebatch AN, Edwards CJ. The influence of early life factors on the risk of developing rheumatoid arthritis. Clin Exp Immunol. 2011;163(1):11–6.
5. Carlens C, Jacobsson L, Brandt L, Cnattingius S, Stephansson O, Askling J. Perinatal characteristics, early life infections and later risk of rheumatoid arthritis and juvenile idiopathic arthritis. Ann Rheum Dis. 2009;68(7):1159–64.
6. Shenoi S, Shaffer ML, Wallace CA. Environmental risk factors and early-life exposures in juvenile idiopathic arthritis: A case-control study. Arthritis Care Res (Hoboken). 2016;68(8):1186–94.
7. Mueller BA, Nelson JL, Newcomb PA. Intrauterine environment and multiple sclerosis: A population- based case-control study. Mult Scler. 2013;19(1):106–11.
8. Nijland MJ, Ford SP, Nathanielsz PW. Prenatal origins of adult disease. Curr Opin Obstet Gynecol. 2008;20(2):132–8.
9. Bach JF. The effect of infections on susceptibility to autoimmune and allergic diseases. N Engl J Med. 2002;347(12):911–20.
10. Miller J, Ponsonby AL, Pezic A, et al. Sibling exposure and risk of juvenile idiopathic arthritis. Arthritis Rheumatol. 2015;67(7):1951–8.
11. Nelson JL. The otherness of self: Microchimerism in health and disease. Trends Immunol. 2012;33(8):421–7.
12. Guthrie KA, Gammill HS, Madeleine MM, Dugowson CE, Nelson JL. Parity and HLA alleles in risk of rheumatoid arthritis. Chimerism. 2011;2(1):11–5.
13. Kekow M, Barleben M, Drynda S, Jakubiczka S, Kekow J, Brune T. Long-term persistence and effects of fetal microchimerisms on disease onset and status in a cohort of women with rheumatoid arthritis and systemic lupus erythematosus. BMC Musculoskelet Disord. 2013;14:325.
14. Rak JM, Maestroni L, Balandraud N, Guis S, Boudinet H, Guzian MC, Yan Z, Azzouz D, Auger I, Roudier C, Martin M, Didelot R, Roudier J, Lambert NC. Transfer of the shared epitope through microchimerism in women with rheumatoid arthritis. Arthritis Rheum. 2009;60(1):73–80.
15. Yan Z, Aydelotte T, Gadi VK, Guthrie KA, Nelson JL. Acquisition of the rheumatoid arthritis HLA shared epitope through microchimerism. Arthritis Rheum. 2011;63(3):640–4.
16. Feitsma AL, Worthington J, van der Helm-van Mil A, Plant D, Thomson W, Ursum J, van Schaardenburg D, van der Horst-Bruinsma I, van Rood JJ, Huizinga T, Toes R, de Vries RRP. Protective effect of noninherited maternal HLA-DR antigens on rheumatoid arthritis development. Proc Natl Acad Sci. 2007;104:19966–70. USA.
17. Stevens AM. Maternal microchimerism in health and disease. Best Pract Res Clin Obstet Gynaecol. 2016;31:121–30 (review).
18. Shenoi S, Bell S, Wallace CA, Mueller BA. Juvenile idiopathic arthritis in relation to maternal prenatal smoking. Arthritis Care Res (Hoboken). 2015; 67(5):725–30.
19. Nielsen HE, Dorup J, Herlin T, Larsen K, Nielsen S, Pedersen FK. Epidemiology of juvenile chronic arthritis: Risk dependent on sibship, parental income, and housing. J Rheumatol. 1999;26(7):1600–5.
20. Prahalad S, Fraser AM, O'Brien E, Kerber RA, Mineau GP, Bohnsack JF. Lack of association between birth order and juvenile idiopathic arthritis. Arthritis Rheum. 2003;48(10):2989–90.
21. Chaudhari M, Moroldo MB, Shear E, et al. Impaired reproductive fitness in mothers of children with juvenile autoimmune arthropathies. Rheumatology (Oxford). 2006;45(10):1282–7.
22. Roohan PJ, Josberger RE, Acar J, Dabir P, Feder HM, Gagliano PJ. Validation of birth certificate data in new york state. J Community Health. 2003;28(5):335–46.

14

Harnessing interactive technologies to improve health outcomes in juvenile idiopathic arthritis

Andrea Coda[1], Dean Sculley[2], Derek Santos[3], Xavier Girones[4], Lucie Brosseau[5], Derek R. Smith[6], Joshua Burns[7], Keith Rome[8], Jane Munro[9] and Davinder Singh-Grewal[7,10*]

Abstract

Background: Children and adolescents with Juvenile Idiopathic Arthritis (JIA) typically have reduced physical activity level and impaired aerobic and anaerobic exercise capacity when compared to their non-JIA counterparts. Low intensity exercise regimens appear to be safe in children with JIA and may results in improvements in overall physical function. Poor adherence to paediatric rheumatology treatment may lead to negative clinical outcomes and possibly increased disease activity. This includes symptoms such as pain, fatigue, quality of life, longer term outcomes including joint damage, as well as increase of healthcare associated costs. Low adherence to medications such as methotrexate and biological-drugs remains a significant issue for paediatric rheumatologists, with alarming reports that less than half of the children with JIA are compliant to drug-therapy.

Main body: The recent advances in interactive technology resulting in a variety of wearable user-friendly smart devices may become a key solution to address important questions in JIA clinical management. Fully understanding the impact that arthritis and treatment complications have upon individual children and their families has long been a challenge for clinicians. Modern interactive technologies can be customised and accessed directly in the hands or wrists of children with JIA. These secured networks could be accessible 'live' at anytime and anywhere by the child, parents and clinicians.

Multidisciplinary teams in paediatric rheumatology may benefit from adopting these technologies to better understand domains such as patient biological parameters, symptoms progression, adherence to drug-therapy, quality of life, and participation in physical activities. Most importantly the use of smart devices technologies may also facilitate more timely clinical decisions, improve self-management and parents awareness in the progression of their child's disease. Paediatric rheumatology research could also benefit from the use of these smart devices, as they would allow real-time access to meaningful data to thoroughly understand the disease-patterns of JIA, such as pain and physical activity outcomes. Data collection that typically occurs once every 1 or 3 months in the clinical setting could instead be gathered every week, day, minute or virtually live online. Arguably, few limitations in wearing such interactive technologies still exist and require further developments.

Conclusion: Finally, by embracing and adapting these new and now highly accessible interactive technologies, clinical management and research in paediatric rheumatology may be greatly advanced.

* Correspondence: davinder.singhgrewal@health.nsw.gov.au
[7]The Children's Hospital at Westmead & the University of Sydney, Hawkesbury Rd & Hainsworth St, Sydney, NSW 2000, Australia
[10]Sydney Children Hospitals Network & Clinical A/Prof- The University of Sydney, Sydney, Australia
Full list of author information is available at the end of the article

Background

Juvenile Idiopathic Arthritis (JIA) incurs a significant burden to patients, their families, and the community [1]. Children with JIA may experience significant issues with school attendance that has a direct impact on their academic performance [2, 3]. Hospitalisation rates in Australia for juvenile arthritis have increased from 14 to 32 per 100,000 population over the past decade [1]. A sharp 118% rise in allied health professional (AHP) involvement has also been recorded in Australia since 2005, including specialist nurses, occupational therapists, physiotherapists, and podiatrists [1]. Some of the prescribed not invasive interventions from AHP, such as regular physical exercises, could be increasingly self-managed by the child and their families and carried out without the need of attending clinics and hospitals, which may positively impact the child's school attendance. Thus, we feel that recent advances in technology resulting in a variety of wearable user-friendly smart devices, capable of providing customised notifications, may become a key instrument in JIA clinical management. Furthermore, data collection and incorporating patient reported outcomes through interactive technologies, may play a significant role in health promotion and self-management of disease into the future [4].

Monitoring symptoms and disease progression using interactive technologies

Understanding the impact that chronic disease and treatment complications have upon children and their families has long been a challenge for clinicians. Typically, practitioners are unable to undertake frequent assessment and so most measures, such as quality of life and disease progression, rely on recall during appointments.

A number of successful attempts have already been made in introducing smart devices to better understand patients' disease, particularly in paediatric oncology, chronic pain, and allergic disease [5, 6]. Cingi et al. (2015), investigated 327 patients diagnosed with mild-to-severe persistent asthma and persistent allergic rhinitis (AR) that were randomised into 2 intervention groups and 2 control groups using a smart mobile platform called POPET. The intervention groups (POPET-AR and POPET-Asthma) received a mobile phone application ("physician on call patient engagement trial" [POPET]), enabling them to interact with their clinicians, and independently record their health status and compliance to their prescribed drugs. Those using the online platform had better health outcomes and quality of life, with a reduction in hospital admissions and number of medical consultations required. Furthermore, improvements were also recorded with regards to activity, productivity, disease perception, and emotion status. Stinson et al. (2015) investigated the validity, reliability, and feasibility of a smartphone pain assessment app among 106 children and adolescent diagnosed with cancer, and concluded that the app had excellent internal consistency, feasibility, and an overall high acceptability amongst patients.

Children and young people with JIA require active involvement in their own health decision-making and lifestyle management [7]. Pilot programs in adult rheumatic disease and other chronic health conditions have already identified the use of modern technology as a possible strategy to improve self-management; however, large scale studies specifically in JIA are still pending [8–10]. The feasibility of online self-assessment system has been performed over a 3-month period using a smart-phone application in only 9 Japanese Rheumatic Arthritis (RA) patients [8]. The smart app provided daily notifications and comments related to the disease activity [8]. The size of this study was very small and 89% of patients were women; however, the results indicated that the app was capable of longitudinally predict the disease activity score in RA patients and it may be an acceptable and useful tool for both patients and healthcare providers [8].

Jongh et al. (2012) published a Cochrane systematic review including four randomised controlled trials, involving 182 participants diagnosed with diabetes, hypertension and asthma. The studies investigated whether mobile phone App, including SMS and MMS, were able to improve self-management by providing medication reminders or supportive notifications to patients to communicate important information to their healthcare providers and exchanged prompt feedback [9]. Although the authors reported that longer studies and larger sample sizes are still necessary, overall moderate quality evidence was found suggesting positive impacts on the health of patients [9].

Majeed-Ariss et al. (2015) conducted a Systematic Review of Adolescents' Use of Mobile Phone and Tablet Apps that Support Personal Management with their Chronic or Long-Term Physical Conditions. It included 4 papers and 46 participants with type 1 diabetes, asthma, and cancer. The authors concluded that smart devices represent a feasible health intervention; however, larger studies are still required in order to determine the Apps' acceptability and effectiveness [10].

Adherence to prescribed medications

Adherence to the prescribed treatment is essential so that children with JIA do not continue to endure joint symptoms, fatigue, reduced physical activity level and lower quality of life [11] and also to avoid rise of healthcare costs through increased frequency of consultations and diagnostic tests [1].

Adherence to medications including methotrexate and biological-drugs remains a significant issue in paediatric rheumatology, with alarming reports that as few as 53% of children with rheumatic disease (RD) have good overall drug-adherence [12]. Bugni et al. (2012) reported that 20 children with RD, equivalent to 20.2% of the participant recruited, had poor medication adherence related to the use of three or more daily medications (p = 0.047). Specifically to children with JIA, 28(51%) patients were not adherent to the prescribed medication [12]. Pelajo et al. (2012) investigated 76 outpatients and the overall rate of non-adherence to methotrexate was 18% amongst American and Portuguese children with JIA, between 1 and 17 years old. The rate of reported non-adherence was 8% in Boston and 24% in Rio de Janeiro (P = 0.012) [13]. Interestingly, the main reason for non-adherence in Boston was "child refused", while in Rio de Janeiro non-adherence was mostly related to an inability to acquire the medication [13]. Multiple reasons should be considered when addressing medication adherence, such as child refusal, adverse effects or lack of medication availability, personal issues, and financial hardship [12]. Another major reason for adherence failure is forgetfulness [12]; therefore, in order to encourage children to take their prescribed drugs, parents/carers are often essential to ensuring adherence. It is possible that smart reminders, accessible directly from the patient's mobile or tablet, may assist medication adherence.

Research in adolescents with asthma has suggested that interactive technologies should be explored as a means of improving medication adherence [14] including customised reminders accessible through a smartphone app and online information [15]. A similar approach, to test medication adherence, was successfully introduced by Crosby et al. [16] in 43 children and adolescents (age range 6–21) with sickle cell disease (SCD) showing 90% satisfaction with patients. This data highlights the potential to integrate smart web-based technology into paediatric clinical care.

Encouraging physical activity

Children with JIA typically have reduced physical activity levels when compared to their non-JIA counterparts [11]. Poor aerobic capacity and low activity detected in children and adolescents with JIA represent a significant clinical concern, as it is likely that the reduced fitness levels will then impact their adulthood [11, 17]. Physical activity is safe in JIA and may results in improvements in physical function [18]. Thus encouraging physical activity in children with JIA is likely to have a beneficial effect. In an age where exercise in children is falling [19], the paediatric rheumatology multidisciplinary team should explore new interactive technologies to increase physical activity adherence.

Modern interactive technologies can be individualised and accessed directly in the hands or on the wrists of children with JIA. Information gathered by smartwatches (or wristbands) that are worn throughout the day by the child, already has the capacity to be wirelessly connected via Cloud networks to databases that collate physical activity data for individual and group analysis. These secured networks could be accessible 'live' at anytime and anywhere by the child, parents and clinicians and allow multidisciplinary teams to better understand domains such as physical activity and energy expenditure. This technology has the potential to facilitate more timely clinical decisions; improve self-management and parent's awareness in the progression of their child's exercise level and physical activity targets.

Smart devices can provide real-time biofeedback; the inbuilt accelerometers and heart rate monitors can measure physical activity intensity, while GPS can be employed to precisely monitor distance of movement throughout the day. As soon as the daily, weekly and/or monthly activity target has been achieved, the child with JIA could be informed (for example with a gentle vibration on the wrist) and recorded for their achievements through messages or 'awards icons' directly on their watch screen. These 'award icons' may serve as incentive and positive reinforcement for participating in a customised management plan, with the ultimate goal of encouraging the child with JIA to be more active and healthier. Future research should investigate the long-term impact of the positive reinforcements and notifications delivered by the smart devices, and possibly develop new methods to promote and sustain long term effectiveness of the interactive technologies.

Access to interactive technologies

Today's children and young adults already have accessible technology integrated into many aspects of their daily life [20]. They are usually comfortable with smart devices, which may engage and motivate them more effectively than traditional methods such as paper-diaries or checklists.

The rapid growth in personal technology such as tablets, smart-phones, and so on, is clearly reflected in daily usage amongst children and adolescents. In 2010, for example, 15% of teenagers in Australia owned a smartphone; and by 2013 users sharply increased to 69% of this population [20]. As smartphones are becoming more accessible and affordable, the number of young consumers is expected to continue growing such that in Australia most adolescents and many younger children are likely to have access to and use smart devices on a regular basis in the future.

Potential new approach to paediatric rheumatology management

With the introduction of already existing interactive technologies as part of the routine paediatric rheumatology care, we feel that new safe and cost effective approaches to care may be possible. Clinicians could connect with the child or family members by providing discreet reminders to inform that a medication is due or if symptom reporting is required. With a simple 'tap' on the smart-watch (or wrist band), the child could confirm when the drug was administered. Similarly, pain levels, physical activity and quality of life data may be recorded weekly, daily or even in real time. Data could be transferred to a secure 'Cloud Platform' for analysis and accessed by patients, their families and clinicians as appropriate. The child with JIA may benefit also from receiving personalised notifications such as text messages, from the clinicians with the aim of promoting positive behavioural changes and encourage daily self-management. The data collected may also facilitate the child, their family and the clinicians to become more aware of disease patterns (Fig. 1).

Data collection that currently occurs once every 1 or 3 months in the clinical setting could instead be gathered constantly and effortlessly, requiring minimal patient and clinician input. In addition to the 'Cloud Platform,' data could also be used to develop logarithms to predict poor outcomes and allow immediate intervention; or foresee early flares of disease and instigate prompt interventions to minimise disruption to the patient's daily life. This new interactive and user-focussed approach has the potential to significantly increase both the child's and family's engagement in their care. The introduction of smart devices to paediatric rheumatology care may provide meaningful improvements in clinical outcomes, patient well-being and engagement, with possible cost reductions for the health care system.

Data protection and limitations

While protecting patient privacy and confidentiality of data remains paramount, many appropriate security protocols already exist amongst the major smart device providers, such as Google™ [21] and Apple™ [22] to ensure constant system security, encryption and data protection, data backup and privacy control, locations services, passwords authentication and intrusion detection. Privacy remains a primary concern for patients, parents and clinicians, especially when it is unclear where the central warehousing of data is installed, who owns the data, and who is responsible for the cost associated with these technologies.

Arguably, there are still challenges in utilising these interactive technologies, such as: the need of evidence regarding feasibility and validity of the apps being utilised and the need for regular software updates by service providers or hospital IT departments, that may impact the reliably of synchronised data transfer. In addition, missing physical activity data may occur during sports such as swimming, when wearing smart watches and wristbands might damage the device. More evidence is required to establish the willingness of children with JIA in interacting with health-related technologies especially at younger age, where children may still exhibit reading difficulties. Finally, these smart technologies might generate few unintended consequences such as increased anxiety, data hyper-vigilance and obsessive tendency in outcome such as physical activity; which need to be monitored by healthcare professionals and family members.

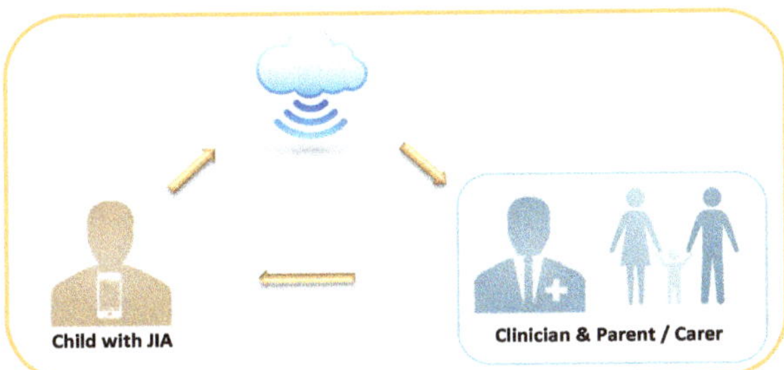

Fig. 1 Data is automatically synchronised to the Cloud Network and instantly available remotely by the multidisciplinary JIA team and their parents/carer

Conclusion

Clearly further studies in paediatric rheumatology are required to critically evaluate the effectiveness and acceptability of available apps in large number of patients and to develop effective apps utilizing valuable input and feedback from patients, carers and clinicians. Overall, by embracing and adapting these new and now highly accessible interactive technologies, clinical management and research progress in paediatric rheumatology could be greatly advanced.

Acknowledgements

The authors would like to thank **Dr. Gabor Major** (*Director of Rheumatology, Bone & Joint Institute Royal Newcastle Centre, Australia*) **Dr. Jeffrey Chaitow** (*Paediatric Rheumatologist; Sydney Children-Hospitals-Network, Australia*) for their kind help and support.

Funding

Not applicable and none to declare.

Authors' contributions

All authors have made substantial contributions to all of the following: -conception and design of the study, –acquisition of information and data. -analysis and interpretation of data, –drafting the article. -critically revising the article for important intellectual content, –all authors read and approved the final manuscript.

Competing interests

The authors declare that they have no competing interests. All authors do not have any financial and personal relationships with other people or organizations that could inappropriately influence this editorial. All authors do not have any potential conflicts of interest such as: employment, consultancies, stock ownership, honoraria, paid expert testimony, patent applications/registrations, and grants or other funding. The work submitted in this editorial is original. The work contained in this editorial has not been previously submitted to meet the requirements for an award at this or any other higher education institution. To the best of my knowledge and belief, the editorial contains no material previously published or written by another person except where due reference is made.

Author details

[1]School of Health Sciences, Faculty of Health and Medicine, The University of Newcastle, Ourimbah, Australia. [2]School of Biomedical Sciences and Pharmacy, Faculty of Health and Medicine, The University of Newcastle, Ourimbah, Australia. [3]School of Health Sciences, Queen Margaret University, Edinburgh, UK. [4]Faculty of Health Sciences at Manresa, University of Vic-Central University of Catalonia, Manresa, Barcelona, Spain. [5]School of Rehabilitation, Ottawa University, Ottawa, Canada. [6]James Cook University, Townsville, Australia. [7]The Children's Hospital at Westmead & the University of Sydney, Hawkesbury Rd & Hainsworth St, Sydney, NSW 2000, Australia. [8]AUT University, Auckland, New Zealand. [9]Department of General Medicine, Royal Children's Hospital, Parkville, VIC, Australia. [10]Sydney Children Hospitals Network & Clinical A/Prof- The University of Sydney, Sydney, Australia.

References

1. Australian Institute of Health and Welfare, [AIHW]. What is juvenile arthritis? 2015. http://www.aihw.gov.au/juvenile-arthritis. Accessed 24 May 2016.
2. Bouaddi I, Rostom S, El Badri D, Hassani A, Chkirate B, Amine B, et al. Impact of juvenile idiopathic arthritis on schooling. BMC Pediatr. 2013; doi:10.1186/1471-2431-13-2.
3. Laila K, Haque M, Islam MM, Islam MI, Talukder MK, Rahman SA. Impact of Juvenile Idiopathic Arthritis on School Attendance and Performance. American Journal of Clinical and Experimental Medicine. 2016; doi:10.11648/j.ajcem.20160406.15
4. Schatz BR. National Surveys of population health: big data analytics for mobile health monitors. Big Data. 2015; 1;3(4):219-229.
5. Cingi C, Yorgancioglu A, Cingi CC, Oguzulgen K, Muluk NB, Ulusoy S, et al. The "physician on call patient engagement trial" (POPET): measuring the impact of a mobile patient engagement application on health outcomes and quality of life in allergic rhinitis and asthma patients. Forum Allergy Rhinol 2015; doi:10.1002/alr.21468.
6. Stinson JN, Jibb LA, Nguyen C, Nathan PC, Maloney AM, Dupuis LL, et al. Construct validity and reliability of a real-time multidimensional smartphone app to assess pain in children and adolescents with cancer. Pain. 2015; doi:10.1097/j.pain.0000000000000385.
7. Tong A, Jones J, Craig JC, Singh-Grewal D. Children's experiences of living with juvenile idiopathic arthritis: a thematic synthesis of qualitative studies. Arthritis Care Res, 2012; doi:10.1002/acr.21695
8. Nishiguchi S, Ito H, Yamada M, Yoshitomi H, Furu M, Shinohara A, et al. Self-assessment of Rheumatoid Arthritis Disease Activity Using a Smartphone Application. Development and 3-month Feasibility Study. J Rheumatol. 2010; doi:10.3899/jrheum.091327.
9. de Jongh T, Gurol-Urganci I, Vodopivec-Jamsek V, Car J, Atun R. Mobile phone messaging for facilitating self-management of long-term illnesses. Cochrane Database Syst Rev. 2012; doi:10.1002/14651858.CD007459.
10. Majeed-Ariss R, Baildam E, Campbell M, Chieng A, Fallon D, Hall A, et al. Apps and Adolescents: A Systematic Review of Adolescents' Use of Mobile Phone and Tablet Apps That Support Personal Management of Their Chronic or Long-Term Physical Conditions. J Med Internet Res. 2015; doi:10.2196/jmir.5043.
11. Szer IS, Kimura Y, Malleson PN, Southwood TR. Arthritis in children and adolescents: juvenile idiopathic arthritis. New York: Oxford University Press; 2006.
12. Bugni VM, Ozaki LS, Okamoto KY, Barbosa CM, Hilário MO, Len CA, et al. Factors associated with adherence to treatment in children and adolescents with chronic rheumatic disease. J Pediatr (Rio J). 2012; doi:10.2223/JPED.2227
13. Pelajo CF, Sgarlat CM, Lopez-Benitez JM, Oliveira SK, Rodrigues MC, Sztajnbok FR, et al. Adherence to methotrexate in juvenile idiopathic arthritis. Rheumatol Int. 2012; doi:10.1007/s00296-010-1774.
14. Nickels A, Dimov V. Innovations in technology: social media and mobile technology in the care of adolescents with asthma. Curr Allergy Asthma Rep. 2012; doi:10.1007/s11882-012-0299-7.
15. Koster ES, Philbert D, de Vries TW, van Dijk L, Bouvy ML. "I just forget to take it": asthma self-management needs and preferences in adolescents. J Asthma. 2015; doi: 10.3109/02770903.2015.1020388.
16. Crosby LE, Barach I, McGrady ME, Kalinyak KA, Eastin AR, Mitchell MJ. Integrating interactive web-based technology to assess adherence and clinical outcomes in pediatric sickle cell disease. Anemia. 2012; doi:10.1155/2012/492428.
17. Lelieveld OT, van Brussel M, Takken T, van Weert E, van Leeuwen MA, Armbrust W. Aerobic and anaerobic exercise capacity in adolescents with juvenile idiopathic arthritis. Arthritis Rheum 2007; doi:10.1002/art.22897
18. Singh-Grewal, D, Schneiderman-Walker, J, Wright, V, Bar-Or, O, Beyene, J, Selvadurai, H, et al. (2007). The Effects of Vigorous Exercise Training on Physical Function in Children With Arthritis: A Randomized, Controlled, Single-Blinded Trial. Arthritis Care and Research. 2007; doi:10.1002/art.23008.
19. Raustorp A, Pagels P, Froberg A, Boldemann C. Physical activity decreased by a quarter in the 11- to 12-year-old Swedish boys between 2000 and 2013 but was stable in girls: a smartphone effect? Acta Paediatr. 2015; doi:10.1111/apa.13027.
20. ACMA, Australia's mobile digital economy – ACMA confirms usage, choice, mobility and intensity on the rise, a.C.A.M: authority editor; 2013.
21. Google. Google Cloud Platform Security [Internet]. Google. 2016. https://cloud.google.com/security. Accessed 13 Oct 2016.
22. Apple. iOS Security - Report No.: 9.3 or Later. 2016; https://www.apple.com/business/docs/iOS_Security_Guide.pdf. Accessed 13 Oct 2016.

15

Access to pediatric rheumatology care for Juvenile Idiopathic Arthritis in the United Arab Emirates

Khulood Khawaja* and Mustafa Al-Maini

Abstract

Background: This study looks at access to care for Juvenile Idiopathic Arthritis through pediatric rheumatology in the UAE, as an example of multi-ethnic society.

Methods: Patients with a diagnosis of Juvenile idiopathic arthritis were identified through the hospital electronic medical records system from January 1st 2011 to December 31st 2014. All residents of the United Arab Emirates hold an Emirates identity card. We divided our patients into two groups: Emirati-Emirates, who are native Emirati children and hold the Emirati nationality, as stated on their Emirates identity card, and who therefore have full, comprehensive access to free medical care; and non-Emirati-Emirates, who represent other nationalities, as stated on their Emirates identity card. The primary objective of this study is to look at access to care for Juvenile idiopathic arthritis through pediatric rheumatology in the two groups. The secondary objective is to look at the effect of having multiple types of healthcare insurance coverage on access to biologics. A retrospective review was carried out.

Results: Sixty-six patients with JIA identified: 33 Emirates and 33 non-Emirates. For Emirates, the mean time from onset to first appointment with pediatric rheumatologist and diagnosis is 9 months (range: 1–48), and for non-Emirates is 12. 4 months (range: 1–96). Among the Emirates, 10 patients are currently on biologic with methotrexate. Among the non-Emirates, 15 are on biologic with methotrexate. Among the Emirates, 12 are currently in remission while on treatment, as are 10 non-Emirates. Regarding disability, one Emirati patient has blindness secondary to noncompliance while under previous treatment. One Non-Emirati developed joint deformities due to periods of noncompliance and no follow up.

Conclusions: Delay in presentation to pediatric rheumatology has been identified as an important factor in our population, which is multi-cultural and multi-ethnic. Type of health care insurance cover did not affect number of patients getting biological therapy once patient seen in the pediatric rheumatology service.

Keywords: Juvenile Idiopathic Arthritis, Access, Care, Pediatric rheumatology

Background

Juvenile Idiopathic Arthritis (JIA) is a chronic inflammatory disease that affects 1 in 1000 children worldwide [1]. It is a heterogeneous group of autoimmune conditions classified into seven different subtypes, based on the clinical features in the first 6 months of presentation, according to International League of Associations of Rheumatology' classification system [2]. UAE's population of 9,346,129 [3] is diverse: 19% of residents are Emirati-Emiratis (EE), who are native Emiratis, which means that they were born in the UAE and originate from the UAE; 81% are non-Emirati-Emiratis (non-EE), who were born in the UAE or other countries and who are originally from outside the UAE, according to their Emirates identity card. The non-EE population includes 23% other Arabs, 50% South Asians, and 8% other expatriates, including Westerners and East Asians [4]. Abu-Dhabi is the capital city of the UAE with a population of 2.3 million [3]. The tertiary Pediatric rheumatology centre is in one of the two main public hospitals in Abu-Dhabi. An out reach clinic provided once weekly to

* Correspondence: kkhawaja@seha.ae
Department of Rheumatology, Allergy and Immunology, Al-Mafraq Hospital, P.O. Box 2951, Abu Dhabi, United Arab Emirates

the other main public hospital in Abu Dhabi. Patients included from both hospitals as the can be seen in either hospital.

There is limited access to pediatric rheumatology care worldwide, and this is particularly true in the United Arab Emirates (UAE). A recent publication by the World Forum on Rheumatic and Musculoskeletal Diseases identified a severe shortage of pediatric rheumatologists both in developed and developing countries [5].

There are also differences in healthcare insurance coverage within the UAE population. It is premium-free and comprehensive for EE children with easy access to public hospitals. For non-EE children health cover is variable from basic emergency cover to full comprehensive treatment. Access to the public hospitals is more difficult for the non-EE due to type of health care insurance cover.

Non-EE child can be referred through "public" primary health care clinic if covered by health insurance or through private sector as pediatric rheumatology considered unique service since it is not available in the private sector. The insurance company still needs to approve the service and treatment. If this is not possible there are government schemes available to fund such treatments once the child seen by the specialist and comprehensive justification for treatment reported.

Our tertiary pediatric rheumatology service is available in the two main public hospitals in the capital city of Abu-Dhabi. The centre is based in one hospital and a weekly outreach clinic is provided in the other public hospital. Referrals are accepted from public and private healthcare providers throughout the country.

The primary objective of this study is to look at access to care for JIA through pediatric rheumatology in the UAE, which is taken as an example of multi-ethnic society. The secondary objective is to look at effect of multiple types of healthcare insurance coverage on access to biologics.

Methods

Patients with a diagnosis of JIA were identified through the hospital electronic medical records system (EMR), which was implemented for all medical documentation in January 2011. Using the International Statistical Classification of Diseases and Related Health Problems (usually referred to by the shorter name "International Classification of Diseases (ICD)), version 9 (ICD 9) (ICD 9 code 714, 714.30,714.89, 696) from January 1st 2011 to December 31st 2014, we sought out all patients under 16 years of age with a diagnosis of JIA. A retrospective review of the electronic medical records (EMR) and paper case notes of the patients who presented to the two main public hospitals in Abu-Dhabi providing tertiary pediatric rheumatology service.

All residents of the UAE hold an Emirates identity card. We divided our patients into two groups: Emirati-Emirates (EE), who are native Emirati children and hold the Emirati nationality, as stated on their Emirates identity card, and who therefore have full, comprehensive access to free medical care; and non-Emirati-Emiratis (non-EE), who represent other nationalities, as stated on their Emirates identity card. Non-EEs can have variable medical insurance coverage as explained in the background.

For the primary objective to look at access to care for JIA through pediatric rheumatology in the UAE we examined the following: percentage of EE children relative to total number of children; subtypes of JIA, according to International League of Associations for Rheumatology (ILAR) classification in each group [2]; time in months (with ranges) from onset to first appointment in pediatric rheumatology and diagnosis, number of health professionals seen prior to referral to pediatric rheumatology, number of self referrals; number of patients on steroids prior to first appointment with rheumatology, number of patients referred to ophthalmology and number of patients with uveitis.

To assess effect of health care insurance coverage on access to biologics we looked at the number of patients on disease-modifying antirheumatic drugs (DMARD) and number of patients on biologics in each group.; number of patients in remission on treatment "Clinical remission on treatment" is defined according to American College of Rheumatology of clinically inactive disease for at least six continuous months while on therapy. (Symptom free, have a CHAQ score of 0, joint count of 0, and normal inflammatory markers). Also number of patients with a disability secondary to JIA.

The information was recorded in a case report form (CRF). Ethical approval was obtained through the hospital's ethics review board.

Data analysis

Data from CRF were entered into a database (Microsoft Office Excel, Microsoft, USA). Descriptive analysis was then performed.

Results

In total, 66 cases with JIA are identified: 33 EE (26 female, 7 male) and 33 non-EE (21 female, 12 male), as seen in Table 1. Of the 33 EEs, the following subtypes of JIA are found: 4 systemic, 10 persistent oligoarticular, 2 extended oligoarticular, 17 polyarticular (7 Rheumatoid factor (RF) + ve, 10 RF-ve).

Among the 33 non-EE cases, the subtypes include 9 systemic, 6 persistent oligoarticular, 1 extended oligoarticular, 15 polyarticular (5 RF + ve, 10 RF-ve), 1 enthesitis related arthritis, 1 psoriatic arthritis).

For EEs, the mean time from onset to first appointment with a pediatric rheumatologist and diagnosis is 9 months, ranging from 1 to 48, while for non-EEs it is

Table 1 Patient Characteristics

	Emirati-Emiratis	Non-Emirati-Emiratis
Total number	33	33
Female/male	26/7	21/12
Systemic	4 (12.2%)	9 (27.3%)
Persistent Oligo JIA	10 (30.3%)	6 (18.2%)
Extended Oligo JIA	2 (6%)	1 (3%)
Poly JIA RF-ve	10 (30.3%)	10 (30.3%)
Poly JIA RF + ve	7 (21.2%)	5 (15.2%)
Enthesitis-related JIA	-	1 (3%)
Psoriatic	-	1 (3%)
Mean time from onset to first appointment with Ped Rheum (months)	9 Range: 1–48	12.4 Range: 1–96
Median time from onset to first appointment with Pediatric rheumatology	10 months	14 months
Oral steroids at diagnosis	31 (94%)	32 (97%)
>2 health professionals seen before pediatric rheumatologist	31 (94%)	25 (75.7%)
Referral to ophthalmology prior to pediatric rheumatology	7 (21.2%)	7 (21.2%)
Uveitis	3 (9%)	2 (6%)
MTX alone	10 (30.3%)	5 (15.2%)
Biologic + MTX treatment	10 (30.3%)	15 (45.5%)
Remission on treatment	12 (36.3%)	10 (30.3%)
Disability	1 blind (uveitis)	1 multiple joint deformities

JIA Juvenile Idiopathic Arthritis, *MTX* Methotrexate

12.4 months, ranging from 1 to 96. Of the 33 EEs, 31 (94%) saw more than two health professionals prior to referral to pediatric rheumatology, as did 25 (75.7%) of the 33 non-EEs.

In each subgroup, 25 patients (75%) had seen two professionals before getting an appointment with a pediatric rheumatologist; 80% saw a pediatrician, 70% an adult rheumatologist, and 60% an orthopedic surgeon. Only 30% of all patients were referred with a possible diagnosis of JIA; the rest were referred with swollen joints query cause or deteriorating function.

For EEs, 30 of the 33 (91%), and for non-EEs, 32 of the 33 (97%), including the persistent oligoarticular subgroup, have received oral steroids.

With regards to uveitis screening, 10 EEs and 7 non-EEs have documented referral to ophthalmology.

Among the EE patients, 15 (45%) of the 33 were self-referrals, as were 13 (39%) of the 33 non-EEs. There was minimum of 4 years of follow up for all patients.

Among the EEs, 10 patients are currently on biologic with methotrexate (4 etanercept, 2 adalimumab, 1 infliximab, 2 tocilizumab, and 1 abatacept), and 10 are on methotrexate alone. Among the non-EEs, 15 are on biologic with methotrexate (7 etanercept, 2 adalimumab, 1 infliximab, and 5 tocilizumab), and 5 are on methotrexate alone.

In each group, 12 are currently in remission on treatment.

Regarding disability, One EE patient with blindness due to periods of non-compliance is under treatment for uveitis. The patient was lost to follow-up for extended periods of time, then returned with complete loss of vision in one eye and limited vision in the other eye.

The non-EE with multiple joint deformities due to periods of non-compliance also had avascular necrosis of one of his hips. He was on long-term oral steroids when he presented to pediatric rheumatology.

Discussion

There are little published data from developing countries on JIA patients' access to tertiary pediatric rheumatology care. Long delays after the onset of JIA in starting definitive treatment remain an important factor, and this is likely to affect the outcome of JIA patients in our region, as is the case in other parts of the world [6–8].

Western literature and one study from Costa Rica offer evidence regarding delays in accessing pediatric rheumatology [9–18] but there is no data available from our country on accessing pediatric rheumatology service.

Our results showed delay for accessing pediatric rheumatology service for both EE and non-EE. Our numbers are small; this in itself reflects the under-referral of JIA patients. According to the population statistics, we should have had more non-EE children presenting with JIA and more South Asian families. For non-EE patients, the type of health insurance coverage might have influenced this and the longer duration of delay in referral compared to EE patients. Patients might have had to go to the private sector because their insurance did not cover care in the public sector. The British Society of Pediatric and Adolescent Rheumatology stressed the importance of early recognition of JIA and prompt referral, with a target of 2 weeks from disease onset to the first appointment in pediatric rheumatology, as this would improve outcomes among JIA patients [19].

There is still lack of awareness among health professionals of the presentations of JIA, hence the lengthy referral time to pediatric rheumatology, lack of referral to opthalmology and multiple professionals assessing the child prior to referral. We know from documented literature in the west that doctors do not feel confident in carrying out musculoskeletal examination [20, 21], as pediatric rheumatology is not part of the core curriculum in most of medical schools [22]. Children with JIA usually present to general pediatricians, orthopedic doctors, and adult rheumatologists, who rely on their experience and teaching during medical school.

We carried out a survey of our group of 40 pediatric residents in training in the two teaching hospitals in the capital city prior to delivering musculoskeletal (MSK) teaching session. The results showed that 39 of the 40 residents did not have a method for MSK screening examination in children and did not feel confident in screening the musculoskeletal system in children presenting with joint pain "unpublished data".

Geographical factors could have been a reason for the delay of presentation for some of our patients. The UAE spans over 83,600 km^2, with a population of 9,346,129 [4], and is made up of seven emirates.

There is a visiting consultant once a month in the private sector and an experienced pediatrician in the public sector providing pediatric rheumatology in other area of the country. This could have partially influenced the results.

We identified more non-EE children than EE children presenting with systemic subtype who were acutely unwell. Non-EE children are more likely to come to the hospital if they are acutely unwell, and they tend to wait longer if presenting with other subtypes of JIA with a chronic history. This has been reported previously in the literature for oligoarticular disease [23], and may explain why we only had six persistent oligoarticular JIA cases in the non-EE group and an equal number of polyarticular JIA in both groups. Oligoarticular patients are not acutely unwell, and non-EE patients dependent on healthcare insurance coverage are more likely to present to private healthcare clinics.

We believe that public awareness is important in our population, as 45% of EE and 39% of non-EE initial appointments were a result of self-referral this can be partly explained by socioeconomic factors. It has been previously reported in the literature that patients from South Asian communities and with a higher level of education are more likely to present early, reflecting the parents' empowerment [24, 25]. However, the majority of non-EE children's parents are migrant workers of less privileged socioeconomic backgrounds, and these families opted to self-refer for their children to get appropriate treatment. More EE patients came through self-referral, which reflects easier access to public sector compared to non-EE patients.

There was significant over use of oral steroids in both groups prior to referral to pediatric rheumatology, including oligoarticular patients, as there was limited access to joint injections with steroids under general anesthetic.

Type of health care insurance cover did not affect type of treatment provided as 10 out of 33 EE patients and 15 out of 33 non-EE patients received biological therapy. This could be due to the fact that we had more systemic and less oligoarticular non-EE patients. For EE patients the government funds biological therapy. For non-EE patients the funding is through insurance cover. There are also government schemes, which can be obtained for children needing biologics with inadequate health insurance cover. However, we believe our numbers might not be a true reflection of the overall care of children needing biologics, as our numbers for non-EE children are lower than what is expected for our population.

We identified two cases with disability, one in each group. The child with blindness had periods of poor compliance and failure to follow up while under treatment. The other child also had periods of non-compliance and sought alternative therapy with over-use of steroids, resulting in avascular necrosis of the hip. The rate of disability is probably underrepresented, in view of the retrospective nature of this work. We found that most children with only uveitis are looked after by ophthalmologists alone, and referral rates from orthopedics to pediatric rheumatology are low. We are conducting two separate studies to look at these issues.

Education is one important aspect to improve access to pediatric rheumatology care over the next 10 years in the UAE. This can possibly be achieved by incorporating musculoskeletal examination in to the core curriculum of our medical students. Foster's pediatric Gait, Arms, Leg and Spine exam is a simple tool that can be used [26]. Also increasing education for resident trainees on musculoskeletal examination, JIA and other rheumatic conditions is needed. Developing postgraduate courses for family doctors, pediatricians, emergency doctors and orthopedic surgeons would potentially improve access to care and reduce delay in referrals. Following these changes our study can be repeated to access improvement of access to care in the UAE.

Comprehensive care for our patients should be provided through multidisciplinary networks, including both public and private, to address all aspects of care for our children with arthritis.

Conclusions

Delay in presentation to pediatric rheumatology have been identified as an important factor in our population, which is multi-cultural and which represents many socioeconomic backgrounds. The reasons for delays are likely multi-factorial. Access to care, lack of awareness, clinical skills, professional networks, and geographical factors all may play a role. Type of health care insurance cover did not affect number of patients getting biological therapy once patient seen in the pediatric rheumatology service. We are currently working with other healthcare providers to address access to care.

Abbreviations

ACR: American College of Rheumatology; CHAQ: Child Health Assessment Questionnaire; CRF: Clinical research form; DMARD: Disease-modifying antirheumatic drug; EE: Emirati-Emiratis (holds Emirati nationality, as stated on Emirates identity card); EMR: Electronic medical records; ICD: International Statistical Classification of Diseases and Related Health Problems; ILAR: International League of Associations for Rheumatology; JIA: Juvenile Idiopathic Arthritis; MSK: Musculoskeletal system; Non-EE: Nationality other than Emiratis stated on Emirates identity card; RF: Rheumatoid factor; UAE: United Arab Emirates

Acknowledgments

We thank all of the children and their families for allowing us to use their data.

Funding

The authors declare they have not received any funding for this study.

Authors' contributions

KK and MM: design of study, data collection, analysis of results, drafting the manuscript, editing the manuscript. Both authors read and approved the final manuscript.

Competing interests

The authors declare they have no competing interests of care.

Consent for publication

Not applicable.

References

1. Ravelli A, Martini A. Juvenile idiopathic arthritis. Lancet. 2007;369:767–78.
2. Petty RE, Southwood TR, Manners P, Baum J, Glass DN, Goldenberg J, et al. International League of Associations for Rheumatology classification of juvenile idiopathic arthritis: second revision, Edmonton 2001. J Rheumatol. 2004;31:390–2.
3. The World Bank, total population data by country. http://data.worldbank.org. Accessed 1 Apr 2016.
4. UAE National Bureau of Statistics. www.scad.ae. Accessed 1 Apr 2016.
5. AlMaini M, Adelowo F, AlSaleh J, AlWeshahi Y, Burmester GR, et al. The global challenges and opportunities in the practice of rheumatology: white paper by the World Forum on Rheumatic and Musculoskeletal Diseases. Clin Rheumatol. 2015;34(5):819–29.
6. Albers HM, Wessels JA, van der Straaten RJ, Brinkman DM, Suijlekom-Smit LW, Kamphuis SS, et al. Time to treatment as an important factor for the response to methotrexate in juvenile idiopathic arthritis. Arthritis Rheum. 2009;61:46–51.
7. Sherry DD, Stein LD, Reed AM, Schanberg LE, Kredich DW. Prevention of leg length discrepancy in young children with pauciarticular juvenile rheumatoid arthritis by treatment with intraarticular steroids. Arthritis Rheum. 1999;42:2330–4.
8. Chia A, Lee V, Graham EM, Edelsten C. Factors related to severe uveitis at diagnosis in children with juvenile idiopathic arthritis in a screening program. Am J Ophthalmol. 2003;135:757–62.
9. Tzaribachev N, Benseler SM, Tyrrell PN, Meyer A, Kuemmerle-Deschner JB. Predictors of delayed referral to a pediatric rheumatology center. Arthritis Rheum. 2009;61:1367–72.
10. Shiff NJ, Abdwani R, Cabral DA, Houghton KM, Malleson PN, Petty RE, et al. Access to pediatric rheumatology subspecialty care in British Columbia, Canada. J Rheumatol. 2009;36:410–5.
11. Adib N, Hyrich K, Thornton J, Lunt M, Davidson J, Gardner-Medwin J, et al. Association between duration of symptoms and severity of disease at first presentation to pediatric rheumatology: results from the Childhood Arthritis Prospective Study. Rheumatology. 2008;47:991–5.
12. Foster HE, Eltringham MS, Kay LJ, Friswell M, Abinun M, Myers A. Delay in access to appropriate care for children presenting with musculoskeletal symptoms and ultimately diagnosed with juvenile idiopathic arthritis. Arthritis Rheum. 2007;57:921–7.
13. Shapiro C, Maenz L, Hossain A, Pahwa P, Rosenberg A. Onset to first visit intervals in childhood rheumatic diseases. J Rheumatol. 2007;34:1913–7.
14. Arguedas O, Fasth A, Andersson-Gare B. A prospective population based study on outcome of juvenile chronic arthritis in Costa Rica. J Rheumatol. 2002;29:174–83.
15. Minden K, Kiessling U, Listing J, Niewerth M, Döring E, Meincke J, et al. Prognosis of patients with juvenile chronic arthritis and juvenile spondyloarthropathy. J Rheumatol. 2000;27:2256–63.
16. Manners PJ. Delay in diagnosing juvenile arthritis. Med J Aust. 1999;171:367–9.
17. Gare BA, Fasth A. The natural history of juvenile chronic arthritis: a population based cohort study. I. Onset and disease process. J Rheumatol. 1995;22:295–307.
18. Shiff NJ, Tucker LB, Guzman J, Oen K, Yeun RA, Duffy C. Factors associated with longer time to access pediatric rheumatologist in Canadian children with Juvenile Idiopathic Arthritis. J Rheumatol. 2010;37(11):2415–21.
19. Davies K, Cleary G, Foster H, Hutchinson E, Baildam E, British Society of Pediatric and Adolescent Rheumatology. BSPAR standards of care for children and young people with juvenile idiopathic arthritis. Rheumatology. 2010;49:1406–8.
20. Jandial S, Myers A, Wise E, Foster HE. Doctors likely to encounter children with musculoskeletal complaints have low confidence in their clinical skills. J Pediatr. 2009;154:267–71.
21. Bonds DE, Mychaleckyj JC, Watkins R, Palla S, Extrom P. Ambulatory care skills: do residents feel prepared? Med Educ Online. 2002;7:7.
22. Jandial S, Rapley T, Foster H. Current teaching of pediatric musculoskeletal medicine within UK medical schools—a need for change. Rheumatology. 2009;48:587–90.
23. Guillaume S, Prieur AM, Coste J, Job-Deslandre C. Long-term outcome and prognosis in oligoarticular-onset juvenile idiopathic arthritis. Arthritis Rheum. 2000;43:1858–65.
24. Foster H, Rapley T. Access to pediatric rheumatology care—a major challenge to improving outcome in Juvenile Idiopathic Arthritis. J Rheumatol. 2015;37(11):2199–202.
25. Dixon-Woods M, Findlay M, Young B, Cox H, Heney D. Parents' accounts of obtaining a diagnosis of childhood cancer. Lancet. 2001;357:670–4.
26. Foster HE, Jandial S. pGALS–paediatric Gait Arms Legs and Spine: a simple examination of the musculoskeletal system. Pediatr Rheumatol. 2013;11:44.

16

Cardiac findings in children with juvenile Dermatomyositis at disease presentation

Serdar Cantez[1], Gil J. Gross[2], Ian MacLusky[3] and Brian M. Feldman[4*]

Abstract

Background: Juvenile Dermatomyositis (JDM) is a pediatric vasculopathy characterized primarily by skin and muscle involvement. Cardiac findings have been reported in children with JDM but have rarely been investigated in detail.

Methods: We aimed to describe the relevant clinical and laboratory cardiac findings of a cohort of patients with JDM, followed at one centre, at disease diagnosis.

Results: We performed a retrospective review of 105 patients with JDM, followed from 1991 to 2007. Six of 70 patients (9%, 6% of the entire cohort) had abnormal electrocardiographic (ECG) findings, while 26 of 54 patients (48%, 25% of the entire cohort) had abnormal echocardiographic (echo) findings. Many of these findings were either mild or unlikely to be a result of JDM.

Conclusions: Our findings suggest that cardiac abnormalities at JDM disease onset are frequently seen, but are rarely significant findings due to disease; however, JDM patients should be considered for screening for cardiac disease as late cardiac complications are well recognized.

Keywords: Juvenile dermatomyositis, Heart disease, Screening

Background

Juvenile Dermatomyositis (JDM) is characterized by a small vessel vasculopathy affecting children, characterized primarily by skin and muscle involvement. The etiology of JDM is not yet known [1]. Typical clinical findings of JDM include proximal muscle weakness, heliotrope rash, Gottron's papules, nail fold capillary changes, skin calcifications and swallowing difficulties [2].

Cardiac abnormalities, sometimes serious, have been reported among the less common findings in JDM patients [2]. For example, Ravelli et al. have published long-term outcome and prognostic factors for JDM patients [3]. From Europe and Latin America 27 centers participated in this multicentre study, and 490 patients' data was collected. They found that the cumulative frequency of damage to the cardiovascular system was 2.9% for 445 patients. Specific cardiac pathology and/or ECG and echo findings were not described in that study. Additionally, Pachman et al. reported a cohort of 21 patients with JDM. They found that 10 of 20 children had ECG abnormalities [4]. ECG changes were also examined in a study of 61 Korean juvenile and adult dermatomyositis patients [5]. In this study, ECG abnormalities were present in 6 of 14 JDM patients (37.5%); 3 patients had right bundle branch block and another 3 had ST changes. In a further study, Rider et al. aimed to validate the myositis damage index (MDI) [6]. In this article, they evaluated both adult polymyositis (PM) patients and JDM patients. Cardiovascular damage was more common in patients with PM than JDM; for the children, 2.8% had hypertension, and 0.7% had ventricular dysfunction.

ECG and echo changes have been recently investigated in a case-control study from Norway [7]. Sixty-one patients with an age and sex matched control group of healthy individuals were enrolled. This study aimed to compare cardiac findings of JDM patients with controls. Patients' ECG and echo findings were investigated an average of 16.8 years after the disease diagnosis. In this study 7 patients developed pericarditis, 12 had hypertension, defined as systolic blood pressure > 140 mmHg, 10

* Correspondence: brian.feldman@sickkids.ca
[4]Department of Pediatrics, Faculty of Medicine, and the Institute of Health Policy, Management & Evaluation, the Dalla Lana School of Public Health,, University of Toronto, Division of Rheumatology, The Hospital for Sick Children, Toronto, Canada
Full list of author information is available at the end of the article

patients had abnormal ECG findings (3 poor R-wave progression, 2 left ventricular hypertrophy, 2 right bundle branch block, one pathological Q-wave, one P pulmonale and one prolonged QTc). Using a similar design, the same group showed that heart rate variability is reduced in JDM patients (followed a median 13.5 years after disease diagnosis) [8], and that long-axis strain was reduced (a marker of systolic dysfunction on echo) in JDM patients followed a median of 16.8 years after diagnosis [9].

Cardiac disease may be serious in JDM and may be a cause of death. In a large series of North American children, heart disease contributed to mortality in 3 of 17 deaths in 329 patients. However, only 1 death (a child with myocarditis) appeared to be directly caused by cardiac disease [10].

Although the Norway studies are very important for demonstrating damage during follow-up, they do not give us information about cardiac findings at onset (the period when disease activity is often the highest). Early cardiac findings in JDM have rarely been investigated in detail; we therefore asked, what is the frequency of ECG and/or echo abnormalities seen at disease diagnosis in children with JDM?

Methods

This study was approved by the Research Ethics Board at The Hospital for Sick Children, Toronto (SickKids). In our institution, every suspected JDM patient undergoes a detailed physical examination and a series of laboratory investigations including, for many, a cardiac work-up with electrocardiogram (ECG) and echocardiogram (echo).

We reviewed 105 patients newly diagnosed and followed at SickKids between 1991 and 2007. At each patient's initial admission and/or first consultation visit, demographic data was noted, detailed physical examination including heart rate, blood pressure, skin examination, muscle weakness assessment and laboratory investigations were recorded, most often including a 12-lead ECG and standard transthoracic two-dimensional, M-mode, and Doppler echo assessment. All patients have been followed by a single pediatric rheumatologist, in a specialized JDM Clinic (BMF), and all have been treated according to our published standardized treatment plan [11].

For this retrospective study, demographic data and clinical findings, ECG and echo findings were obtained from clinical charts, rheumatology and cardiology clinic databases. All ECG and echo findings were reviewed by a single experienced pediatric cardiologist (GG). Heart rhythm, PR interval, corrected QT interval (QTc) and QRS duration were re-measured.

A standardized protocol had been used for all echocardiographic examinations [12]. For interpretation, we used institutional standardized z-scores, similar to those published [13], which our group has used in many publications. ECG standards followed previously published guidelines [14].

Descriptive statistics have been used to present our findings (proportions for categorical variables, means and medians with measures of spread as appropriate). Calculations were done with DataDesk 8.0.0 (Data Description, Inc., Ithaca, NY) and Microsoft Excel 15.35 (Microsoft, Redmond, WA).

Results

105 patients (72 female) were included. Median age at the time of diagnosis was 6.9 years (range 2.0–17.6 years). Median time of follow up, at the time of our review, was 10.2 years (7 months – 15.8 years). (Table 1).

Electrocardiograms were available for 69 patients. Thirty-six patients either did not have ECGs done, or the ECG was no longer retrievable.

Six patients had abnormal ECG findings (9%). QTc findings for all 69 patients were as follows: mean 416 ms, range of values 370–509 ms. QTc was abnormally prolonged in 5 patients. (Mean abnormal QTc was 462 ms.) Mean PR interval was 131 ms (94–214 ms). Mean QRS duration was 78.3 ms (56–112 ms). One patient had prolonged PR interval and wide QRS. (This patient also had moderate pulmonary insufficiency and mitral regurgitation by echo.)

Echo was available for 52 patients, of which 26 were normal (Table 2). Three patients had pericardial effusions; one of them was small and one was considered "trivial". Isolated tricuspid regurgitation was seen in 3 patients. Six patients had tricuspid regurgitation combined with

Table 1 Demographics

N	105 (72 girls)
Median (range of values) age at diagnosis, years	6.9 (2.0–17.6)
Median (range of values) follow-up time, years	10.2 (0.6–15.8)
Diagnosis	
JDM	102
Hypomyopathic JDM	1
Overlap myositis	1
Polymyositis	1
Number of Patients with ECG	69
Normal	63
Abnormal	6
Number of Patients with ECHO	52
Normal	26
Abnormal	26

Table 2 ECG and ECHO Abnormalities

Abnormality	Number	Percent
ECG		
Normal	63	91.3
Prolonged QTc	5	7.2
Prolonged PR + wide QRS	1	1.4
ECHO		
Normal	26	50.0
THLAA	1	1.9
PER EFF	3	5.8
TR + PI	6	11.5
TR + PI + MR	1	1.9
TR	3	5.8
ASD	1	1.9
VSD	1	1.9
AI + PI	1	1.9
PDA + DIL LA + LV	1	1.9
PI	3	5.8
MVP + MR + PI	1	1.9
↑RVED dimension	1	1.9
↑ IVRT + TR + PI	1	1.9
PI + MR	1	1.9
↓ PV D wave vel.	1	1.9

pulmonary insufficiency. One patient had both aortic and pulmonary insufficiency. Isolated pulmonary insufficiency was seen in 3, all considered trivial. One patient had mitral valve prolapse and mild mitral regurgitation and pulmonary insufficiency. Mitral regurgitation with pulmonary insufficiency was seen in one patient. One patient was found to have increased right ventricular end diastolic dimension. Another patient had decreased pulmonary vein D-wave velocity. Four patients had conditions that are almost certainly incidentally identified congenital abnormalities, and therefore unrelated to JDM: patent ductus arteriosus (PDA) with dilated left atrium and left ventricle, tubular hypoplasia of left aortic arch (THLAA), atrial septal defect, and ventricular septal defect. Ventricular function (left ventricular ejection fraction) was normal in all.

The cardiac findings are listed along with the clinical features of JDM at diagnosis in Table 3.

Discussion

Our results suggest that many JDM patients have abnormal ECG and echo results at first presentation. Some of the findings, though, were mild and unlikely to be related to the underlying disease; for example, mild tricuspid regurgitation and/or pulmonary insufficiency are common and not necessarily abnormal. Although none of our patients presented with clinically serious cardiac dysfunction, and many of our patients had findings commonly seen in children without JDM, we believe that the high incidence of abnormalities is a reasonable justification for a cardiac work-up at disease onset. This, coupled with the reported accumulation over time of cardiac damage, suggests to us that careful cardiac monitoring over the disease course should be carried out in JDM patients [6, 7, 9].

We found more abnormalities at the outset of disease than other authors have seen over the course of the illness.[3] This is likely because we used laboratory examinations to determine cardiac abnormalities; none of our patients were symptomatic, and none developed clinically meaningful cardiac disease during follow-up (although few had detailed laboratory examinations repeated over time as most were both asymptomatic and had normal heart rates and normal blood pressures for the duration of follow-up).

Our study should be interpreted in the light of possible limitations. Because our cohort goes back to the early 1990s, we have been unable to find some ECG and echo data; some patients did not have these investigations and others went missing. The implications of these

Table 3 JDM measures sorted by cardiac abnormality

		Manual Muscle Testing (/10)[a] [15]					Heliotrope rash			Gottron's sign/papules			Other skin rash			Nail fold capillaries		
		n	median	IQR	min	max	n	Abnormal	%	n	Abnormal	%	n	Abnormal	%	n	Abnormal	%
ECHO	All (*n* = 105)	98	8	2	0	10	105	69	65.7	104	79	76.0	98	76	77.6	97	82	84.5
	Abnormal (*n* = 26)	26	8	3.75	0	10	26	19	73.1	26	21	80.8	25	19	76.0	24	21	87.5
	Normal (*n* = 26)	26	8	2.5	2	10	26	18	69.2	25	18	72.0	26	21	80.8	25	23	92.0
	Not done (*n* = 53)	46	8	1	2	10	53	32	60.4	53	40	75.5	47	36	76.6	48	38	79.2
ECG	All (*n* = 105)	98	8	2	0	10	105	69	65.7	104	79	76.0	98	76	77.6	97	82	84.5
	Normal (*n* = 63)	60	8	2.25	0	10	63	45	71.4	62	49	79.0	62	51	82.3	61	55	90.2
	Abnormal (*n* = 6)	6	8	1.5	5	10	6	4	66.7	6	6	100.0	6	5	83.3	6	5	83.3
	Not done (*n* = 36)	32	8	1.25	2	10	36	20	55.6	36	24	66.7	30	20	66.7	30	22	73.3

[a]As determined by the weakest muscle group at presentation using the 10-point Kendall scale

missing data are unclear; however, as described above, none of these patients has gone on to have important cardiac morbidity.

Conclusion

In conclusion, children with new onset JDM have a high frequency of cardiac abnormalities, mostly minor, as determined by ECG and echocardiography. We recommend that a cardiac workup should be considered in the initial workup for every suspected JDM patient.

Abbreviations

ECG: Electrocardiogram; Echo: Echocardiogram; JDM: Juvenile dermatomyositis; MDI: Myositis damage index; PDA: Patent ductus arteriosus; PM: Polymyositis; QTc: Corrected QT interval; THLAA: Tubular hypoplasia of left aortic arch

Acknowledgements

Not applicable.

Funding

Not applicable.

Authors' contributions

SC and BF contributed to data collection. All authors gave input with design of the study, interpretation of the data, as well as drafting, reviewing and approval of the final manuscript.

Consent for publication

Not applicable.

Competing interests

The authors declare that they have no competing interests.

Author details

[1]Department of Pediatrics, Istanbul University, Istanbul Faculty of Medicine, Istanbul, Turkey. [2]Department of Pediatrics, University of Toronto, Division of Cardiology, The Hospital for Sick Children, Toronto, Canada. [3]Department of Pediatrics, University of Ottawa; Division of Respirology, the Childrens' Hospital of Eastern Ontario, Ottawa, Canada. [4]Department of Pediatrics, Faculty of Medicine, and the Institute of Health Policy, Management & Evaluation, the Dalla Lana School of Public Health,, University of Toronto, Division of Rheumatology, The Hospital for Sick Children, Toronto, Canada.

References

1. Feldman BM, Rider LG, Reed AM, Pachman LM. Juvenile dermatomyositis and other idiopathic inflammatory myopathies of childhood. Lancet. 2008 Jun 28;371(9631):2201–12.
2. Ramanan AV, Feldman BM. Clinical features and outcomes of juvenile dermatomyositis and other childhood onset myositis syndromes. Rheum Dis Clin N Am. [Review]. 2002 Nov;28(4):833-857.
3. Ravelli A, Trail L, Ferrari C, Ruperto N, Pistorio A, Pilkington C, et al. Long-term outcome and prognostic factors of juvenile dermatomyositis: a multinational, multicenter study of 490 patients. Arthritis Care Res (Hoboken). [Comparative Study Multicenter Study Research Support, Non-U. S. Gov't]. 2010 Jan 15;62(1):63-72.
4. Pachman LM, Cooke N. Juvenile dermatomyositis: a clinical and immunologic study. J Pediatr. [Research Support, U.S. Gov't, P.H.S.]. 1980 Feb;96(2):226-234.
5. Na SJ, Kim SM, Sunwoo IN, Choi YC. Clinical characteristics and outcomes of juvenile and adult dermatomyositis. J Korean Med Sci. [Case Reports]. 2009 Aug;24(4):715-721.
6. Rider LG, Lachenbruch PA, Monroe JB, Ravelli A, Cabalar I, Feldman BM, et al. Damage extent and predictors in adult and juvenile dermatomyositis and polymyositis as determined with the myositis damage index. Arthritis Rheum. [Comparative Study Research Support, N.I.H., Extramural Research Support, Non-U.S. Gov't]. 2009 Nov;60(11):3425-3435.
7. Schwartz T, Sanner H, Husebye T, Flato B, Sjaastad I. Cardiac dysfunction in juvenile dermatomyositis: a case-control study. Ann Rheum Dis. [Research Support, Non-U.S. Gov't]. 2011 May;70(5):766-771.
8. Barth Z, Nomeland Witczak B, Schwartz T, Gjesdal K, Flato B, Koller A, et al. In juvenile dermatomyositis, heart rate variability is reduced, and associated with both cardiac dysfunction and markers of inflammation: a cross-sectional study median 13.5 years after symptom onset. Rheumatology (Oxford). 2016;55(3): 535-43. doi:10.1093/rheumatology/kev376. Epub 2015 Oct 24.
9. Schwartz T, Sanner H, Gjesdal O, Flato B, Sjaastad I. In juvenile dermatomyositis, cardiac systolic dysfunction is present after long-term follow-up and is predicted by sustained early skin activity. Ann Rheum Dis. 2014;73(10):1805–10.
10. Huber AM, Mamyrova G, Lachenbruch PA, Lee JA, Katz JD, Targoff IN, et al. Early illness features associated with mortality in the juvenile idiopathic inflammatory myopathies. Arthritis Care Res (Hoboken). 2014;66(5):732–40.
11. Ramanan AV, Campbell-Webster N, Ota S, Parker S, Tran D, Tyrrell PN, et al. The effectiveness of treating juvenile dermatomyositis with methotrexate and aggressively tapered corticosteroids. Arthritis Rheum. 2005;52(11):3570–8.
12. Lai WW, Geva T, Shirali GS, Frommelt PC, Humes RA, Brook MM, et al. Guidelines and standards for performance of a pediatric echocardiogram: a report from the task force of the pediatric Council of the American Society of echocardiography. J Am Soc Echocardiogr. 2006;19(12):1413–30.
13. Daubeney PE, Blackstone EH, Weintraub RG, Slavik Z, Scanlon J, Webber SA. Relationship of the dimension of cardiac structures to body size: an echocardiographic study in normal infants and children. Cardiol Young. 1999;9(4):402–10.
14. Davignon A, Rautaharju P, Boisselle E, Soumis F, Megelas M, Choquette A. Normal ECG standards for infants and children. Pediatr Cardiol. 1980;1(2):123–31.
15. IMACS. Manual muscle testing procedures. [cited 2017 June 29]; Available from: https://www.niehs.nih.gov/research/resources/assets/docs/muscle_grading_and_testing_procedures_508.pdf. Accessed 7 July 2017.

Telemedicine and other care models in pediatric rheumatology: an exploratory study of parents' perceptions of barriers to care and care preferences

Danielle R. Bullock[1*], Richard K. Vehe[1], Lei Zhang[2] and Colleen K. Correll[1]

Abstract

Background: The United States pediatric rheumatology workforce is committed to a mission of providing children access to pediatric rheumatology care. With a limited number and distribution of pediatric rheumatologists, telemedicine has been proposed as one way to meet this mission, yet the adoption of this modality has been slower than expected. The purpose of this study was to explore the parent perspective on barriers to accessing pediatric rheumatology care and to explore the acceptability of telemedicine and other alternative care models.

Methods: Over a period of six weeks, all new and return English-speaking parents/guardians of patients visiting a single center were offered an opportunity to complete a survey which assessed barriers to care and interest in alternative models of care. Responses were analyzed using descriptive statistics.

Results: Survey response rate was 72% (159/221). Twenty-eight percent (45/159) traveled more than three hours to the pediatric rheumatology clinic, and 43% (65/152) reported travel as inconvenient. An overwhelming majority of respondents (95%, 144/152) reported a preference for in-person visits over the option of telemedicine. This preference was similar regardless of whether respondents reported travel to the clinic as inconvenient vs convenient (inconvenient 92%, 60/65; convenient 97%, 84/87; $p = 0.2881$) and despite those reporting travel as inconvenient also reporting greater difficulty with several barriers to care. Those familiar with telemedicine were more likely to report a preference for telemedicine over in-person visits (27%, 3/11 vs 3%, 4/140; $p = 0.0087$). The option of an outreach clinic was acceptable to a majority (63%, 97/154); however, adult rheumatology and shared-care options were less acceptable (22%, 35/156 and 34%, 53/156 respectively).

Conclusion: Among survey respondents, in-person visits were preferred over the option of telemedicine, even when travel was noted to be inconvenient. Telemedicine familiarity increased its acceptability. Outreach clinics were acceptable to a majority. Ultimately, the parent perspective can shape acceptable ways to address barriers and provide accessible care.

Keywords: Access, Barriers, Outreach, Pediatric rheumatology, Telemedicine

* Correspondence: brue0190@umn.edu
[1]Division of Pediatric Rheumatology, Department of Pediatrics, University of Minnesota, East Bldg Rm M668, 2450 Riverside Ave, Minneapolis, MN 55454, USA
Full list of author information is available at the end of the article

Background

The pediatric rheumatology (PR) workforce is committed to a mission of providing children with access to care and superior clinical outcomes [1]. With rheumatic diseases affecting more than 300,000 children in the United States (US), the PR workforce of approximately 300 pediatric rheumatologists, primarily concentrated at academic institutions, faces many challenges in achieving this mission [2]. Recognizing a clear deficit in the number and distribution of pediatric rheumatologists, a 2007 report to Congress recommended several remedies, including piloting telemedicine networks [2]. This was echoed in a more recent 2011 examination of the PR workforce [1], and telemedicine has also been viewed as a promising solution to access concerns in adult rheumatology [3]. Other solutions, such as shared-care, in which patients are co-managed with community-based physicians, have also been proposed [2].

Despite probable benefits, telemedicine adoption has been slower than expected. Studies in other areas of medicine, including but not limited to adult rheumatology and other pediatric subspecialties, have reported high levels of satisfaction with telemedicine [3–5]; however, the acceptability is not universal. A recent survey which sampled households in rural Montana reported that a high percentage of respondents were unequivocally averse to using telemedicine for their healthcare, despite the inconvenience of in-person visits [6]. Additional concerns include the clinical effectiveness of telemedicine in a specialty highly dependent on the physical examination, cost effectiveness, and the quality of the patient-physician relationship, all of which would need to be addressed for successful adoption in the PR community [7–9].

Few PR clinics currently use telemedicine, and there is only one publication describing its use for PR patients [10]. This study found that telemedicine interest was greater for those living further from the tertiary care center and among those spending more time away from work [10]. As additional PR clinics consider telemedicine adoption, more research is needed to understand how certain factors might contribute to or hinder telemedicine success. In other areas of medicine, various predictors of and barriers to telemedicine adoption have been explored (e.g. age, Internet use, digital literacy, rural residence, perceived privacy), yet conclusive evidence on many of these remains elusive [11, 12]. Additionally, because telemedicine is unlikely to be appropriate for all patients, the acceptability of other care models should also be explored.

The purpose of this survey study was to delineate barriers to PR care and to explore the acceptability of alternative PR care models, with an emphasis on telemedicine, among a population of PR patients in the Upper Midwest. Specific objectives were 1) to explore the parent/guardian perspective on barriers to accessing PR care and to identify factors associated with discrepant barrier perceptions, 2) to assess whether a telemedicine option, if available, might be preferred over in-person care, 3) to identify factors influencing opinions about telemedicine use, and 4) to examine the acceptability of other care models, including outreach clinics, adult rheumatology care, and shared-care.

Methods

Patients

All new or return English-speaking parents/guardians of patients who visited the University of Minnesota PR Clinic during a six-week period in 2015 were eligible. This was a convenience sample since only those coming to the clinic during this time period were offered the survey. Patients 18 years of age or older were allowed to complete the survey independently.

Survey design and administration

Review of the PR workforce literature, barriers to accessing care, and telemedicine informed development of the survey, which was deemed exempt by the University of Minnesota Institutional Review Board (IRB). Parents/guardians were given a paper copy of the survey at the time of their child's PR appointment. Survey responses included multiple choice answers as well as "choose all that apply" options. A five dollar gift card was given for survey completion.

Survey questions included demographics as well as the child's diagnosis, length of time the child was a patient in the clinic, and travel time to the clinic. A subjective assessment of whether travel was convenient vs inconvenient was also included. Eleven potential barriers to accessing care were assessed: availability of appointment dates/times, travel time/distance, need for lodging, adequate transportation, driving in the metropolitan, direct costs (medical bills, medications, etc.), indirect costs (gas, hotel, food, etc.), child missing school, parent/guardian missing work, arranging care for other children, and insurance approval for visits. These were scored on a 0 (no difficulty) to 10 (difficult enough to stop you from getting health care for your child) scale. Visit preference (in-person vs telemedicine), familiarity with telemedicine (personal telemedicine use and/or having a close family member or friend who had used telemedicine), and subjective assessment of telemedicine quality were examined. Finally, the acceptability of outreach clinics, adult rheumatology, and shared-care were explored. Since the care model for the University of Minnesota PR Division at the time of this survey consisted of only in-person visits at the academic center, the respondent assessment of alternative care models was based on a brief description of these modalities and any personal experience outside of the clinic. A copy of the survey can be viewed as an additional file (see Additional file 1).

Survey analysis

Responses were summarized using descriptive statistics, expressed as frequencies and percent, or mean ± standard deviation (SD)/median and interquartile range (IQR). Due to small, non-normally distributed data or small sample size, Kruskal-Wallis test was used for group comparisons of continuous variables. For categorical variables, Fisher's exact test was used to compare groups. All analyses were done using the SAS system (v. 9.3; SAS Institute, Cary, NC). *P*-values were two-sided with <0.05 considered statistically significant. Bonferroni adjustment was applied for multiple comparisons. Missing data were excluded from analyses using pairwise deletion, and the values in the reported results reflect that some respondents did not answer all survey questions.

Results

Patient characteristics

The response rate was 72% (159/221). Twenty-four percent (38/159) of the respondents were parents/guardians of new patients to the clinic; the remainder were follow-up visits. Patient characteristics are listed in Table 1. The majority were parents/guardians of adolescent Caucasian patients and had private insurance. Most patients carried a diagnosis of juvenile idiopathic arthritis (JIA). Geographic distribution of patients included Minnesota, Wisconsin, North Dakota, and South Dakota with 52% (82/159) traveling more than one hour and 28% (45/159) traveling more than three hours to the clinic. Due to survey anonymity, characteristics of non-responders could not be assessed.

Table 1 Patient characteristics

Characteristic	Classification	N (%)[a]
Age	< 6	15 (9.4)
	6–12	65 (40.9)
	≥ 13	76 (47.8)
Ethnicity	White	136 (85.5)
	Non-white	21 (13.2)
Insurance	Private	113 (71.1)
	Public	43 (27.0)
	None	1 (0.6)
Primary diagnosis	Juvenile idiopathic arthritis	90 (56.6)
	Not yet determined	26 (16.4)
	Other	10 (6.3)
	Juvenile dermatomyositis	7 (4.4)
	Uveitis/iritis	6 (3.8)
	Chronic recurrent multifocal osteomyelitis	4 (2.5)
	Spondyloarthropathy	3 (1.9)
	Systemic lupus erythematosus	3 (1.9)
	Mixed connective tissue disease	3 (1.9)
	Periodic fever	2 (1.3)
	Psoriasis	1 (0.6)
	Reactive arthritis	1 (0.6)
	Behcet's disease	1 (0.6)
	Amplified musculoskeletal pain	1 (0.6)
Travel time	≤ 1 h	76 (47.8)
	> 1 h - ≤ 3 h	37 (23.3)
	> 3 h - ≤ 6 h	37 (23.3)
	> 6 h	8 (5.0)

[a]Percentages are out of 159 survey respondents. Some respondents did not answer all questions

Barriers to accessing care

The highest scoring barrier (0 being none and 10 being great) was the child missing school with a median of 2.50 (IQR 0.50–5.00), followed by travel time/distance and parent/guardian missing work, each with a median of 2.00 (IQR 0.50–5.00 and 0.00–5.00, respectively). Other median scores were as follows: availability of appointment dates/times (median 0.50, IQR 0.00–2.00), need for lodging (0.00, 0.00–1.00), adequate transportation (0.00, 0.00–0.50), driving in the metropolitan (0.50, 0.00–3.00), direct costs (0.50, 0.00–3.00), indirect costs (0.50, 0.00–3.00), arranging care for other children (0.00, 0.00–1.50), insurance approval for visits (0.00, 0.00–1.00).

Pairwise comparison revealed a statistically significant difference in arranging care for other children, with families whose child was less than six years old reporting a higher score (median 1.50, IQR 0.00–6.00) compared to families whose child was 13 years or older (0.00, 0.00–0.50; $p = 0.016$). Those with non-private insurance scored travel time/distance as a greater barrier than those with private insurance (median 3.75, IQR 0.75–5.50 vs 2.00, 0.50–5.00; $p = 0.0398$). Other pairwise comparisons between barrier scoring and patient factors (age, insurance, ethnicity, and diagnosis) revealed no significant differences.

Those who indicated travel as inconvenient vs convenient reported significantly greater difficulty with several barriers: travel time/distance (median 5.00, IQR 2.50–6.00 vs 1.00, 0.00–2.50; $p < 0.0001$), need for lodging/housing (0.25, 0.00–4.00 vs 0.00, 0.00–0.50; $p = 0.0047$), driving in the metropolitan (2.75, 0.00–5.00 vs 0.00, 0.00–1.00; $p < 0.0001$), indirect costs (2.50, 0.00–5.00 vs 0.00, 0.00–1.00; $p < 0.0001$), parent missing work (3.00, 1.00–6.00 vs 1.00, 0.00–3.00; $p < 0.0001$), child missing school (4.00, 1.25–6.25 vs 2.00, 0.50–3.50;

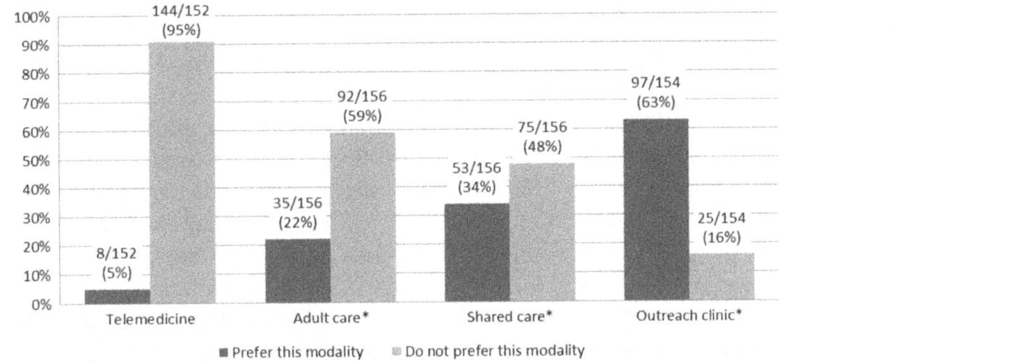

Fig. 1 Acceptability of alternative care models. Legend: * Respondents with neutral interest in these alternative care models are not represented in this figure

p = 0.0008), and arranging care for other children (0.25, 0.00–5.00 vs 0.00, 0.00–0.50; p = 0.0219). The overall distribution of travel times was different depending on whether care was perceived as inconvenient vs convenient (p < 0.0001). For those reporting travel as convenient, 71% traveled an hour or less, 17% traveled more than an hour to 3 h or less, 10% traveled more than 3 h to 6 h or less, and 1% traveled more than 6 h. For those reporting travel as inconvenient, 18% traveled an hour or less, 34% more than an hour to 3 h or less, 37% more than 3 h to 6 h or less, and 11% more than 6 h.

Telemedicine

An overwhelming majority of respondents (95%, 144/152) reported a preference for in-person visits over the option of telemedicine (Fig. 1). This preference was similar regardless of whether travel was inconvenient (inconvenient 92%, 60/65 vs convenient 97%, 84/87; p = 0.2881) and despite the inconvenient group reporting greater difficulty with several barriers.

Only 8% (13/158) of respondents reported familiarity with telemedicine. The majority of respondents (75%, 115/154) felt that they had inadequate knowledge about telemedicine to compare its quality to in-person visits; however, those familiar with telemedicine were more likely to report it as equal to or better than in-person visits (42%, 5/12 vs 8%, 11/142; p = 0.0033) and were also more likely to report a preference for telemedicine over in-person visits (Fig. 2).

The small number of respondents preferring a telemedicine option scored travel time/distance as a greater barrier compared to those preferring in-person visits (median 5.00, IQR 4.00–6.25 vs 2.00, 0.50–5.00; p = 0.0142). No other differences in barrier scores were detected between those preferring the option of telemedicine visits over in-person visits.

Neither views on telemedicine quality compared to in-person visits nor preference for in-person visits significantly differed by patient demographics, insurance type, length of time the child was a patient in the clinic, or travel time. Additionally, there was no detectable difference in median days of internet or video chat use between groups.

Other care models

Interest in adult rheumatology care (22%, 35/156) and shared-care management with an adult rheumatologist or primary physician (34%, 53/156) was low (Fig. 1). In contrast, 63% (97/154) indicated that outreach clinics would be an acceptable alternative to current tertiary center care (Fig. 1). There was no detectable difference in willingness to participate in a shared-care model of care based on the perceived comprehensiveness of the child's primary care clinic.

Travel time/distance was consistently scored as a significantly greater barrier among those interested vs not interested in alternative care models – adult rheumatology care (median 5.00, IQR 2.00–6.00 vs 1.75, 0.00–5.00; p = 0.0054), shared-care (4.50, 1.00–5.00 vs 1.00, 0.00–5.00; p = 0.0031), and outreach clinics (4.25, 1.00–5.50 vs 0.00, 0.00–1.00; p < 0.0001). Direct costs, indirect

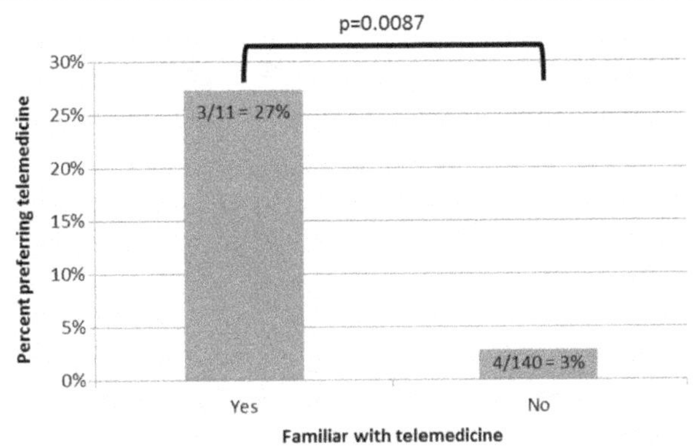

Fig. 2 Respondents familiar with telemedicine more accepting of this modality

costs, driving in the metropolitan, parent missing work, and child missing school were also scored as greater barriers among those interested in certain alternative care models (Additional file 2).

Separate from the travel time/distance barrier assessment, self-reported total travel time was also examined. Interest in adult rheumatology care did not differ based on travel time. For shared care and outreach clinics, the distribution of self-reported travel times differed depending on interest in these care models (Table 2).

Discussion

Health care access is a complex issue with many contributing factors. Availability and accessibility are just part of a bigger picture [13], yet clearly affect PR referral decisions among primary pediatricians, as shown in two recent survey studies [14, 15]. While solutions have been recommended to help remedy these concerns [1, 2], including piloting telemedicine networks and enhancing the rheumatology training of adult rheumatologists and primary care providers, no previous studies have examined the parent perspective on barriers to PR care or the perceived acceptability of proposed solutions.

We found that respondents in this survey reported few barriers to PR care. Certain features, such as having younger children or viewing travel as inconvenient, may affect barrier perceptions and should certainly be taken into account when considering a family's needs. This does not, however, necessarily translate into acceptance of alternative models. While some barriers, such as travel time/distance, were scored higher among those interested in alternative models, a majority of respondents still preferred the current care model. Even when travel was inconvenient, respondents strongly preferred in-person visits over the idea of telemedicine, and this was true even though several barriers were scored higher by those reporting travel as inconvenient. With limited resources, we must question whether improving care for children with rheumatic diseases should focus on expanding the reach of care or enriching current care models. It remains to be seen what barriers would truly be lessened by different alternative care models. As models are implemented, further research is needed to better quantify the trade-offs. A recent PR telemedicine study, for example, showed patients and families using telemedicine missed less time from school or work compared to usual tertiary center care [10]. Understanding, quantifying, and transparently sharing the ways in which alternative care models may reduce such barriers will be vital to gaining acceptability.

While most families scored barriers to care relatively low and reported a preference for the current care model, it is imperative to recognize that these preferences do not apply to all families. We should not underestimate the role that accessibility might play for some families. Though not a majority, accessibility was still a notable barrier among our survey respondents and specifically addressing this concern could contribute to the success of alternative models for certain families. Travel time/distance – an accessibility issue – was reported as a greater barrier among those who expressed interest in telemedicine, adult rheumatology care, shared-care, and outreach clinics. Further work is needed to understand what contributes to these barrier perceptions and when such perceptions are enough to tip the balance toward acceptance of alternative care models. Furthermore, it is easy to assume that an objective measure of access, such as distance from a care center, determines barriers and informs potential solutions. Our results demonstrate that such an approach fails to account for differences between parent perspective and objective measures. As mentioned, the acceptability of all alternative care models varied based on *parent-reported* barriers in travel time/distance. Actual travel times, however, gave more varied results. While there were differences in the actual travel time distribution for shared care and outreach clinics, we were unable to identify variations in acceptability of telemedicine and adult rheumatology care based on travel time. Additionally, while identifying travel time/distance as a barrier seemed to be one factor contributing to perceptions of whether travel was convenient vs inconvenient, other barriers also seemed to contribute to this perception. Parent perceptions about care accessibility and what contributes to this, then, are equally as important as the objective measures we often use as a proxy, and we need to be cautious about how

Table 2 Interest in shared care and outreach according to travel time

Care Model	Agree or Disagree[a]	Travel Time ≤ 1 h N (%)	> 1 - ≤ 3 h N (%)	> 3 - ≤ 6 h N (%)	> 6 h N (%)	*P*-value
Shared Care	Agree	17 (32)	17 (32)	16 (30)	3 (6)	0.0387
	Disagree	43 (58)	12 (16)	14 (19)	5 (7)	
Outreach	Agree	38 (40)	23 (24)	31 (32)	4 (4)	0.0041
	Disagree	16 (64)	7 (28)	0 (0)	2 (8)	

[a]Those with neutral interest are not displayed in this table

we apply such proxies. For example, providers sometimes refer patients to specialties more geographically accessible than PR due to the provider-perceived barrier of a long travel distance [14]. It is not clear that all parents would perceive this barrier in the same way, and we must consider the shortcoming of making such assumptions and find more effective ways to include family perspective in care decisions.

The assessment of additional alternative care models revealed that a majority of respondents were agreeable to outreach clinics. Adult rheumatology and shared-care, on the other hand, were not preferable by the majority, but some respondents were still agreeable to these. Our survey also revealed low preference for telemedicine overall; however, familiarity positively influenced both a preference for a telemedicine option and the assessment of telemedicine quality. We were unable to identify other potential predictors of telemedicine success. These findings, together with the fact that most respondents felt that they had inadequate knowledge about telemedicine to comment on its quality, highlights the vital need to focus on buy-in from those who might use this technology. Low preference does not exclude telemedicine use but informs us that acceptance may not be as quick or easy as anticipated. In thinking about telemedicine adoption, then, it is imperative to tailor implementation accordingly. A rapid expansion without the necessary buy-in and exposure may result in a telemedicine failure. In contrast to other predictors of and barriers to telemedicine adoption [10–12], telemedicine familiarity is modifiable and should be a focus of future access efforts. Studies suggest that among those actually using the technology, acceptance is high [3, 4, 10], and hesitation is a characteristic of those not necessarily familiar with telemedicine [6]. The initial barrier seems to be convincing those who are unfamiliar that telemedicine is an acceptable and effective alternative. High quality research in this area is lacking [7, 9], and as we strive to increase telemedicine familiarity, we have an obligation to ensure that convenience does take precedence over quality. It will also be critical for the PR community to consider how additional technologies, such as platforms which capture patient-reported outcomes and wearable devices, might be integrated into patient care.

An important limitation of our survey is sample bias since only those who came to our PR clinic were surveyed. These families may have different views on barriers to care and acceptable alternatives than those who never make it to our clinic. Potentially, those who could be helped most by alternative care models were not captured in this study because they never made it to the PR clinic. There is unfortunately no way to accurately identify such patients. While this sample bias is an important consideration when it comes to the generalizability of results, the intent of this survey was to capture the views of a population of already established PR patients in the Upper Midwest and to demonstrate how such views might be used, in conjunction with the literature and other objective measures, to inform thinking about care expansion. It is possible that the preference for current care at our center could be due to our sampling and/or inexperience with the other care modalities. Survey results were not intended to preclude use of other care modalities but to highlight the importance of knowing where current preferences lie, to understand where there may be resistance to care expansion, and to appreciate factors which might make expansion of alternative care models more acceptable. It is important to note that the entirety of factors which contribute to parent perceptions of care cannot be captured in a single survey. To more completely understand parent perceptions, it will be helpful in future studies to also include qualitative methods. Additionally, given limited experience with telemedicine among respondents in our survey, it will be useful to also assess telemedicine perceptions at a clinic where patients are more familiar with this modality. This, too, could include qualitative methods to identify themes around telemedicine acceptance and/or hesitation.

We had a relatively homogenous group of patients that may not be representative of other PR centers. Centers with demographics differing greatly from ours, such as centers caring primarily for patients with public insurance, could find differing preferences. The wide catchment area and long travel times for many patients coming to our clinic makes exploration of alternative care models particularly relevant for our center. This may not be the case for other centers, although it is interesting that our survey identified parent-reported travel barriers and travel inconvenience as more meaningful than actual travel time. Thus, barrier perceptions and acceptability of alternative care models can be a useful assessment at any center and can help shape expansion of care. PR centers might also consider what modalities best fit with their intended mission. Telemedicine, for example, might be implemented in parts of the world where there are no pediatric rheumatologists, and some PR centers may have interest in developing such partnerships.

Finally, small numbers, such as the small number of respondents preferring telemedicine, made it difficult to detect differences between groups in our survey. Certain distributions were weighted unevenly, such as a large percentage of patients traveling less than one hour and only a few traveling more than six hours, thus skewing median barrier scores.

Conclusions

Effectively deploying a limited workforce is an enduring issue and requires appropriately guided stewardship of valuable resources. As we seek to remedy the PR access concerns, we must assess the readiness to engage the solutions. Given a strong preference for current care at our center, it is important that any alternative models compliment rather than detract from current offerings. Of several alternatives offered to bridge pediatric rheumatology access gaps, outreach clinics were the most preferred option at our center. While not a majority, a portion of respondents also expressed interest in adult rheumatology care and shared care. Moving forward, it will be important to gain a better understanding of what factors, in addition to the barriers to care assessed here, might cause patients to favor certain modalities over others. Telemedicine was a less favored option which, again, would not exclude its use, but further work should be done to understand which types of patients are the best fit for this modality and how exposure to this technology might change perceptions over time. It will also be important to explore the possibility of combined models (e.g. alternating current care and telemedicine visits) and assess what visit types (e.g. new encounter vs return) or diagnoses might be more amendable to alternative care models. As our center plans and pilots both outreach clinics and telemedicine, we are reminded that our mission is multifaceted – providing children with access to care as well as ensuring superior clinical outcomes [1]. In accomplishing this mission, it will be important to measure alternative models against current care, both in terms of family perceptions and objective clinical measures.

Abbreviations
IQR: Interquartile range; IRB: Institutional review board; JIA: Juvenile idiopathic arthritis; PR: Pediatric rheumatology; SD: Standard deviation; US: United States

Acknowledgements
Thank you to Dr. Eileen Harwood for assistance with survey development. Thank you to the University of Minnesota Explorer Clinic staff for assistance with survey distribution and collection.

Funding
Research reported in this publication was supported by the National Center for Advancing Translational Sciences of the National Institutes of Health Award Number UL1TR000114. The content is solely the responsibility of the authors and does not necessarily represent the official views of the National Institutes of Health.

Authors' contributions
DRB was responsible for study conception, survey design, survey administration, and manuscript preparation. RKV assisted with study design and manuscript revisions. LZ analyzed patient data and assisted with manuscript revisions. CKC assisted with study conception, study design, and manuscript revisions. All authors read and approved the final manuscript.

Consent for publication
Not applicable.

Competing interests
The authors declare that they have no competing interests.

Author details
[1]Division of Pediatric Rheumatology, Department of Pediatrics, University of Minnesota, East Bldg Rm M668, 2450 Riverside Ave, Minneapolis, MN 55454, USA. [2]Clinical and Translational Sciences Institute, University of Minnesota, 717 Delaware Street SE, Minneapolis, MN 55414, USA.

References
1. Henrickson M. Policy challenges for the pediatric rheumatology workforce: part II. Health care system delivery and workforce supply. Pediatr Rheumatol Online J. 2011;9:24. eCollection 2011
2. Department of Health and Human Services. Report to Congress - The Pediatric Rheumatology Workforce: A Study of the Supply and Demand for Pediatric Rheumatologists - pedrheumatology.pdf. 2007. https://pdfs.semanticscholar.org/4f1d/41eec3b2ecbe7e529efb169cdb0d82c0a951.pdf.
3. Ward IM, Schmidt TW, Lappan C, Battafarano DF. How critical is tele-medicine to the rheumatology workforce? Arthritis Care Res (Hoboken). 2016;68:1387–9.
4. Leggett P, Graham L, Steele K, Gilliland A, Stevenson M, O'Reilly D, et al. Telerheumatology–diagnostic accuracy and acceptability to patient, specialist, and general practitioner. Br J Gen Pract. 2001;51:746–8.
5. Marcin JP, Ellis J, Mawis R, Nagrampa E, Nesbitt TS, Dimand RJ. Using telemedicine to provide pediatric subspecialty care to children with special health care needs in an underserved rural community. Pediatrics. 2004;113(1 Pt 1):1–6.
6. Call VR, Erickson LD, Dailey NK, Hicken BL, Rupper R, Yorgason JB, et al. Attitudes toward telemedicine in urban, rural, and highly rural communities. Telemed J E Health. 2015;21:644–51.
7. Dorsey ER, Campion EW, Topol EJ. State of telehealth. N Engl J Med. 2016; 375:154–61. doi:10.1056/NEJMra1601705.
8. Workforce C on P, Marcin JP, Rimsza ME, Moskowitz WB. The use of telemedicine to address access and physician workforce shortages. Pediatrics. 2015;136:202–9.
9. McDougall JA, Ferucci ED, Glover J, Fraenkel L. Telerheumatology: a systematic review. Arthritis Care Res (Hoboken) 2016. doi:10.1002/acr.23153.
10. Kessler EA, Sherman AK, Becker ML. Decreasing patient cost and travel time through pediatric rheumatology telemedicine visits. Pediatr Rheumatol Online J. 2016;14:54.
11. Zanaboni P, Wootton R. Adoption of telemedicine: from pilot stage to routine delivery. BMC Med Inform Decis Mak. 2012;12:1.
12. O'Connor S, Hanlon P, O'Donnell CA, Garcia S, Glanville J, Mair FS. Understanding factors affecting patient and public engagement and recruitment to digital health interventions: a systematic review of qualitative studies. BMC Med Inform Decis Mak. 2016;16:120.
13. McLaughlin CG, Wyszewianski L. Access to care: remembering old lessons. Health Serv Res. 2002;37:1441–3. doi:10.1111/1475-6773.12171.
14. Correll CK, Spector LG, Zhang L, Binstadt BA, Vehe RK. Barriers and alternatives to pediatric rheumatology referrals: survey of general pediatricians in the United States. Pediatr Rheumatol Online J. 2015;13:32.
15. AAP State Pediatrician Workforce Survey Committee on Pediatric Workforce. 2015;2016 7/20/2016. https://www.aap.org/en-us/Documents/members_aap_state_pediatrician_workforce_survey_n.pdf.

18

Assessment, classification and treatment of calcinosis as a complication of juvenile dermatomyositis: a survey of pediatric rheumatologists by the childhood arthritis and rheumatology research alliance (CARRA)

A. B. Orandi[1*], K. W. Baszis[1], V. R. Dharnidharka[2], A. M. Huber[3], and M. F. Hoeltzel[4] for the CARRA Juvenile Myositis subgroup

Abstract

Background: There is no standardized approach to the management of JDM-associated calcinosis and its phenotypes. Current knowledge of treatment outcomes is confined to small series and case reports. We describe physician perspectives toward diagnostic approach, classification and treatment directly targeting calcinosis, independent of overall JDM therapy.

Methods: An electronic survey of 22 questions was organized into sections regarding individual practices of assessment, classification and treatment of calcinosis, including perceived successes of therapies. Invitations to complete the survey voluntarily and anonymously were sent to CARRA physician members and the Pediatric Rheumatology Bulletin Board, an electronic list-serv. Results were analyzed by descriptive statistics and chi-square analyses.

Results: Of 139 survey responses, 118 were included in analysis. Of these, 70% were based in the USA and 88 (75%) were CARRA members. Only 17% of responders have seen more than 20 cases of calcinosis, and only 28% perform screening imaging studies on new JDM diagnoses. Increasing systemic immunosuppression is first-line therapy for 67% of respondents. Targeted therapy against calcinosis is most often instituted for symptomatic patients. IVIG and bisphosphonates are most frequently used and considered most successful, but many other agents are used. Experienced physicians are more likely to use bisphosphonates, calcium channel blockers and topical sodium thiosulfate ($p < 0.002$ or lower).

Conclusions: Coexisting JDM disease activity influences whether calcinosis is considered active disease or targeted directly. Experience treating JDM-related calcinosis is low, as are rates of formal screening for calcinosis. Experienced physicians are more likely to use non-immunosuppressive treatments.

Keywords: Juvenile dermatomyositis, Calcinosis, Survey, CARRA, Treatment

* Correspondence: aorandi@wustl.edu
[1]Department of Pediatrics, Division of Rheumatology, Washington University School of Medicine, 660 S. Euclid Ave, Campus Bo 8116, St. Louis, Missouri 63110, USA
Full list of author information is available at the end of the article

Background

Juvenile dermatomyositis (JDM) is the most common inflammatory myopathy of childhood, though still rare, with an estimated incidence of 3.2 children per million per year [1]. The cardinal features include proximal muscle weakness and characteristic rash, but multiple other organs can be involved and contribute to morbidity and mortality, including the gastrointestinal, cardiac and pulmonary systems. With improved disease understanding and treatments, mortality has been significantly reduced [2, 3], but long-term morbidity and treatment toxicity remain as challenges [4]. A prominent contributor to overall morbidity is calcinosis, the accumulation of dystrophic carbonate apatite [5] in skin and soft tissues, both a trademark and feared complication whose presence has been unyielding in the face of other advances. Its staying power is owed to an incomplete understanding of both its pathogenesis and actionable risk factors that could support alterations in management [6–8]. Although it is reported that early aggressive treatment can prevent the development of calcinosis [9–11], the incidence continues to remain at an estimated 30–40% of patients through various cohort and registry studies [12–15].

To date, there are no randomized controlled trials or standardized recommendations for the treatment of calcinosis as it occurs in JDM. Many therapeutic agents with different mechanisms of action have been used, with none showing a consistently positive response. In a recent review, nearly 20 different therapies have been described to have positive responses in published cases [15]. Further complicating the management of this condition are the varying phenotypes [16, 17], such as circumscripta, tumoral, universalis and exoskeleton lesions, as well as the inconsistent timing of calcinosis respective to other disease features [18–20]. While the ultimate goal is to improve outcomes of patients with calcinosis, our aim is to describe the current practices of pediatric rheumatologists, including approaches to assessment, classification and treatment, thereby consolidating consensus opinions that can be formally studied. This technique has been successfully implemented in the overall treatment of JDM by the Childhood Arthritis and Rheumatology Research Alliance (CARRA), whose consensus treatment plans are currently being instituted and analyzed [21–24].

Methods

Using the REDCap platform, an electronic survey was created, consisting of 22 questions divided into four sections: demographic characteristics, assessment, classification and treatment (Additional file 1). For phenotype classification questions, calcinosis phenotypes were described as follows: Circumscripta; superficial plaques or nodules. Tumoral; larger nodules that extend into deeper layers. Universalis; involvement along fascial planes of muscles or tendons. Exoskeleton; hardened deposits over a surface area. For treatment choice-related questions, 'immunomodulatory' agents are those which directly suppress or modulate the immune system whereas 'alternative' agents are those with non-immunosuppressive actions, such as altering calcium and/or phosphorous metabolism. Any treatment success-related questions are defined as physician perceived success. For questions related to situational treatment, 'targeted treatment' refers to a treatment chosen for calcinosis specifically and not any other co-existing JDM disease activity.

Physicians, including fellows-in-training, who specialize in pediatric, adult, combined rheumatology or immunology were invited by e-mail to complete the survey. Participants were asked to respond according to their personal experience, not that of institution or group practices or based on the medical literature. Respondents were asked to quantify their experience by years of practice and lifetime cases seen of JDM-associated calcinosis. In January 2016, the survey was electronically sent to 303 voting and trainee physician members of CARRA; a North American collaborative research organization and to the Pediatric Rheumatology Bulletin Board, an international electronic list-serv. Members of CARRA who are also on the Bulletin Board were asked to only respond once. All respondents voluntarily and anonymously completed the survey.

Physicians of different experience levels, determined by years of practice and by number of cases seen, were captured, and the discrepancy between experience levels highlighted an important finding: because of the rare incidence of JDM, even some seasoned physicians had seen few cases of calcinosis. Because of this finding, the number of cases seen was used as the metric of experience instead of years in practice. Therefore, a physician who is experienced with treating JDM-associated calcinosis was defined as having seen greater than 10 cases. The results of the survey were analyzed by descriptive statistics and chi-square analyses for comparisons between physicians who have seen greater and less than 10 cases. Analysis was performed using IBM SPSS Statistics (version 24), Armonk, NY.

Results

A total of 139 individuals accessed the survey with 5 individuals excluded for not answering any questions. Four respondents were excluded for no personal experience with JDM patients less than 21 years of age, and 3 were excluded for no personal experience treating JDM-associated calcinosis. An additional 9 were excluded for only completing the demographic section. A total of 118 respondents completed at least one full survey section in addition to demographic characteristics, qualifying for analysis, with a total of 103 respondents completing the survey entirely (Fig. 1). CARRA members constituted 75% (88/118) of the analyzed responses and based on the number of CARRA members who received the survey invitation the CARRA response rate is estimated at 30% (88/303).

Less than 5% of respondents practiced something other than pediatric rheumatology. Approximately 70% of respondents were based in the United States, with Europe the next most common location at 14%. The distribution of experience by years showed nearly equal young providers (current fellow to 5 years) and those with more than 20 years experience, at 27% for both, with lesser numbers in between. When experience was measured by number of cases seen, the majority, 62%, have seen between 1 and 10 cases, with only 17% having seen greater than 20 cases. Of these who have seen more than 20 cases, 16 (80%) have more than 15 years experience. However, of those with more than 15 years experience, 39% had seen less than 10 cases. Complete respondent characteristics are detailed in Table 1.

Assessment

When evaluating a new JDM diagnosis, 60% use only history and/or physical exam to screen for calcinosis. If history and physical exam are negative, 33 (28%) perform imaging studies. Only 11% perform no formal assessment. For presence or suspicion of calcinosis, radiographs are the initial imaging studies for 88%, whereas 18% use ultrasound, 17% MRI and 4% computed tomography. If calcinosis is suspected or found, nearly equal numbers send laboratory studies evaluating calcium and vitamin D levels or no labs at all (45% each). Once treatment is initiated, 95% use physical exam to monitor response to therapy (if phenotype is able to be examined), whereas 70% use imaging. Of these, plain radiographs are used by 72% of respondents, 15% use MRI, 7% use ultrasound and 4% use computed tomography.

Classification–Calcinosis phenotype

Two-thirds of respondents believed it was important to classify the phenotype of calcinosis lesions, with selected

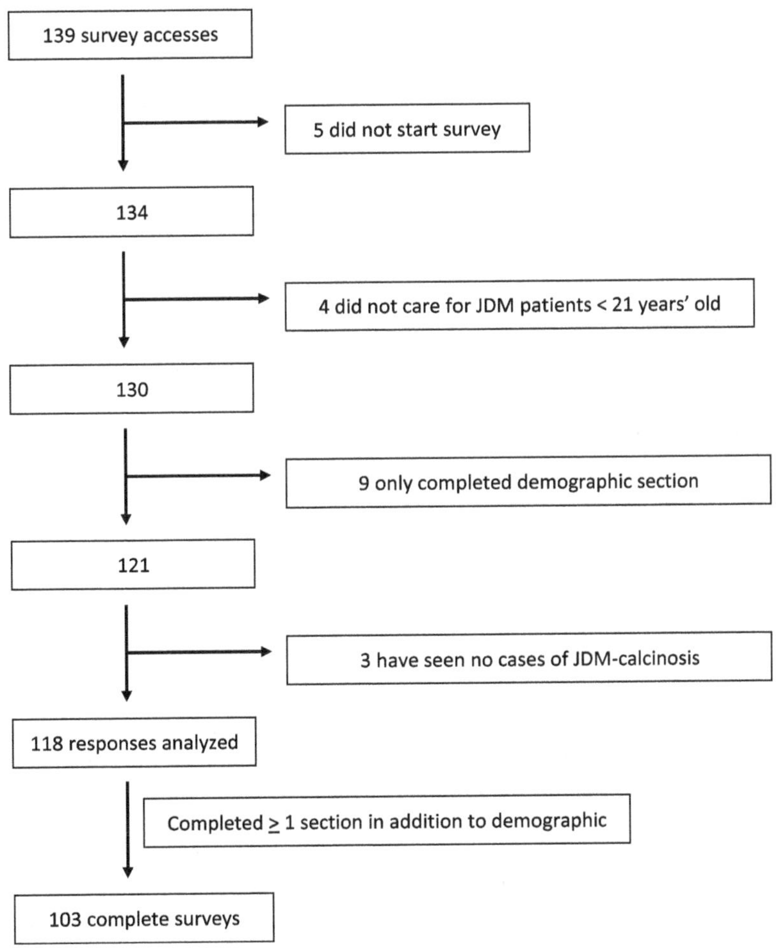

Fig. 1 Number of survey respondents

Table 1 Respondent characteristics

Characteristic	n (%)
Practice scope	
Pediatric Rheumatology	114 (96.6)
Adult Rheumatology	1 (0.8)
Combined adult/pediatric Rheumatology	3 (2.5)
Immunology	0 (0)
Practice location	
United States	82 (69.5)
Canada	8 (6.8)
Central/South America	9 (7.6)
Europe	16 (13.6)
Asia/India	1 (0.8)
Other (Turkey, Kenya)	1, 1 (0.8)
CARRA Member	
Yes	88 (74.6)
No	30 (25.4)
Experience (by years of practice)	
Current fellow to 5 years	32 (27.1)
6 to 10 years	30 (25.4)
11 to 15 years	10 (8.5)
16 to 20 years	14 (11.9)
More than 20 years	32 (27.1)
Experience (by # of JDM-calcinosis cases seen)	
1 to 10 cases	74 (62.7)
11 to 20 cases	24 (20.3)
21 to 50 cases	18 (15.3)
More than 50	2 (1.7)

Demographic characteristics of all survey respondents included in analysis

rationale of the phenotype affecting treatment type (surgical or medical), treatment aggression or predicting response to treatment. Others listed different expected morbidity or severity from specific phenotypes. Opponents of classification believed that only the presence of calcinosis was important, regardless of phenotype. When asked to rate phenotypes by perceived severity or worse prognosis, 65% listed universalis, followed by exoskeleton lesions at 57% and tumoral at 42%.

Classification–Disease activity

When asked to characterize "active JDM disease", nearly all respondents reported the presence of skin and muscle disease (defined as presence of rash, nail fold capillary changes, muscle weakness, elevation of muscle enzymes, abnormal muscle imaging or EMG findings) as active JDM disease, opinions that were unchanged by the presence of new or persistent/refractory calcinosis. However, in the absence of skin and muscle disease, 73% reported new onset calcinosis as active JDM disease, while only 14% regarded absent skin and muscle disease with persistent/refractory calcinosis as active JDM disease. Given the same scenarios of JDM disease states, respondents were asked to consider *targeted* treatment of calcinosis, independent of therapy prescribed for overall JDM disease activity. The rates of consideration for targeted treatment were higher in scenarios where skin and muscle disease activity were decreased and persistence of calcinosis increased, such that only 56% would consider targeted treatment of calcinosis for active skin and muscle disease with new calcinosis, but 80% would consider targeted treatment of calcinosis for absent skin and muscle disease with persistent/refractory calcinosis. Only 43% would consider targeted treatment of calcinosis in all scenarios, and 9% would not consider targeted therapy in any scenario.

The features of calcinosis lesions that increase the likelihood of targeted therapy, independent of overall JDM therapy, are more likely to be symptomatic features as follows: Functional impairment and pain were listed by 97% of respondents, whereas threat to adjacent organs and recurrent infections were listed by 89 and 80%, respectively. Cosmesis (or psychosocial impact) was listed by 71%. Only 29% listed calcinosis phenotype, and 8% listed presence of certain myositis antibodies (listed as Jo-1, MDA-5 and NXP2) that would increase the likelihood of targeted treatment. When these features were ranked in order of importance to considering targeted treatment, functional impairment was ranked highest by 41%, pain ranked second by 40%, and location (as threatening to other organs) third at 37%.

Treatment–Surgical

As first line therapy, only 5% of respondents would refer for surgical excision. However, if the type of lesion is amenable to surgical removal, 24% believed every such case should have a surgical evaluation. Further, 60% would consider surgery if the lesion(s) caused significant limitation in mobility or significant pain, but 38% believe it should be used only if medical therapy failed. Only 4% believe there is no role for surgery in the management of calcinosis.

Treatment–Medical

Therapies were separated into two categories: immunomodulatory and alternative agents, the latter including drugs with non-immunosuppressive actions, such as altering calcium and phosphorus metabolism. The drugs in each category and their frequencies of use are displayed in Fig. 2. For the patient developing or presenting with calcinosis, increasing or adding systemic immunosuppression was first line therapy for 67% of respondents, followed by alternative agents at 13%. A total of

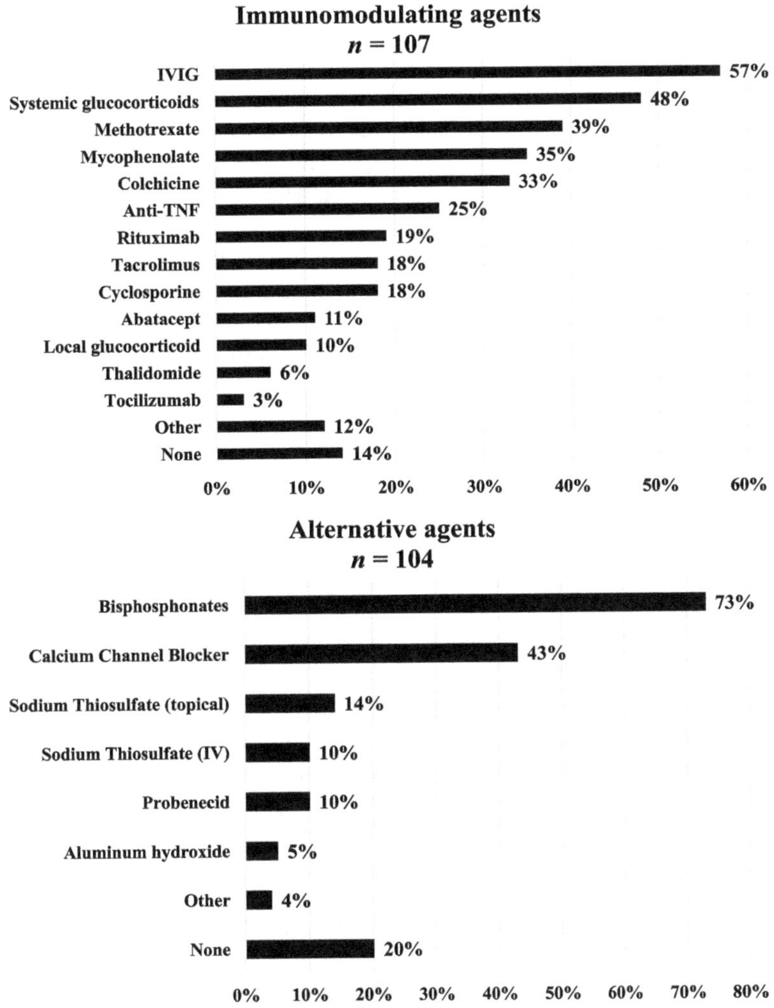

Fig. 2 Treatment categories and frequency of use among all respondents

14 (13%) would prescribe no specific treatment other than 'standard' therapy for overall JDM activity.

Of the immunomodulatory agents listed, the most frequently used include IV immune globulin (IVIG) by 61 (57%), systemic glucocorticoids by 48% and methotrexate (specifically for calcinosis) at 40%. Less frequently used agents include TNF-alpha inhibitors at 25%, rituximab at 19% and abatacept at 11%. Other immunomodulatory agents that were not listed, but totaled 12%, included anakinra, cyclophosphamide, lenalinomide and sirolimus.

When asked to rank which treatment was perceived to be most successful against calcinosis, IVIG was ranked first by 30% of users and second by 26% of users, whereas systemic glucocorticoids were ranked first by 32% of users and second by 17%. Methotrexate was ranked first by 24% and second by 9% of respondents. Only mycophenolate, tacrolimus, colchicine and cyclosporine were ranked in the top three by greater than 10% of respondents; they were listed second by 20, 12, 12%, and third by 10% respectively.

For alternative agents, bisphosphonates were the most frequently used (73% of respondents), followed by calcium channel blockers at 43%. Intravenous sodium thiosulfate was used by 10%, with 14% using the topical formulation. Other agents not listed that were used include warfarin and minocycline (totaling 4%). Of note, 20% of respondents have not used any of the alternative agents.

When ranked according to perceived success against calcinosis, approximately 60% ranked bisphosphonates most effective, whereas only 15% ranked calcium channel blockers highest, with an additional 30% ranking second most effective. Although few respondents have used intravenous sodium thiosulfate, it was perceived as most effective by three individuals (30%).

Experience differences

Separating experience by those who have seen more or less than 10 cases, there was no statistically significant difference regarding certain assessment and classification practices (Fig. 3). Roughly equal numbers screen new diagnoses with imaging or have no formal screening process. Neither group was more or less likely to consider new or stable calcinosis as active JDM disease in the absence of skin and muscle disease. Similarly, there was no difference in the consideration to target treatment against calcinosis in the absence of skin and muscle activity.

Examining the differences in treatment use, both groups reported highest use of the same top three immunomodulatory agents: IVIG, systemic glucocorticoids and methotrexate (Fig. 4). For every agent except local glucocorticoids, the more experienced respondents reported greater frequency of use, but only colchicine (19/40 versus 16/67, Pearson chi-square value = 6.348, p = 0.012) and tacrolimus reached statistical significance (11/40 versus 8/67, Pearson chi-square value = 4.152, p = 0.042). Regarding alternative medications, again each group had the same top two most frequently used agents: bisphosphonates and calcium channel blockers (Fig. 5). However, the increased use by more experienced respondents reached statistical significance for bisphosphonates (37/40 versus 39/64, Pearson chi-square value = 12.464, $p< 0.001$), calcium channel blockers (25/40 versus 20/64, Pearson chi-square value = 9.793, p = 0.002) and topical sodium thiosulfate (10/30 versus 4/60, Pearson chi-square value = 7.429, p = 0.006).

Discussion

Calcinosis remains a significant source of morbidity for many JDM patients, yet it is poorly understood and lacks uniform treatment approaches compared to other aspects of JDM. This survey describes the approach and management of calcinosis by a large number of pediatric rheumatologists.

The inconsistency in the published literature regarding therapeutic effectiveness can be explained by the relative inexperience of physicians and the multitude of different treatments and treatment scenarios. To date there have been no published reports comparing therapeutic effectiveness against calcinosis when there is active versus absent skin and muscle disease. Additionally, not all published reports list failed therapies prior to success or concurrent background medications [25]. Part of the discrepancy between number of cases seen and experience is owed to practice type (size, university affiliation) and location (city, region, competing practices), which was not assessed in this survey. However, another potential contributor is the low percentage of physicians who routinely screen for calcinosis beyond patient history and physical examination. Based on our results, only 28% perform additional imaging if history and exam are negative for calcinosis while 11% perform no formal screening. This low frequency may be in part due to the lack of any studied screening methods. It is well-

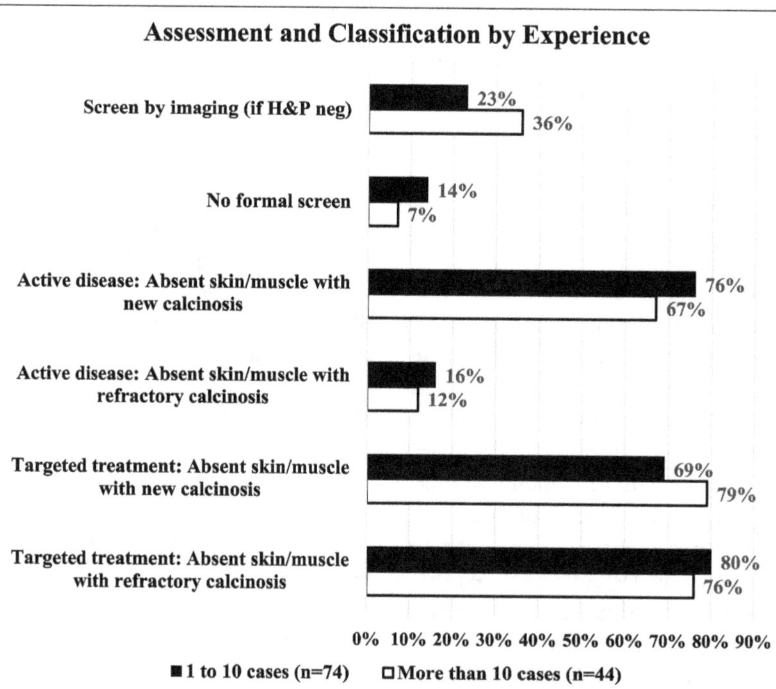

Fig. 3 Assessment and classification by experience in regards to using imaging to screen for calcinosis if none is apparent by history or physical exam or if no formal screen is done. Respondent opinion of what constitutes active disease based on the presence or absence of skin/muscle disease with or without new or refractory calcinosis; and if they would consider targeted treatment against calcinosis irrespective of other disease activity in the same scenarios

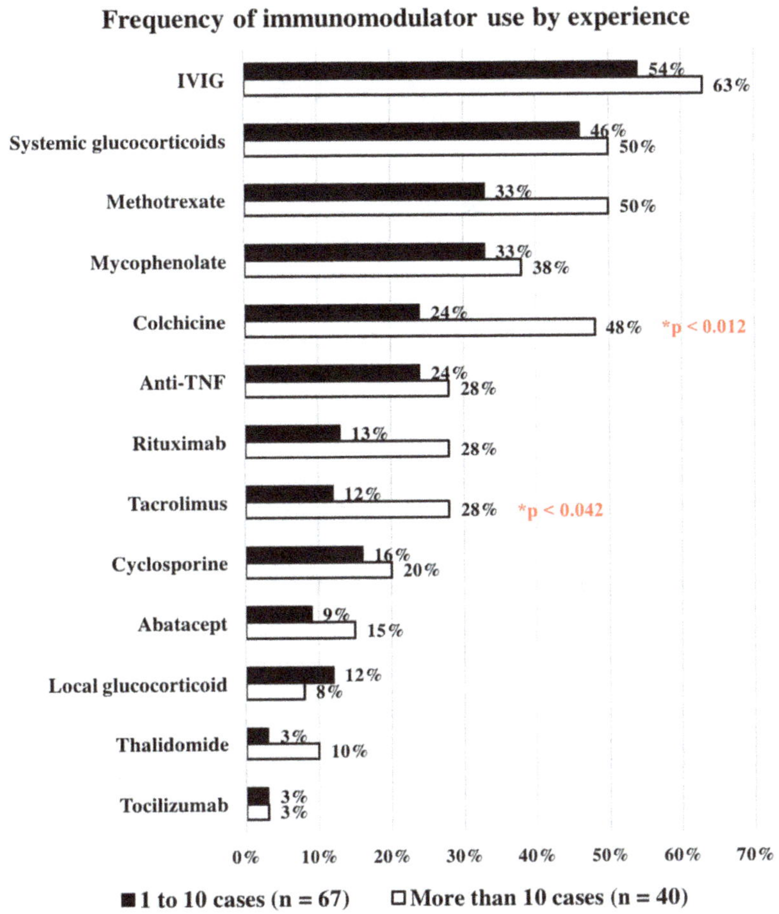

Fig. 4 Frequency of immunomodulatory use by experience

reported that lesions can be present at diagnosis or much later [26]. Deeper lesions such as exoskeleton and universalis phenotypes may not be apparent until a critical size or mass effect is reached. A lack of screening is unique to calcinosis when compared to other JDM complications, such as interstitial lung disease, where screening with pulmonary function testing and/or CT imaging is routinely performed since it is known that even asymptomatic children can have long-term sequelae [27–29].

Also revealing was the expressed understanding of the role calcinosis plays in active disease and the decision to treat with therapies targeted at calcinosis. It was clear that respondents believed the new development of calcinosis with otherwise absent skin and muscle disease represents active disease (73%), however, only 56% would consider targeted treatment of calcinosis in the most agreed upon active systemic disease state. Combining these results provides stark evidence that the majority (80% combined) prefer to prescribe either systemic immunosuppression or a regimen based on overall JDM activity with only symptomatic complaints prompting targeted treatment against calcinosis. Importantly, none of the above showed significant differences among physicians of different experience levels. The results showed, however, that experienced physicians may be more willing to use unconventional therapies in the treatment of this complication. Colchicine and tacrolimus were two immunomodulatory agents used significantly more by experienced physicians for treatment of calcinosis, but they are not mainstays of immunosuppressive treatment of JDM as a whole. Similarly, although both groups used alternative agents, experienced physicians were significantly more likely to use bisphosphonates, calcium channel blockers and topical sodium thiosulfate.

Our study has several limitations, including the relatively low response rate for CARRA members. In addition, the majority of respondents were from North America and/or CARRA members. Although our intent to include the pediatric rheumatology bulletin board community was to obtain a broad scope of practice across the field, the results cannot be reliably generalized to the field at-large and perhaps more accurately represent North American and CARRA members with an interest in JDM. It is possible that many chose not to

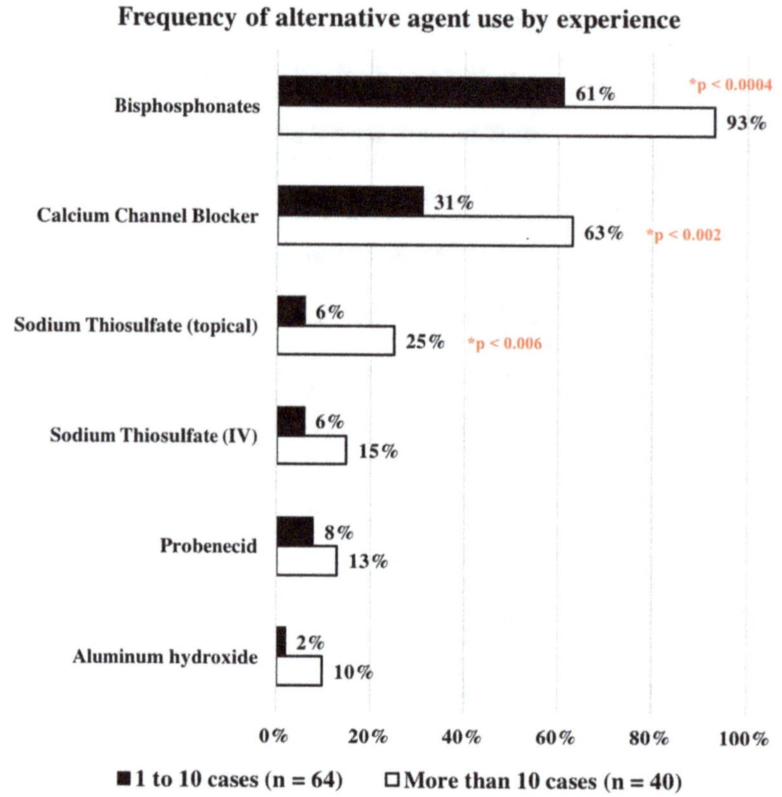

Fig. 5 Frequency of alternative agent use by experience

complete the survey due to a lack of experience with JDM-associated calcinosis. Thus, an increase number of respondents with only a few cases seen may not significantly alter the results. Another limitation of our survey (and others that attempt to describe practice), is that physicians may answer based on information other than personal experience and duplicate their responses despite instructions to discourage these types of responses. Many of the questions were based on hypothetical situations, without complete details that would be present in case-based surveys. This survey did not directly address the successes of each physician's practices, complications of treatment or cost-effectiveness. Finally, this study is not intended to recommend specific treatment(s) for JDM-associated calcinosis but to describe the current trends in management and highlight the need for increased evidence in assessment and treatment efficacy.

Conclusion

Calcinosis is considered a major source of morbidity, but often excluded as a metric of clinically active or inactive disease [30], leaving many physicians with limited experience. There is a lack of formal screening, and most direct treatment decisions are based on symptomatic complaints, which is at odds with the moderate numbers who consider it a component of active disease. Increased formal research is needed, which could include screening methods, consensus treatment plans that incorporate disease activity, and the study of combination therapies in different patient subgroups.

Abbreviations

CARRA: Childhood arthritis and rheumatology research alliance; IVIG: Intravenous immune globulin; JDM: Juvenile dermatomyositis.

Acknowledgements

The authors wish to acknowledge CARRA, and the ongoing Arthritis Foundation financial support of CARRA. The authors would also like to thank Noor Al-Hammadi for assistance with statistical analysis.

Funding

Grant Number T32 HD043010, from the NIH Eunice Kennedy Shriver Institute of Child Health and Human Development. Training of the Pediatric Physician-Scientist. Grant Number UL1 TR000448 from the NIH National Center for Advancing Translational Sciences (NCATS), components of the National Institutes of Health (NIH), and NIH Roadmap for Medical Research.

Authors' contributions

AO, KB, VR, AH and MH developed the study and methodology. AO collected and analyzed the data and drafted the manuscript. AO, KB, VR, AH and MH analyzed the data and provided critical revisions for the manuscript. All authors read and approved the final manuscript.

Consent for publication

Not applicable

Competing interests

The authors declare that they have no competing interests.

Author details

[1]Department of Pediatrics, Division of Rheumatology, Washington University School of Medicine, 660 S. Euclid Ave, Campus Bo 8116, St. Louis, Missouri 63110, USA. [2]Department of Pediatrics, Division of Nephrology, Washington University School of Medicine, St. Louis, Missouri, USA. [3]Department of Pediatrics, Division of Rheumatology, IWK Health Centre and Dalhousie University, Halifax, Nova Scotia, Canada. [4]Department of Pediatrics, Division of Rheumatology, University of Michigan Medical School, Ann Arbor, Michigan, USA.

References

1. Mendez EP, Lipton R, Ramsey-Goldman R, Roettcher P, Bowyer S, Dyer A, Pachman LM, Group NJDRPR. US incidence of juvenile dermatomyositis, 1995-1998: results from the National Institute of Arthritis and Musculoskeletal and Skin Diseases Registry. Arthritis Rheum. 2003;49(3):300–5. doi: 10.1002/art.11122.
2. Shah M, Mamyrova G, Targoff IN, Huber AM, Malley JD, Rice MM, Miller FW, Rider LG, Childhood Myositis Heterogeneity Collaborative Study G. The clinical phenotypes of the juvenile idiopathic inflammatory myopathies. Med (Baltimore). 2013;92(1):25–41. doi: 10.1097/MD.0b013e31827f264d.
3. Hashkes PJ, Wright BM, Lauer MS, Worley SE, Tang AS, Roettcher PA, Bowyer SL. Mortality outcomes in pediatric rheumatology in the US. Arthritis Rheum. 2010;62(2):599–608. doi: 10.1002/art.27218.
4. Huber AM, Lang B, LeBlanc CM, Birdi N, Bolaria RK, Malleson P, MacNeil I, Momy JA, Avery G, Feldman BM. Medium- and long-term functional outcomes in a multicenter cohort of children with juvenile dermatomyositis. Arthritis Rheum. 2000;43(3):541–9. doi: 10.1002/1529-0131(200003)43:3<541::AID-ANR9>3.0.CO;2-T.
5. Eidelman N, Boyde A, Bushby AJ, Howell PG, Sun J, Newbury DE, Miller FW, Robey PG, Rider LG. Microstructure and mineral composition of dystrophic calcification associated with the idiopathic inflammatory myopathies. Arthritis Res Ther. 2009;11(5):R159. doi: 10.1186/ar2841.
6. Pachman LM, Liotta-Davis MR, Hong DK, Kinsella TR, Mendez EP, Kinder JM, Chen EH. TNFalpha-308A allele in juvenile dermatomyositis: association with increased production of tumor necrosis factor alpha, disease duration, and pathologic calcifications. Arthritis Rheum. 2000;43(10):2368–77. doi: 10.1002/1529-0131(200010)43:10<2368::AID-ANR26>3.0.CO;2-8.
7. Hoeltzel MF. Race is a risk factor for calcinosis in patients with JD - early results from the CARRAnet registry study. Pediatr Rheumatol. 2012;10(Suppl 1):A65. doi: 10.1186/1546-0096-10-S1-A65.
8. Pachman LM, Abbott K, Sinacore JM, Amoruso L, Dyer A, Lipton R, Ilowite N, Hom C, Cawkwell G, White A, Rivas-Chacon R, Kimura Y, Ray L, Ramsey-Goldman R. Duration of illness is an important variable for untreated children with juvenile dermatomyositis. J Pediatr. 2006;148(2):247–53. doi: 10.1016/j.jpeds.2005.10.032.
9. Bowyer SL, Blane CE, Sullivan DB, Cassidy JT. Childhood dermatomyositis: factors predicting functional outcome and development of dystrophic calcification. J Pediatr. 1983;103(6):882–8.
10. Kim S, El-Hallak M, Dedeoglu F, Zurakowski D, Fuhlbrigge RC, Sundel RP. Complete and sustained remission of juvenile dermatomyositis resulting from aggressive treatment. Arthritis Rheum. 2009;60(6):1825–30. doi: 10.1002/art.24571.
11. Fisler RE, Liang MG, Fuhlbrigge RC, Yalcindag A, Sundel RP. Aggressive management of juvenile dermatomyositis results in improved outcome and decreased incidence of calcinosis. J Am Acad Dermatol. 2002;47(4):505–11.
12. Ramanan AV, Feldman BM. Clinical features and outcomes of juvenile dermatomyositis and other childhood onset myositis syndromes. Rheum Dis Clin N Am. 2002;28(4):833–57.
13. McCann LJ, Juggins AD, Maillard SM, Wedderburn LR, Davidson JE, Murray KJ, Pilkington CA, Juvenile Dermatomyositis Research G. The Juvenile Dermatomyositis National Registry and Repository (UK and Ireland)–clinical characteristics of children recruited within the first 5 yr. Rheumatol (Oxford). 2006;45(10):1255–60. doi: 10.1093/rheumatology/kel099.
14. Clemente G, Piotto DG, Barbosa C, Peracchi OA, Len CA, Hilario MO, Terreri MT. High frequency of calcinosis in juvenile dermatomyositis: a risk factor study. Rev Bras Reumatol. 2012;52(4):549–53.
15. Robinson AB, Hoeltzel MF, Wahezi DM, Becker ML, Kessler EA, Schmeling H, Carrasco R, Huber AM, Feldman BM, Reed AM, Juvenile Myositis Carra Subgroup ftCRI. Clinical characteristics of children with juvenile dermatomyositis: the Childhood Arthritis and Rheumatology Research Alliance Registry. Arthritis Care Res (Hoboken). 2014;66(3):404–10. doi: 10.1002/acr.22142.
16. Blane CE, White SJ, Braunstein EM, Bowyer SL, Sullivan DB. Patterns of calcification in childhood dermatomyositis. AJR Am J Roentgenol. 1984; 142(2):397–400. doi: 10.2214/ajr.142.2.397.
17. Sanyal S, Atwal SS, Mondal D, Garga UC. Radiographic patterns of soft tissue calcinosis in juvenile dermatomyositis and its clinical implications. J Clin Diagn Res. 2014;8(12):RD08–11. doi: 10.7860/JCDR/2014/10787.5321.
18. Efthimiou P, Kukar M, Kagen LJ. Images in rheumatology. Severe adult-onset calcinosis in a patient with a history of juvenile dermatomyositis. J Rheumatol. 2010;37(1):194. doi: 10.3899/jrheum.090628.
19. Tugnet N, Rees DH. Calcinosis in juvenile dermatomyositis. Postgrad Med J. 2010;86(1018):510. doi: 10.1136/pgmj.2010.101170.
20. Mathiesen P, Hegaard H, Herlin T, Zak M, Pedersen FK, Nielsen S. Long-term outcome in patients with juvenile dermatomyositis: a cross-sectional follow-up study. Scand J Rheumatol. 2012;41(1):50–8. doi: 10.3109/03009742.2011.608376.
21. Stringer E, Bohnsack J, Bowyer SL, Griffin TA, Huber AM, Lang B, Lindsley CB, Ota S, Pilkington C, Reed AM, Scuccimarri R, Feldman BM. Treatment approaches to juvenile dermatomyositis (JDM) across North America: The Childhood Arthritis and Rheumatology Research Alliance (CARRA) JDM Treatment Survey. J Rheumatol. 2010;37(9):1953–61. doi: 10.3899/jrheum.090953.
22. Huber AM, Giannini EH, Bowyer SL, Kim S, Lang B, Lindsley CB, Pachman LM, Pilkington C, Reed AM, Rennebohm RM, Rider LG, Wallace CA, Feldman BM. Protocols for the initial treatment of moderately severe juvenile dermatomyositis: results of a Children's Arthritis and Rheumatology Research Alliance Consensus Conference. Arthritis Care Res (Hoboken). 2010; 62(2):219–25. doi: 10.1002/acr.20071.
23. Huber AM, Robinson AB, Reed AM, Abramson L, Bout-Tabaku S, Carrasco R, Curran M, Feldman BM, Gewanter H, Griffin T, Haines K, Hoeltzel MF, Isgro J, Kahn P, Lang B, Lawler P, Shaham B, Schmeling H, Scuccimarri R, Shishov M, Stringer E, Wohrley J, Ilowite NT, Wallace C, Juvenile Dermatomyositis Subcommittee of the Childhood A, Rheumatology Research A. Consensus treatments for moderate juvenile dermatomyositis: beyond the first two months. Results of the second Childhood Arthritis and Rheumatology Research Alliance consensus conference. Arthritis Care Res (Hoboken). 2012; 64(4):546–53. doi: 10.1002/acr.20695.
24. Reed AM, Huber AM, Tomlinson G, Pullenayegum E, Matelski J, Goh Y, Schanberg L, Feldman BM. CARRA dermatomyositis CTP pilot study. Pediatr Rheumatol. 2016;14(Suppl 1):P23. doi: 10.1186/s12969-016-0098-0.
25. Touimy M, Janani S, Rachidi W, Etaouil N, Mkinsi O. Calcinosis universalis complicating juvenile dermatomyositis: improvement after intravenous immunoglobulin therapy. Joint Bone Spine. 2013;80(1):108–9. doi: 10.1016/j.jbspin.2012.07.001.
26. Sato JO, Sallum AM, Ferriani VP, Marini R, Sacchetti SB, Okuda EM, Carvalho JF, Pereira RM, Len CA, Terreri MT, Lotufo SA, Romanelli PR, Ramos VC, Hilario MO, Silva CA, Corrente JE, Saad-Magalhaes C, Rheumatology Committee of the Sao Paulo Paediatrics S. A Brazilian registry of juvenile

dermatomyositis: onset features and classification of 189 cases. Clin Exp Rheumatol. 2009;27(6):1031–8.
27. Sanner H, Aalokken TM, Gran JT, Sjaastad I, Johansen B, Flato B. Pulmonary outcome in juvenile dermatomyositis: a case-control study. Ann Rheum Dis. 2011;70(1):86–91. doi: 10.1136/ard.2010.131433.
28. Mathiesen PR, Buchvald F, Nielsen KG, Herlin T, Friis T, Nielsen S. Pulmonary function and autoantibodies in a long-term follow-up of juvenile dermatomyositis patients. Rheumatology (Oxford). 2014;53(4):644–9. doi: 10.1093/rheumatology/ket380.
29. Trapani S, Camiciottoli G, Vierucci A, Pistolesi M, Falcini F. Pulmonary involvement in juvenile dermatomyositis: a two-year longitudinal study. Rheumatol (Oxford). 2001;40(2):216–20.
30. Almeida B, Campanilho-Marques R, Arnold K, Pilkington CA, Wedderburn LR, Nistala K, Juvenile Dermatomyositis Research G. Analysis of Published Criteria for Clinically Inactive Disease in a Large Juvenile Dermatomyositis Cohort Shows That Skin Disease Is Underestimated. Arthritis Rheumatol. 2015;67(9):2495–502. doi: 10.1002/art.39200.

19

Pigmented villonodular synovitis in pediatric population

Mohsen Karami*, Mehryar Soleimani and Reza Shiari

Abstract

Background: Pigmented villonodular synovitis (PVNS) is a rare proliferative process in children that mostly affects the knee joint.

Case Presentation: The study follows the case of a 3-year-old boy presenting recurrent patellar dislocation and PVNS. Due to symptoms such as chronic arthritis, he had been taking prednisolone and methotrexate for 6 months before receiving a definitive diagnosis. After a period of showing no improvements from his treatment, he was referred to our center and was diagnosed with local PVNS using magnetic resonance imaging (MRI). The patient was treated for his patellar dislocation by way of open synovectomy, lateral retinacular release, and a proximal realignment procedure, with no recurrence after a 24-month follow-up.

Conclusion: PVNS may appear with symptoms resembling juvenile idiopathic arthritis, thus the disease should be considered in differential diagnosis of any inflammatory arthritis in children. PVNS may also cause mechanical symptoms such as patellar dislocation. In addition to synovectomy, a realignment procedure can be a useful method of treatment.

Keywords: Juvenile idiopathic arthritis, Patellar dislocation, Pigmented villonodular synovitis

Background

Pigmented villonodular synovitis (PVNS) is a rare proliferative process that affects the synovial joint, tendon sheaths, and bursa membranes [1]. The estimated incidence of PVNS is around 1.8 cases per million people in a population [1]. PVNS is usually found in adults aged 20–50 years, but it may also be found in children [2–4].

The youngest patient reported with PVNS was 12 months old [5]. Knee involvement is common in pediatric PVNS, although other affected areas have been reported, such as the foot and ankle, elbow, hip, sacroiliac joint, and multiple joint involvements [3, 5–32]. Some authors have determined that there is no sex predilection in PVNS, while other reports have shown a male or female predominance [1, 2, 33].

The etiology of PVNS is unknown, but chronic inflammation, a tumor-like disorder with chromosomal aberrations that cause hemorrhagic tendencies, as well as genetic factors, have been proposed as potential causes [2, 3]. Trauma and rheumatoid arthritis association have also been considered [14, 15, 33].

The following study reports on a 3-year-old boy with a 4-month-long history of pain and swelling in the right knee. The patient was initially treated for juvenile idiopathic arthritis (JIA) and growth retardation.

Case Presentation

This study follows the case of a 3-year-old boy with a 4-month-long history of pain and swelling in the right knee and no history of trauma. The patient had been taking prednisolone and methotrexate for a period of 6 months in response to signs and symptoms very similar to juvenile idiopathic arthritis (JIA). Previously, he had also received a yearlong growth hormone treatment, for which the medical reason is unknown. He had no familial history of rheumatological conditions.

A physical examination of the patient revealed swelling and a limited range of motion in the knee. It was

* Correspondence: mnkarami@gmail.com
Mofid Children Hospital, Shahid Beheshti University of Medical Sciences, Shariati Ave., Tehran 15514-15468, Iran

clinically evident that the patella had been dislocated. The results of laboratory tests did not suggest that the patient suffered from JIA. Radiography images depicted soft tissue swelling around the knee joint. An MRI showed a large signal mass of synovium posterior to the lateral patellar facet, which caused lateral dislocation of the patella (Fig. 1).

The chosen method of treatment for the patient was surgery, consisting of an open excisional biopsy and a proximal realignment procedure (vastus medialis obliquus advancement) through medial parapatellar incision. A histologic examination of the tissue exposed hyperplasia of the synovium, foamy macrophage, spindle cells, multinucleated giant cells and a considerable amount of hemosiderin deposits, all of which supported the diagnosis of PVNS (Fig. 2).

After the open surgical synovectomy and 3 months of physiotherapy, the swelling of the knee lessened and the range of motion in the knee returned to normal. The patient was followed for 24 months without any signs of recurrence.

Discussion

This study reviews and summarizes 29 articles, published between 1975 and 2016, in which 42 cases of pediatric PVNS were reported [3, 5–32] (Table 1). Because of the impossibility to retrieve pediatric data, the articles representing mixed adult and pediatric cases were excluded from the review [34]. The mean age of the reported cases was 8.9 years. Sixty-two percent ($n = 26$) was female and 38% ($n = 16$) was male. PVNS affected only one joint in all but 6 cases, and the main localization was the knee joint ($n = 23$, 64%).

Approximately 81% ($n = 34$) of patients presented joint pain and swelling. This entity may have been misdiagnosed with other causes of arthritis such as rheumatoid arthritis, hemophilic arthropathy, tuberculosis, and neoplastic processes [3, 15].

A localized intra-articular form of PVNS that causes mechanical symptoms, such as anterior knee pain, meniscal injury, and patellar dislocation has been reported in adult PVNS [35–39]. Mechanical symptoms are extremely rare in pediatric cases of PVNS [3, 5–32]. Recurrent patellar dislocation is a rare presentation of PVNS that was previously only reported in adult cases [38]. This study presents a 3-year-old boy with patellar dislocation caused by PVNS, an unusual demonstration of PVNS at an unusual age. To the best of our knowledge, this is the first report of patellar dislocation in pediatric PVNS.

Joint aspiration fluid in PVNS is usually serosanguinous and, without a history of trauma, can be nearly diagnostic [2]. Initial stages of radiography may show an increasing density or radiolucent defect with a thin sclerotic rim [2, 3]. Only 33% of reported cases of pediatric PVNS produced positive findings on the initial X-ray [3]. In the present case, radiography images showed nothing more than swelling of the soft tissue. CT-scans are useful in determining the severity of bone loss in large joints such as the hip and knee. Medium-contrast enhanced CT-scans may also be worthwhile in detecting recurrent lesions [2]. The most effective screening method for diagnosis of PVNS is the MRI. MRIs can reveal scattered low-signal intensity areas in the synovial membrane, representing hemosiderin deposits on T2-weighted images, and dotted areas of low-signal intensity, representing fibrous components of the lesion on T1-weighted images [1–3] (Fig. 1).

There is not a standard method of treatment for PVNS, especially in pediatric patients [1–3]. The aim of treatment for PVNS is to remove all abnormal tissue in order to relieve pain, lower the risk of joint destruction,

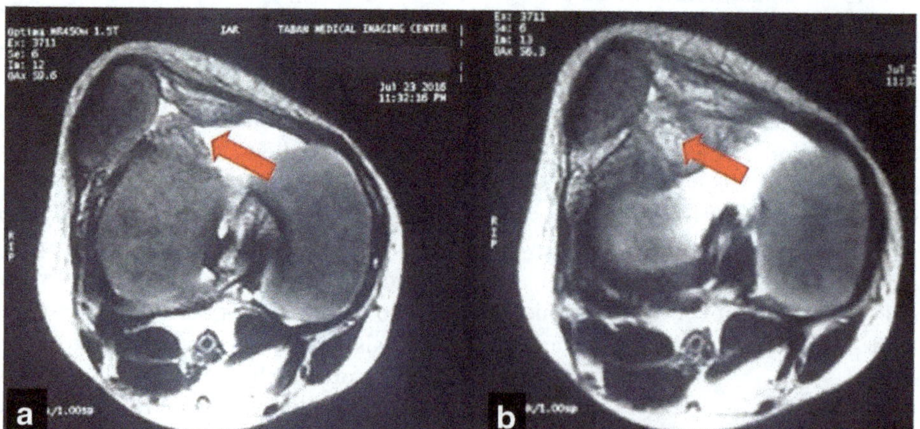

Fig. 1 MR image. **a** Arrow showes synovial proliferation on T2-Weighted image. Note patellar dislocation and joint effusion. **b** Arrow indicates scattered low-signal intensity areas in the synovial membrane, representing hemosiderin deposits on T2-weighted images

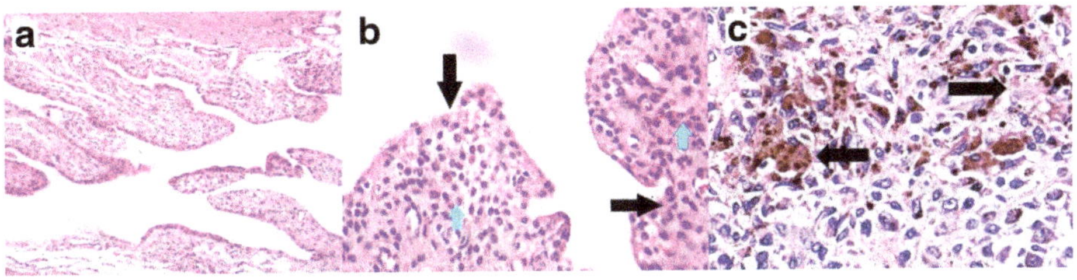

Fig. 2 Microscopic section of the synovial biopsy, Pigmented Villonodular Synovitis, **a.** Villous and nodular configuration. Note the hypertrophied synovium. (×4 and ×10, Hematoxylin-Eosin), **b.** Hypertrophied synovium (black arrows) and histiocytes, Hemosiderin-laden macrophages and osteoclast-like giant cells (blue arrowheads) are visible. (×40, Hematoxylin-Eosin), **c.** This section shows admixture of hemosiderin-laden and lipid-laden macrophages

and avoid local recurrence. The localized form of PVNS tends to be episodic and result in a good prognosis, while the diffuse form tends to progress gradually and recur more frequently [1, 4, 33]. Though there are several therapeutic solutions, the most common treatment is surgery [3]. Open or arthroscopic subtotal synovectomy is the most widely accepted surgery [1–3]. Some authors prefer arthroscopy to treat the localized form because this method results in less morbidity and a similar outcome as open surgery [1]. Some others

Table 1 Clinical presentations reported in literatures

Clinical presentation	Number of patients	Age (years)	Sex	Treatment (OS[a]/AS[b])	Follow up	Recurrence	Authors
Knee pain and swelling	21	1–15 (mean 9.1)	10 M[c], 11 F[d]	12 OS, 7 AS, 1 OS + AS, 1 injection	5 month-2 years	None	Baroni [3], Neubauer [12], Bruns [11], Jawadi [5], Deepak [14], Hong [6], Saulsburg [7], Jha [9], Maric [15], Nizam [13]
Painless swelling of knee	1	5	1 M	AS	2 years	None	Van Emelen [10]
Politeal cyst	1	12	1 M	OS + AS	–	–	Meehan [8]
Foot and ankle pain and swelling	4	3–14 (mean 10.3)	3 M 1 F	OS	6 month-2 years	None	Neubauer [12], Aghasi [24], Freedman [23], Kaneko [26]
Painless mass of foot and ankle	3	11–12 (mean 11.7)	1 M 2 F	OS	1–4 years	None	Zambakides [25], Sofier [21], Duncan [22]
Elbow	1	8	1 F	AS	–	–	Hsiu Su [19]
Non tender mass or swelling of elbow	2	6 (mean 6)	2 F	OS	2 years	None	Sekiya [18], Aydingoz [17]
Multifocal involvement	6	4.5–7 (mean 5.8)	1 M 5 F	OS	6 month-25 years	3 cases	Mukhopadhyay [28], Tavangar [27], Vedantam [29], Zhao [30], Walls [32], Leszczynski [31]
Hip pain	1	7	1 F	AS + OS	–	Not reported	Higuchi [20]
Sacral joint involvement	1	12	1 F	OS	–	–	Kang [20]
Hand swelling	1	7	1 F	OS	7 year	1 case	Neubauer [12]
Average	3.8	8.9	F/M: 1.6/1	OS 69%, AS 21.5%, OS + AS 7%, Injection 2.5	4.9 years	9.5%	

[a]Open synovectomy
[b]Arthroscopic synovectomy
[c]Male
[d]Female

prefer open surgery to arthroscopy because of the latter's disadvantages, such as the risk of recurrence and the possibility of portal contamination [3].

The literature reported 3 recurrences in cases in which the large joints were affected in multifocal form, and one recurrence in a case affecting the small hand joints (Table 1). The present case was treated with open synovectomy, lateral release, and a proximal realignment procedure and did not show any signs of recurrence during the 24 months following the treatment.

Radiotherapy and isotopic synoviorthesis have been used in adults for relapse cases or as adjuvant modality, but the use of radiotherapy in children is controversial, due to the possibility of post-irradiation sarcoma and damage to the physis [1–4]. Because PVNS, or tenosynovial giant cell tumor (TGCT), has characteristic cytogenetic abnormalities resulting in the overexpression of colony stimulating factor 1 (CSF1), systemic medication targeting the CSF1/CSF1R axis (imatinib, nilotinib, emactuzumab, and PLX3397) has been proposed in patients with diffuse, relapsed, or multifocal PVNS/TGCT [40]. The results from related studies will need to be confirmed in larger, ideally randomized clinical trials [41].

Conclusion

Although PVNS is a rare condition in pediatric patients, it can occur with symptoms resembling juvenile idiopathic arthritis, therefore it should be considered in differential diagnosis of any arthritis in children. PVNS in children may cause mechanical symptoms such as patellar dislocation. In these cases, lateral release and a proximal realignment procedure, in addition to synovectomy, can be useful methods of treatment.

Abbreviations

JIA: Juvenile idiopathic arthritis; MRI: Magnetic resonance imaging; PVNS: Pigmented villonodular synovitis; VMO: Vastus Medialis Obliquus

Acknowledgments

The authors wish to express their thanks to all hospital personnel involved in this study.

Funding

The study was performed without any funding.

Authors' contributions

MK designed the study and carried out the surgery for the patient. MS participated in data collection and wrote the article. RS carried out the rheumatologic consultation and reviewed articles on the subject. All authors read and approved the final manuscript.

Consent for publication

Consent to publish the manuscript has been obtained from the patient.

Competing interests

The authors declare that they have no competing interests.

References

1. Ottaviani S, Aryal X, Dougados M, Gossec L. Pigmented villonodular synovitis: a retrospective single center study of 122 cases and review of literature. Semin Arthritis Rheum. 2011;40(6):539–46.
2. Rydholm U. How I do it pigmented villonodular synovitis. Acta Orthop Scand. 1998;69(2):203–10.
3. Baroni E, Russo BD, Masquijo JJ, Bassini O, Miscione H. Pigmented villonodular synovitis of the knee in skeletally immature patients. J Child Orthop. 2010;4(2):123–7.
4. Flandry F, Hughston JC. Current concepts review: pigmented villonodular synovitis. J Bone Joint Surg Am. 1987;69:942–9.
5. Jawadi AH. Pigmented villonodular synovitis of the knee in a 12-month-old girl. J Taibah Univer Med Sci. 2014;9(4):335–7.
6. Man Hong C, TunHing L. Acute knee pain in a child due to pigmented Villonodular Synovitis. J Orthop Case Rep. 2015;5(3):78–80.
7. Saulsbury FT. Pigmented villonodular synovitis of the knee in a 9-year-old child. South Med J. 2004;97(1):80–2.
8. Meehan PL, Daftari T. Pigmented villonodular synovitis presenting as a popliteal cyst in a child. A case report. J Bone Joint Surg. 1994;76(4):593–5.
9. Jha SC, Nishisho T, Matsuura T, Takeuchi M, Miyagi R, Takao S, et al. Pigmented villonodular synovitis of the knee joint in a 5-year-old girl treated with combined open and arthroscopic surgery: a case report. J Ped Orthop. 2016;25(6):564–9.
10. Van Emelen K, Moens P, Wouters K, Fabry G. Villonodular synovitis of the knee in a 5-year-old child. Apropos of a case. Rev Chir Orthop Reparatrice Appar Mot. 1999;85(6):621–6.
11. Bruns J, Schubert T, Eggers-Stroeder G. Pigmented villonodular synovitis in children. A case report. Arch Orthop Trauma Surg. 1993;112:148–51.
12. Neubauer P, Weber K, Miller NH, McCarthy EF. Pigmented Villonodular Synovitis in children: a report of six cases and review of the literature. Iowa Orthop J. 2007;27:90–4.
13. Shand N, Hordon LD. Diffuse pigmented villonodular synovitis in a child – what is the best management? BMC Musculoskelet Disord. 2013;14(Suppl 1):A6.
14. Deepak S, Warrier K, Kerslake R, Rangaraj S. Knee swelling in a teenager - infection, inflammation or malignancy? Int J Clin Med Imaging. 2016;3:482.
15. Maric D, Vokovic N, Gajdobranski D, Draskovic B, Bekic V, Jovanovic M, et al. Pigmented villonodular synovitis of the knee in a child - case report. Arch of Oncol. 2004;12(1):75–7.
16. Higuchi C, Ohno I, Yoshikawa H. Hip joint pigmented villonodular synovitis in a young girl: a case report. J Ped Ortho B. 2012;21(4):335–8.
17. Aydingöz U, Leblebicioglu G, Gedikoglu G, Atay OA. Pigmented villonodular synovitis of the elbow in a 6-year-old girl. J Shoulder Elb Surg. 2002;11(3): 274–7.
18. Sekiya H, Ozawa H, Sugimoto N, Kariya Y, Hoshino Y. Pigmented villonodular synovitis of the elbow in a 6- years- girl: a case report. J Orthop Surg. 2007;15(1):106–8.
19. Su H, Gould E, Penna J, Meng H. A rare manifestation of pigmented Villonodular Synovitis of the elbow in a child. Radiol Case Rep. 2008;3(2):156.
20. Kang GH, Chi JG, Choi IH. Pigmented villonodular synovitis in the sacral joint with extensive bone destruction in a child. Pediatr Pathol. 1992;12(5): 725–30.
21. Soifer T, Guirguis S, Vigorita VJ, Bryk E. Pigmented villonodular synovitis in a child. J Ped Surg. 1993;28(12):1597–600.
22. Duncan N, Rajan R. Case report of pigmented villonodular synovitis arising from the calcaneocuboid joint in a 12 year old male. Foot. 2015;25:59–61.
23. Freedman BA, Lin DL, Tis JE. Pigmented Villonodular Synovitis of the Calcaneocuboid joint in an 11-year-old child with Subtalar coalition. Foot Ankle Int. 2007;28(4):511–5.
24. Aghasi MK, Robinson D, Reif RM, Halperin N. Pigmented Villonodular Synovitis of the talus in a child. Foot Ankle. 1988;9(3):139–42.
25. Christos Z, Stavros C, Vasileios S, Lampros MG, Panagiota G, et al. Pigmented Villonodular Synovitis emerging from the calcaneocuboid joint in a 12-year-old female child: a case report and review of the literature. Orthop Rheumatol. 2016;4(2):555–632.
26. Kaneko K, Nakahara D, Tobe M, Iwase H, Inoue Y, et al. Pigmented villonodular synovitis of the ankle in an adolescent. Intern Orthop (SICOT). 2000;24:234–7.

27. Tavangar SM, Ghafouri M. Multifocal pigmented villonodular synovitis in a child. Singap Med J. 2005;46(4):193.
28. Mukhopadhyay K, Smith M, Hughes PM. Multifocal PVNS in a child – followed over 25 years. Skelet Radiol. 2006;35(7):539–42.
29. Vedantam R, Strecker W, Schoenecker P, Salinas-Madrigal L. Polyarticular pigmented Villonodular Synovitis in a child. Clinical Ortho Related Res. 1998; 348:208.
30. Zhao L, Zhou K, Hua Y, Li Y, Mu D. Multifocal pigmented villonodular synovitis in a child: a case report. Medicine. 2016;95(33):e4572.
31. Leszczynski J, Huckell JR, Percy JS, LeRiche JC, Lentle BC. Pigmented villonodular synovitis in multiple joints. Occurrence in a child with cavernous haemangioma of lip and pulmonary stenosis. Ann Rheum Dis. 1975;34(3):269–72.
32. Walls J, Nogi J. Multifocal pigmented Villonodular Synovitis in a child. J Ped Orthop. 1985;5(2):229–31.
33. Myers BW, Masi AT, Feigenbaum SL. Pigmented villonodular synovitis and tenosynovitis: a clinical epidemiologic study of 166 cases and literature review. Medicine. 1980;59:223–38.
34. Xie GP, Jiang N, Liang CX, Zeng JC, Chen ZY, Xu Q, et al. Pigmented villonodular synovitis: a retrospective multicenter study of 237 cases. PLoS One. 2015;10(3):e0121451.
35. Flandry FC, Jacobson KE, Andrews JR. Localized pigmented villonodularsynovitis of the knee mimicking meniscal injury. Arthroscopy. 1986;2:217–21.
36. Özalay M, Tandogan RN, Akpınar S, Cesur N, Hersekli MA, Özkoç G, Uysal M. Arthroscopic treatment of solitary benign intra-articular lesions of the knee that cause mechanical symptoms. Arthroscopy. 2005;21(1):12–8.
37. Delcogliano A, Galli M, Menghi A, Belli P. Localized pigmented Villonodular Synovitis of the knee: report of two cases of fat pad involvement. Arthroscopy. 1998;14(5):527–31.
38. Edwards MR, Tibrewal S. Patello-femoral joint pain due to unusual location of localized pigmented villonodular synovitis: a case report. Knee. 2004;11:327–9.
39. Bartlett MJ, Lavelle J. Localized pigmented villonodular synovitis presenting as recurrent dislocation of the patella. Arthroscopy. 2000;16(7):767–9.
40. Temple HT. Pigmented villonodular synovitis therapy with MSCF-1 inhibitors. Curr Opin Oncol. 2012;24(4):404–8.
41. Brahmi M, Vinceneux A, Cassier PA. Current systemic treatment options for tenosynovial giant cell tumor/pigmented villonodular synovitis: targeting the CSF1/CSF1R axis. Curr Treat Options in Oncol. 2016;17(2):10.

20

Is palindromic rheumatism amongst children a benign disease?

Yonatan Butbul-Aviel[1,2,3], Yosef Uziel[4,5], Nofar Hezkelo[4], Riva Brik[1,2,3,4] and Gil Amarilyo[4,6*]

Abstract

Background: Palindromic rheumatism is an idiopathic, periodic arthritis characterized by multiple, transient, recurring episodes. Palindromic rheumatism is well-characterized in adults, but has never been reported in pediatric populations. The aim of this study was to characterize the clinical features and outcomes of a series of pediatric patients with palindromic rheumatism.

Methods: We defined clinical criteria for palindromic rheumatism and reviewed all clinical visits in three Pediatric Rheumatology centers in Israel from 2006through 2015, to identify patients with the disease. We collected retrospective clinical and laboratory data on patients who fulfilled the criteria, and reviewed their medical records in order to determine the proportion of patients who had developed juvenile idiopathic arthritis.

Results: Overall, 10 patients were identified. Their mean age at diagnosis was 8.3 ± 4.5 years and the average follow-up was 3.8 ± 2.7 years. The mean duration of attacks was 12.2 ± 8.4 days. The most frequently involved joints were knees. Patients tested positive for rheumatoid factor in 20% of cases.
One patient developed polyarticular juvenile idiopathic arthritis after three years of follow-up, six patients (60%) continued to have attacks at their last follow-up and only three children (30%) achieved long-term remission.

Conclusions: Progression to juvenile idiopathic arthritis is rare amongst children with palindromic rheumatism and most patients continued to have attacks at their last follow-up. Longer follow-up periods are required to predict the long-term outcomes of pediatric patients with palindromic rheumatism.

Keywords: Palindromic rheumatism, Children, Juvenile, Idiopathic, Arthritis, Palindromic

Background

Palindromic rheumatism (PR), originally described in 1944 by Hench and Rosenberg, is an idiopathic, periodic arthritis characterized by multiple, transient, recurring episodes of mono- or oligo-arthritis, associated with tissue swelling around the involved joints [1]. Episodes last from a few hours to a few days and then resolve spontaneously. Between episodes, there is no residual joint damage.

The condition involves little or no constitutional symptoms or abnormalities in laboratory tests, and no significant functional, pathologic, or radiological changes, even after years of disease.

* Correspondence: gamarilyo@clalit.org.il
[4]Sackler Faculty of Medicine, Tel Aviv University, Ramat Aviv, Israel
[6]Pediatric Rheumatology Unit, Schneider Children's Medical Center of Israel, 14 Kaplan St., 4920235 Petach Tikva, Israel
Full list of author information is available at the end of the article

In 1986, Pasero and Barbieri proposed five criteria for the diagnosis of PR, which include: (1) at least a six-month history of brief, recurrent episodes of mono-arthritis or polyarthritis with sudden onset, (2) direct observation by a physician of at least one attack, (3) involvement of three or more joints, although they could be involved at different times, (4) complete absence of radiographic findings, and (5) exclusion of all other arthritides [2].

Estimated prevalence is 1/8 to 1/20 compared to rheumatoid arthritis (RA) cases [2, 3]. Female predominance is similar to that observed among RA patients [4, 5], and cases were reported in persons 20 to 80 years-of-age [4]. Except for one recent case report, no cases have been described to date in the pediatric population [5]. There is no known ethnic predisposition to the disease.

The differential diagnosis of PR is broad and includes rheumatoid arthritis; crystalline arthropathies, such as gout; seronegative spondyloarthropathies, such as reactive arthritis or inflammatory bowel disease-related arthritis; Whipple's disease; Behcet's syndrome; relapsing polychondritis; intermittent hydrarthrosis and familial Mediterranean fever (FMF).

The aim of this study was to describe the clinical and laboratory features, therapies and follow-up outcomes of a series of pediatric patients with PR.

Methods

This cross-sectional, retrospective study was based on a review of medical records from patients referred to three, large, tertiary academic hospitals in Israel. To identify cases, a preliminary search of the electronic medical records of the outpatient pediatric rheumatology clinics (run by the authors YB, RB, YU, GA) was conducted. The search included the words arthropathy OR juvenile OR arthritis in the field "diagnosis" during the 10-year period from March 2006 to May 2016. The study was approved by the local Institutional Review Board of each participating hospital. Informed consent was waived.

Inclusion criteria were based on the Pasero and Barbieri criteria with some modifications, and included: age 1–16 years at presentation, recurrent attacks (at least three) of sudden-onset monoarthritis, polyarthritis or periarticular tissue inflammation lasting from a few hours to 5 weeks, verification of at least one attack by a physician and exclusion of all other forms of arthritides [2].

Retrieved data included demographic characteristics, age at onset of the disease, family history, attack frequency, triggering factors, duration of attacks, involved joints, and symptoms between attacks (if any). Laboratory tests included complete blood count, erythrocyte sedimentation rate (ESR), C-reactive protein (CRP), rheumatoid factor (RF), anti-CCP, anti-nuclear antibody (ANA), anti-double stranded DNA antibody (anti-dsDNA) and imaging data. When available, results from other diagnostic tests, such as the pathergy test, human leukocyte antigen (HLA)-B27/B5 test, radiography of other parts, genetics for common MEFV mutations and ophthalmologic examination data were collected.

Results

Among 630 records identified, 11 matched the inclusion criteria and were reviewed thoroughly. One patient was excluded due to sparse follow-up data. Ten pediatric patients with palindromic rheumatism were diagnosed from March 2006 to May 2016. Demographic characteristics of the patients are presented in Table 1.

Five patients (50%) had a family history of rheumatic disease, including two with a family history of Crohn's disease, one of RA and two patients of psoriasis.

Table 1 Demographic data of pediatric patients with palindromic rheumatism

Age at diagnosis (years ± SD)	8.3 ± 4.5
Male/female (N)	6/4
Number of episodes during follow up (N ± SD); (range)	11.3 ± 8.8; (4–29)
Length of follow-up [a] (years ± SD)	3.8 ± 2.7
Total number of involved joints (no. ± SD)	3.1 ± 1.6
Systemic symptoms during attacks (%)	20
Average duration of episodes (days)	12.2 ± 8 .4
Morning stiffness during attacks (%)	50

[a]Defined as the time from first presentation to last follow-up

The duration of follow-up ranged from 6 months to 9.9 years (median 3.5 years) and the number of episodes ranged from 3 to 29 (median 9.5 episodes).

Except for arthritis, no patients had any other systemic manifestations (including fevers) during flares. The knee was the joint most frequently involved and all patients had knee arthritis at least once. The second most frequently involved joints were the wrists and ankles in three patients, each (30%) (Table 2). In nine patients (90%), flares were monoarticular or oligoarticular.

Laboratory and radiographic findings

During flares, C-reactive protein (CRP) was elevated in four patients (40%), the average value was 21.5 mg/dl (median 2.5 mg/dl, range 0.5–120 mg/dl). The erythrocyte sedimentation rate (ESR) measured in eight patients was higher than 30 mm/h in half of the cases. No leukocytosis was noted in any patient.

RF was measured in nine patients and was positive, albeit in low titers, in two patients (22%). Antinuclear antibodies (ANA) were measured in nine patients and were positive (defined as a titer higher than 1:80) in three patients (33%). HLAB27 antigen was measured in three patients and was negative in all cases.

Table 2 Prevalence of involved joints during attacks in pediatric patients with palindromic rheumatism

Joints	Percentage
Knees	100
Wrists	30
Ankles	30
Hips	20
Elbows	10
Fingers	10

Genetics for the most common MEFV mutations were evaluated in six patients, none of whom was found to be a carrier. The affected joints were x-rayed at least once in eight patients; no erosions, joint space narrowing, or subchondral cyst erosions were observed. One patient had a bone scan that showed evidence of arthritis. Two patients had US of the affected joint (2 knees and 1 elbow) during flare, which demonstrated evidence of synovitis with variable degrees of synovial effusion. Six patients were examined by an ophthalmologist and had normal results.

Six children had joint aspiration. Only one had a markedly elevated synovial white blood cell count ($57.300 \times 10^9/l$). Synovial fluid cultures were negative in all cases.

Medications and long-term follow-up

Three patients were treated during flares with a short course of systemic corticosteroids, all with good response. One patient received a local corticosteroid joint injection with flare resolution.

A trial of a prophylactic agent was administered to six patients: colchicine to four with partial response, and two patients were treated with NSAIDS for long periods with no response.

Patients were asymptomatic between flares, and only one developed fever during a portion of the episodes.

Long-term remission was defined as at least six months with no flares. and was achieved in three patients (30%) during the follow-up period. These included one who was treated with prophylactic colchicine, but eventually developed JIA.

In addition, one patient developed polyarticular JIA 3 years after experiencing palindromic flares in his knee and wrists. Six patients (60%) continued to have attacks and never achieved long-term remission (followed for 5.3 ± 2.7 years).

Discussion

Although PR is well-described in the adult population, to the best of our knowledge it has never been reported in the pediatric population, except for one recent case report [5]. The definition of PR in adults is not well-established and a few criteria have been suggested. In 1987, Hannonen et al. [2] suggested criteria that included: (1) recurrent attacks of sudden-onset monoarthritis, polyarthritis or periarticular tissue inflammation, lasting from a few hours to one week; 2) verification of at least one attack by a physician; 3) subsequent attacks in at least three different joints; and 4) exclusion of other forms of arthritides [6]. This set of criteria has not been adopted by the American Rheumatism Association or by the American College of Rheumatology.

The criteria used in this study were based on the Hannonen criteria [6], as in our experience, some of the attacks lasted longer than one week. The length of episodes in most of the patients ranged from a few days to two weeks. The first presenting episode ranged from 2 days to 2 weeks.

Unlike JIA, which affects mostly females, men were more commonly affected in our series. The literature provides mixed information as to whether there is a sex difference in adult PR, and a report which suggests male predominance [7].

In terms of joints affected, knee, wrists, and small joints of the hand have been reported in the literature as most commonly affected in adult PR. In our series, most of the patients experienced involvement of the large joints and all had knee arthritis at least once [3].

Unlike in the adult population, the differential diagnosis of pediatric PR may include a number of unique clinical entities, such as sport and playground injuries; joint hypermobility/Ehlers-Danlos; transient hip synovitis; post-infectious arthritis, (such as post streptococcal reactive arthritis); osteochondrosis, and pain amplification syndromes. These possibilities, as well as others were carefully ruled out by the treating pediatric rheumatologists after extensive workup.

Family history of rheumatic disease was relatively common in our series (45%), and most of the reported family diseases were of psoriasis and inflammatory bowel disease. This finding has not been reported previously.

Cañete, et al. found a high frequency of MEFV mutations in Spanish PR patients with anti-citrullinated protein antibody-negative PR, compared with those with positive anti-citrullinated protein antibody (22.2% vs. 5.3%) [8]. FMF is not a rare disease in the Israel population, and although PR is not a typical presentation of FMF, six patients had negative tests for the common MEFV mutation. Four patients were treated with colchicine and all exhibited only partial response.

Inflammatory markers were elevated in 40% of our patients (40% to 50%), comparable to adult PR. RF is usually found in 40% to 65% of adult PR, and its presence has been associated with a more severe form of the disease, as well as with a higher probability of eventually developing classic RA [6]. In our series, only two patients (ages 9 and 15) had low, positive RF titers, and anti-CCP levels were not examined in these patients.

Although most of the patients in our series did not achieve long-term remission, only one child developed JIA after 3 years of PR. In adults, it has been reported that at one-year follow-up, 27.5% of patients with PR developed RA and 3% developed systemic lupus erythematosus, while 50% of the patients developed different types of chronic arthritis [9]. The outcomes in our series were better than that in adults, but a longer follow-up period is required to determine the percentage of pediatric PR patients who will develop chronic arthritis. The literature reports only one case of progression of PR to JIA, that occurred in a Japanese girl carrying heterozygous L110P-E148Q substitutions of the MEFV gene [5].

Limitations of our study include its retrospective nature, the paucity of described cases and a short follow-up period of 0.5–9.9 years. Moreover, since FMF is relatively common in the Israeli population and the MEFV gene is not fully screened, some of our patients may have an unusual presentation of FMF. Nonetheless, Israeli rheumatologists are very familiar with FMF and in all cases where FMF was suspected, even with a negative genetic test, a colchicine trial was initiated. No patient displayed a prominent response to colchicine therapy.

Conclusion

This is the first case series reported of a pediatric population with PR which summarizes clinical follow-up of 10 patients from 3 large Israeli tertiary pediatric medical centers. Progression to juvenile idiopathic arthritis in this children was found to be uncommon and most patients continued to have attacks at their last follow-up. Clinicians should be aware of this disease in children and it should be considered in the differential diagnosis of any child who presents with recurrent acute arthritis and negative work-up for autoimmune or autoinflammatory disease. Additional studies are needed to better describe PR and its long-term outcomes, and to determine optimal treatments for this syndrome.

Acknowledgements
Faye Schreiber edited the manuscript.

Funding
None to declare.

Authors' contributions
ABY conceptualized and designed the study, drafted the initial manuscript, participated in data collection, and reviewed and revised the manuscript. YU participated in data collection, and reviewed and revised the manuscript. NH participated in data collection, and reviewed and revised the manuscript. RB participated in data collection, and reviewed and revised the manuscript. GA conceptualized and designed the study, participated in data collection, and reviewed and revised the manuscript. All authors read and approved the final manuscript.

Competing interests
The authors declare that they have no competing interests.

Author details
[1]Department of Pediatrics B, Ruth Rappaport Children's Hospital, Rambam Medical Center, Haifa, Israel. [2]Pediatric Rheumatology Service, Ruth Rappaport Children's Hospital, Rambam Medical Center, Haifa, Israel. [3]The Ruth and Bruce Rappaport Faculty of Medicine, The Technion - Israel Institute of Technology, Haifa, Israel. [4]Sackler Faculty of Medicine, Tel Aviv University, Ramat Aviv, Israel. [5]Pediatric Rheumatology Unit, Department of Pediatrics, Meir Medical Center, Kfar Saba, Israel. [6]Pediatric Rheumatology Unit, Schneider Children's Medical Center of Israel, 14 Kaplan St., 4920235 Petach Tikva, Israel.

References

1. Hench PS, Rosenberg EF. Palindromic Rheumatism. Arch Intern Med. 1944; 73:293–321.
2. Pasero G, Barbieri P. Palindromic rheumatism: you just have to think about it!. Clin Exp Rheumatol. 4(3):197–9. Available from: http://www.ncbi.nlm.nih.gov/pubmed/3490340. [cited 2017 Apr 1].
3. Powell A, Davis P, Jones N, Russell AS. Palindromic rheumatism is a common disease: comparison of new-onset palindromic rheumatism compared to new-onset rheumatoid arthritis in a 2-year cohort of patients. J Rheumatol. 2008;35(6):992–4. Available from: http://www.ncbi.nlm.nih.gov/pubmed/18412310. [cited 2017 Apr 1].
4. Gonzalez-Lopez L, Gamez-Nava JI, Jhangri GS, Ramos-Remus C, Russell AS, Suarez-Almazor ME. Prognostic factors for the development of rheumatoid arthritis and other connective tissue diseases in patients with palindromic rheumatism. J Rheumatol. 1999;26(3):540–545. Available from: http://www.ncbi.nlm.nih.gov/pubmed/10090159. [cited 2017 Apr 1].
5. Kobayashi I, Yamazaki Y, Tozawa Y, Ueki M, Takezaki S, Yamada M, et al. Progression of palindromic rheumatism to juvenile idiopathic arthritis in a Japanese girl carrying heterozygous L110P-E148Q substitutions of MEFV gene. Mod Rheumatol. 2015;1–4. Available from: http://www.tandfonline.com/doi/full/10.3109/14397595.2015.1106639. [cited 2017 Apr 1].
6. Hannonen P, Möttönen T, Oka M. Palindromic rheumatism. A clinical survey of sixty patients. Scand J Rheumatol. 1987;16(6):413–20. Available from: http://www.ncbi.nlm.nih.gov/pubmed/3423751. [cited 2017 Apr 1].
7. Khabbazi A, Hajialiloo M, Kolahi S, Soroosh M, Esalatmanesh K, Sharif S. A multicenter study of clinical and laboratory findings of palindromic rheumatism in Iran. Int J Rheum Dis. 2012;15(4):427–430. Available from: http://doi.wiley.com/10.1111/j.1756-185X.2012.01739.x. [cited 2017 Apr 1].
8. Cañete JD, Arostegui JI, Queiró R, Gratacós J, Hernández MV, Larrosa M, et al. An unexpectedly high frequency of MEFV mutations in patients with anti-citrullinated protein antibody-negative palindromic rheumatism. Arthritis Rheum. 2007 Aug;56(8):2784–8. Available from: http://doi.wiley.com/10.1002/art.22755. [cited 2017 Apr 1].
9. Tamai M, Kawakami A, Iwamoto N, Arima K, Aoyagi K, Eguchi K. Contribution of anti-CCP antibodies, proximal interphalangeal joint involvement, HLA-DRB1 shared epitope, and PADI4 as risk factors for the development of rheumatoid arthritis in palindromic rheumatism. Scand J Rheumatol. 2010;39(4):287–91. Available from: http://www.tandfonline.com/doi/full/10.3109/03009741003604534. [cited 2017 Apr 1].

21

Development of practice and consensus-based strategies including a treat-to-target approach for the management of moderate and severe juvenile dermatomyositis in Germany and Austria

Claas H. Hinze[1*], Prasad T. Oommen[2], Frank Dressler[3], Andreas Urban[4], Frank Weller-Heinemann[5], Fabian Speth[6,7], Elke Lainka[8], Jürgen Brunner[9], Heike Fesq[10], Dirk Foell[1], Wolfgang Müller-Felber[11], Ulrich Neudorf[8], Christoph Rietschel[12], Tobias Schwarz[13], Ulrike Schara[14] and Johannes-Peter Haas[10]

Abstract

Background: Juvenile dermatomyositis (JDM) is the most common inflammatory myopathy in childhood and a major cause of morbidity among children with pediatric rheumatic diseases. The management of JDM is very heterogeneous. The JDM working group of the Society for Pediatric Rheumatology (GKJR) aims to define consensus- and practice-based strategies in order to harmonize diagnosis, treatment and monitoring of JDM.

Methods: The JDM working group was established in 2015 consisting of 23 pediatric rheumatologists, pediatric neurologists and dermatologists with expertise in the management of JDM. Current practice patterns of management in JDM had previously been identified via an online survey among pediatric rheumatologists and neurologists. Using a consensus process consisting of online surveys and a face-to-face consensus conference statements were defined regarding the diagnosis, treatment and monitoring of JDM. During the conference consensus was achieved via nominal group technique. Voting took place using an electronic audience response system, and at least 80% consensus was required for individual statements.

Results: Overall 10 individual statements were developed, finally reaching a consensus of 92 to 100% regarding (1) establishing a diagnosis, (2) case definitions for the application of the strategies (moderate and severe JDM), (3) initial diagnostic testing, (4) monitoring and documentation, (5) treatment targets within the context of a treat-to-target strategy, (6) supportive therapies, (7) explicit definition of a treat-to-target strategy, (8) various glucocorticoid regimens, including intermittent intravenous methylprednisolone pulse and high-dose oral glucocorticoid therapies with tapering, (9) initial glucocorticoid-sparing therapy and (10) management of refractory disease.

Conclusion: Using a consensus process among JDM experts, statements regarding the management of JDM were defined. These statements and the strategies aid in the management of patients with moderate and severe JDM.

Keywords: Dermatomyositis, Child, Consensus, Diagnosis, Antirheumatic agents, Comparative effectiveness research

* Correspondence: claas.hinze@ukmuenster.de
[1]Department of Pediatric Rheumatology and Immunology, University Hospital Münster, Albert-Schweitzer-Campus 1, Building D3, 48149 Münster, Germany
Full list of author information is available at the end of the article

Background

Juvenile dermatomyositis (JDM) is the most common inflammatory myopathy of childhood and a major cause of morbidity and mortality among patients with pediatric rheumatic diseases [1]. The management of JDM is highly variable internationally [2, 3]. Few controlled trials have been performed on the treatment of JDM, e.g. on methotrexate (MTX), cyclosporin A (CSA) and rituximab (RTX) [4, 5]. The type of glucocorticoid regimen used is especially variable, with many centers using high-dose oral glucocorticoid therapy while others use intermittent intravenous methylprednisolone pulse therapy [6–10]. Multiple smaller open label or retrospective studies have been performed, e.g. on cyclophosphamide (CYC), tumor necrosis factor inhibitors (TNFi), high-dose intravenous immune globulins (IVIG), or mycophenolate mofetil (MMF) [9, 11–13]. Frequently, treatment is based on expert opinion [1, 6, 14]. Notably, only few formally approved treatment options exist for the treatment of dermatomyositis (DM), in Germany, including various glucocorticoids (methylprednisolone, prednisolone, prednisone, dexamethasone, triamcinolone), azathioprin [AZA], and, under certain conditions, IVIG) [15]. However, none of these medications have been specifically approved for the use in JDM. Recently, consensus treatment plans have been established in North America by the Childhood Arthritis & Rheumatology Research Alliance (CARRA) and consensus-based treatment recommendations were developed by the Single Hub and Access point for pediatric Rheumatology in Europe (SHARE) initiative [16, 17]. The role of biologic agents in the management of JDM is less well defined, even though they are frequently used as outlined by a recent survey among CARRA members [18]. However, there is evidence that treatment approaches for JDM in Germany vary in several aspects from those used in other countries, including the choice of glucocorticoid therapy regimens [19]. Lately, the concept of treat-to-target and tight control has been a cornerstone of current treatment recommendations for rheumatoid arthritis, systemic lupus erythematosus and gout, and has been discussed for pediatric rheumatic diseases as well [20–24].

The PRO-KIND (PROjekte zur Klassifikation, Überwachung und Therapie in der KINDerrheumatologie; projects for the classification, monitoring and therapy in pediatric rheumatology) initiative is a sub-committee of the Society for Pediatric Rheumatology (GKJR) in Germany and Austria and aims to define consensus-based plans to harmonize diagnostic and treatment approaches. This initiative was started since it was perceived that children with juvenile rheumatic diseases in Germany and Austria often are either treated too late or not treated with the most up-to-date therapeutic regimens. To meet this challenge, the goal of the PRO-KIND initiative is to foster the use of harmonized diagnostic and treatment plans with defined targets [25, 26]. Previously, the JDM working group had identified current practice patterns in Germany and Austria among pediatric rheumatologists and neurologists [19].

As a next step, the goal of the PRO-KIND working group on JDM was to harmonize previously identified patterns into plans and statements.

Methods

PRO-KIND JDM working group and expert panel

The JDM working group was formed in April 2015, initially comprised of 12 pediatric rheumatologists with clinical expertise in the management of patients with JDM. Identification of project goals took place via a formal online survey using the web-based program SurveyMonkey (SurveyMonkey Inc.; San Mateo, California, USA; www.surveymonkey.com). Nine pediatric rheumatologists participated in an initial face-to-face meeting in January 2016. There was consensus that the expert panel should also include expert pediatric neurologists. Therefore, 2 pediatric neurologists with special expertise in managing JDM (W. M-F. and U.S.) were also invited to join the group, forming an extended interdisciplinary expert panel.

Consensus conference

An extended expert panel with 13 voting members (11 pediatric rheumatologists, 2 pediatric neurologists) and a non-voting dermatologist experienced in the care of children with JDM participated in a final face-to-face consensus meeting on January 13, 2017. The extended expert panel overlapped with but was not identical with the members of the initial working group. Prior to the consensus conference, the voting members had received access to various essential data via sciebo, a cloud service hosted by the state of Northrhine-Westphalia. The data provided included detailed results of previous online surveys, previous meeting protocols, essential literature obtained via an extensive literature search (but not formally graded), including the 112 papers that were scored by SHARE [16]. The process was guided by a psychologist trained as a professional moderator. We used nominal group technique for consensus building. For each individual statement, the following procedures were performed: the statement and its background were presented by one of the co-authors (C.H.) who had formulated the statement in question. Subsequently, every participant of the consensus conference had 1 min of time available to raise issues with the statement being discussed. These issues were recorded on a flip-chart. Then there was a 15-min open discussion of these items to further improve the statement. Changes to the statement were made ad hoc by another co-author (P.O.) using the PowerPoint presentation program, visible to all participants. Finally, anonymous voting took place during which each participant could either accept or reject the respective statement via an electronic audience response system. Consensus was considered to be present if at least 80% of experts supported a statement.

Results

Expert panel

The expert status of the panel members is demonstrated by the fact that centers represented in the panel contributed more than half of all patients (for example, in 2016: 72 out of 127 [57%]) with JDM documented within the National Pediatric Rheumatic Disease Database ("Kerndokumentation rheumakranker Kinder und Jugendlicher").

Diagnosis and case definition

Regarding the diagnosis of JDM, there was consensus that the conventional Bohan and Peter criteria should be modified. In particular, there was consensus that typical magnetic resonance imaging (MRI) findings represented an important finding for establishing a diagnosis of JDM. Furthermore, electromyography was removed from the list of findings. The finding of symmetric proximal muscle weakness was modified to also include myalgia as a possible criterion (Table 1). Concerning the statements developed and the resulting treatment strategies, the group devised a case definition for moderate and severe JDM, similar to an existing CARRA definition (Table 1) [17]. According to the consensus, all patients with active moderate or severe JDM may be treated with strategies outlined here. Regarding this manuscript, we will from now on simply refer to JDM, indicating moderate or severe JDM. Additionally, the group developed a list of diagnostic tests that may be useful in patients with JDM. While some of the tests may be useful for establishing a diagnosis of JDM, others may be useful to rule out alternative diagnoses or to assess for potential organ involvement or complications. Also, myositis-specific antibodies were felt to be an important aspect of the work-up.

Disease monitoring

It was felt to be important to define a minimum dataset that should be routinely collected on all patients with at least moderate JDM (Table 2). The group discussed the various validated parameters, taking into account the familiarity of practitioners in Germany with the respective investigations based on a recently performed online survey among pediatric rheumatologists and neurologists in Germany [16, 19, 27–30]. The investigations include measurements of global, muscular and extramuscular disease activity, functional impairment, quality of life and disease damage.

Treatment strategy and treatment targets

The group defined a treat-to-target strategy, which means treatment to be adjusted according to the achievement of previously defined targets (Table 3). It was felt that generally, the initial phase of therapy should be more intensive in order to quickly achieve improvement ("remission induction") and avoid undertreatment, with the aim to reduce damage, such as contractures, calcinosis and chronic muscle weakness. The reason for this notion was two-fold: first, there is a high risk of complications in the acute phase of the disease, and, second, there is an increased risk for disease damage with longer duration of active disease [31–34]. Concerning treatment targets, there was consensus that at least a moderate improvement should be observed within 6 weeks after implementing a major change in therapy and at least a major improvement within 12 weeks after a major change in therapy, with improvement defined according to the American College of Rheumatology/European League Against Rheumatism criteria (Table 3) [35]. The consensus on the 12-month goal was to achieve a glucocorticoid-free treatment regimen. This is similar to what the CARRA consensus treatment plans state [17].

Specific therapies for juvenile dermatomyositis

Supportive therapies

There was consensus that all patients with JDM should receive supportive therapy including physical therapy to prevent contractures, muscle weakness, de-conditioning and disability. Early return to sports activities is encouraged as long as it is safely possible. Effective sun and/or ultraviolet light protection using avoidance, textile protection or sunscreen is strongly suggested. Additional supportive therapies may include hydroxychloroquin (HCQ), vitamin D or calcium supplementation (Table 4). It was debated whether HCQ constituted a supportive therapy or a disease-modifying antirheumatic drug (DMARD) in the context of JDM, i.e. a medication that may fundamentally alter the course of disease, in the context of JDM. Eventually, there was consensus that there is not enough evidence to consider HCQ a DMARD sensu stricto. Therefore, in order to avoid the (mis)use of HCQ in case of refractory disease as a means to intensify therapy, it was opted to define HCQ as a supportive agent for the purpose of this project.

Glucocorticoid therapies

Different glucocorticoid regimens were preferred by experts within the panel. Based on the results of a previous survey [19], 3 glucocorticoid regimens have been listed which were generally acceptable to the group members in the treatment of patients with new-onset JDM. The regimens included an intermittent intravenous methylprednisolone pulse (IVMP) therapy in combination with either low-to-moderate (prednisone/prednisolone [PDN] equivalent 0.2–0.5 mg/kg/day) or moderate-to-high-dose (PDN equivalent 0.5–2 mg/kg max. 60–80 mg/day) glucocorticoids, or conventional high-dose oral glucocorticoids (PDN equivalent 2 mg/kg max. 60–80 mg/day) with or without a single IVMP pulse (Table 4).

Table 1 Diagnosis of juvenile dermatomyositis and case definitions

Statements	Consensus
Diagnosis	100%
For the diagnosis of juvenile dermatomyositis, the following findings should be present prior to age 18 years: • Typical skin finding (heliotrope and/or Gottron-sign/–papules) Additional criteria: • Symmetric proximal muscle weakness and/or myalgia • Increased muscle-related enzymes (creatine kinase, glutamate oxaloacetate transaminase, lactate dehydrogenase and/or aldolase) • Typical findings on muscle biopsy • Typical findings on magnetic resonance imaging Other possible etiologies should be excluded. Probable JDM: Skin findings and at least 2 additional criteria Definite JDM: Skin findings and at least 3 additional criteria	
Case definition	92%
The treatment strategies discussed below apply to patients with active moderately severe or severe juvenile dermatomyositis. Patients with severe juvenile dermatomyositis fulfill at least one of the following characteristics and none of these characteristics is present in patients with moderate JDM: • Age < 1 year • Requirement for intensive care therapy • Marked disability as measured by being bedridden, childhood myositis assessment scale (CMAS) < 15 or manual muscle testing (MMT)8 < 30 • Relevant pulmonary disease • Myocarditis • Vasculitis with organ involvement (gastrointestinal tract, kidney, lungs or central nervous system) • Aspiration or marked dysphagia • Severe cutaneous ulceration • Significant calcinosis	
Diagnostic work-up	100%
Obtaining the following parameters may be useful in case of probable or definite JDM: • Laboratory tests: o Enzymes (creatine kinase, glutamate oxaloacetate transaminase, glutamate pyruvate transaminase, lactate dehydrogenase, aldolase) o Complete blood count with differential count o Routine serum chemistry panel o Inflammatory markers (C-reactive protein, erythrocyte sedimentation rate) o Antinuclear antibody (ANA) o In case of positive ANA: anti-ds-DNA, anti-PM-Scl, Sm antibodies, anti-SS-A, anti-SS-B and anti-U1RNP antibodies o Extended myositis-blot/myositis-specific antibody (incl. Anti-synthetase, anti-MDA5, anti-Mi-2, anti-NXP-2, anti-SRP, anti-TIF-1-γ antibodies) o Immunoglobulin (Ig)G, IgA, IgM o Complement (CH50) o Von Willebrand factor-antigen o Troponin o TSH o Immunization status o Urinalysis o Stool for occult blood • Further testing: o Electrocardiography o Echocardiography o Magnetic resonance imaging (incl. Short tau inversion recovery or equivalent sequences) o Chest X-ray o Abdominal ultrasound o Muscle ultrasound o Muscle biopsy o Bodyplethysmography with CO-diffusion capacity o Capillary microscopy	

Tapering of glucocorticoids

No consensus was found concerning a specific tapering protocol for glucocorticoids. However, the group defined landmarks for the glucocorticoid taper, i.e. the aim to discontinue glucocorticoids after 12 months of therapy, and, in case of initial high-dose oral glucocorticoid therapy, PDN doses of 50, 25 and 12.5% 2 months, 4 months and 6 months after initiation of therapy, respectively (Table 4).

Choice of initial disease-modifying antirheumatic drug therapy

There was consensus that all patients with at least moderate JDM should receive MTX therapy, preferentially subcutaneously, or, if there was intolerance to MTX, an alternative disease-modifying antirheumatic drug (DMARD) therapy, such as AZA, CSA or MMF. Furthermore, there was consensus that high-dose IVIG may be used in conjunction with DMARD therapy, especially in case of severe JDM (Table 4). However, specific regimens of IVIG therapy were not addressed.

Treatment of refractory disease

The expert group considered refractory disease to be present if the predefined treatment targets were not reached. Furthermore, patients with longstanding (i.e. not new-onset) JDM may be treated according to strategies outlined here. The group considered two options to be viable under these circumstances: (1) Additional therapy with another DMARD, specifically, AZA, calcineurin inhibitos (CSA or tacrolimus), CYC, IVIG, MMF, RTX or TNFi, or (2) changing therapy to one of these medications. However, there was no consensus on which specific sequence of medications would be preferred. In order to reflect this uncertainty, the medications or medication classes are simply listed alphabetically (Table 4).

Developing a treatment strategy

The statements developed are condensed in Fig. 1. Patients with JDM may enter the treatment strategies outlined before either with new-onset disease or with existing long-standing disease. Patients with new-onset JDM are treated with one of the glucocorticoid regimens and a DMARD, preferentially MTX, whereas treatment

Table 2 Monitoring parameters for patients with juvenile dermatomyositis

Statement	Consensus
Disease monitoring tools	100%
In order to monitor disease activity and disease damage over time, the regular measurement of the following parameters may be useful (initially every 6 weeks, later every 3 months): • Length, weight, blood pressure • Physician global assessment of disease activity (visual analog scale 0–10) • Parent/Patient global assessment of disease activity (visual analog 0–10) • Manual muscle testing (MMT)8 and/or Childhood Myositis Assessment Scale (CMAS) • Childhood Health Assessment Questionnaire (CHAQ) • A validated Quality of life instrument • Muscle enzymes • Extramuscular disease activity, e.g. via Disease Activity Score, Myositis Disease Activity Assessment Tool or Visual Analog Scale • Myositis damage index (annually)	

with existing and active JDM may enter the strategies later. An essential part of the treatment strategies is the treat-to-target concept, i.e. the need for frequent monitoring of disease activity and adjustment of treatment if treatment targets are not reached.

Discussion

Based on data on the current clinical practice in Germany we defined consensus-based statements and strategies supporting the diagnosis and the management of JDM. The expert panel consisted both of pediatric neurologist and rheumatologists with all of them having practical experience in managing JDM. The group supports the use of "adapted" Bohan and Peter criteria for the diagnosis of JDM, including the use of specific MRI findings as a Bohan and Peter "equivalent" criterion, similar to what others have proposed in the past [2]. There are a variety of diagnostic tests that are frequently employed in Germany to assist in the diagnosis and assessment of patients with JDM, and therefore are represented here. More recent developments, such as the discovery of myositis-specific antibodies (MSAs) that may be rather specific to JDM when compared to adult DM are also included, and it is felt that these antibodies may have diagnostic and prognostic value [36–39]. We defined, to our knowledge for the first time, an explicit treat-to-target strategy for the management of JDM using the recently developed ACR/EULAR response criteria indicating absent, minimal, moderate or major improvement for formal assessment of treatment response [35]. Notably, others have shown that aggressive therapy of JDM using treatment targets may lead to improved outcome [8]. Similarly, the North American CARRA plans guide treatment decisions based on whether patients are unchanged, worsening, or experiencing medication side effects or disease complications [17]. The European SHARE recommendations focus on whether improvement is present or absent to guide treatment decisions but does not precisely delineate time frames for improvement [16]. The treat-to-target concept focusses on strategy rather than on specific treatment modalities which, for example, has been proven superior to conventional therapy in rheumatoid arthritis [40]. While the overall goal of therapy was defined as clinical inactive disease, we did not define this further during the consensus conference. However, we think that it would be reasonable to apply the validated set of criteria by either IMACS or PRINTO [41, 42].

Table 3 Treatment targets and treatment strategy

Statements	Consensus
Treatment targets	100%
The overall goal is clinical inactive disease within 1 year after initiation of therapy, ideally under a glucocorticoid-free treatment regimen. Under some circumstances, low-dose glucocorticoids or intermittent intravenous methylprednisolone pulse therapy may be acceptable. The following interim improvement[a] is targeted: • At least a moderate improvement within 6 weeks after initiation or substantial change in therapy. • At least a major improvement within 3 months after initiation or substantial change in therapy.	
General treatment strategy	92%
The consensus treatment strategies for JDM serve to harmonize existing therapies in clinical practice. The treatment strategy generally consists of a treat-to-target strategy, i.e. therapies are modified according to reaching or failing previously established targets. In addition, there is a more intensive first (induction) treatment phase (6–8 weeks) and a less intensive subsequent (maintenance) phase. Components of the initial therapy include glucocorticoids and glucocorticoid-sparing DMARDs.	

[a] American College of Rheumatology/European League Against Rheumatism criteria (categories: no, minimal, moderate, major improvement) [34]

Since there is a relative lack of data from randomized controlled clinical trials (RCTs), and since it is unlikely that large-scale RCTs for JDM will take place, one possible solution to gather more information on the efficacy or inefficacy of various treatments may be to collect "real life" data on disease outcome, i.e. to pursue comparative effectiveness research [43]. An important prerequisite for comparative effectiveness research is the application of uniform and harmonized treatments. Therefore, the harmonization of existing clinical practice has been an important goal for this project. Furthermore, the regular collection of a dataset in patients with JDM is of utmost importance to allow comparison of clinical outcomes, not only nationally but also internationally. Consequently, our statements include the minimal dataset agreed upon by international experts [29].

These harmonized consensus strategies overall fit rather well into the above-mentioned framework set up by the CARRA consensus treatment plans and the SHARE

Table 4 Therapies used in juvenile dermatomyositis

Statements	Consensus
Supportive therapy	100%
Early and intensive physical therapy is essential in order to avoid contractures and improve/maintain muscle strength, even during active myositis. Participation in sports is desirable after individual counseling. Effective sun protection is essential, incl. textile protection and sunscreen. The following treatments may be considered individually: • Supplementation of vitamin D, e.g. depending on 25-OH vitamin D level, glucocorticoid treatment and/or bone mineral density • Supplementation of calcium, e.g. in case of insufficient intake • Hydroxychloroquin	
Initial glucocorticoid therapy	92%
The principal glucocorticoid strategy options include • Intermittent intravenous methylprednisolone pulse (IVMP) therapy + moderate-to-high-dose daily glucocorticoids (prednisone equivalent 0.5–2 mg/kg [max. 80 mg] daily) • Intermittent IVMP therapy + lower-to-moderate dose daily glucocorticoids (prednisone equivalent 0.2–0.5 mg/kg daily) • High-dose daily glucocorticoid therapy (2 mg/kg [max. 60–80 mg] daily) +/− initial single IVMP pulse	
Glucocorticoid tapering	92%
The following landmarks may be applied when tapering glucocorticoids, assuming an adequate treatment response (i.e. treatment targets are reached): • IVMP o 20–30 mg/kg (max. 1000 mg) daily × 3 days o At 2 and 4 weeks, subsequently every 4–6 weeks × 6–12 months • High-dose daily glucocorticoids (prednisone or prednisolone) o 2 mg/kg (max. 60–80 mg) × 1 month, then start taper o 50% of initial dose at 2 months, 25% at 4 months, 12.5% at 6 months, discontinue at 12 months • Moderate-dose daily glucocorticoids (0.5–2 mg/kg daily, < 60 mg daily) o Stop within 12 months • Lower-dose daily glucocorticoids (< 0.5 mg/kg daily) o Stop within 12 months	
Glucocorticoid-sparing therapies	100%
The following glucocorticoid-sparing therapies are used in the initial treatment: • Methotrexate (MTX) 15–20 mg/m^2 (max. 30 mg) once weekly (s.c. preferred) • MTX 15–20 mg/m^2 (max. 30 mg) once weekly (s.c. preferred) + intravenous immune globulins (IVIG) (especially in case of severe juvenile dermatomyositis) In case of MTX intolerance, MTX can be replaced by azathioprin (AZA), cyclosporin A (CSA) or mycophenolate mofetil (MMF).	
Refractory disease	92%
In case of not reaching predefined targets (Table 3) or disease flare, a change in therapy is required. In this situation, current therapies should be intensified, exchanged and/or another therapy added.	
Further treatment should be discussed individually with experts. The following agents are generally used: AZA, calcineurin inhibitors, cyclophosphamide, IVIG, MMFmycophenolate mofetil, rituximab, tumor necrosis factor inhibitors	

Abbreviations: *AZA* azathioprin, *CSA* cyclosporin A, *IVIG* intravenous immune globulins, *IVMP* intravenous methylprednisolone pulse, *JDM* juvenile dermatomyositis, *MTX* methotrexate, *MMF* mycophenolate mofetil, *s.c.* subcutaneously

recommendations which had been developed previously or simultaneously, respectively. However, there are important differences in clinical practice in Germany when compared to this framework. For example, practitioners in Germany have a strong preference to choose a glucocorticoid regimen consisting of ongoing intermittent IVMP therapy in combination with low-to-moderate dose glucocorticoids instead of conventional daily high-dose glucocorticoid regimens [19]. There is surprisingly little data available on this important question. Proponents of intermittent IVMP pulse therapy suspect similar efficacy to high-dose daily glucocorticoids but less adverse effects, whereas other data suggest it may be less efficacious [7, 44, 45]. However, there are no definitive data that demonstrate superiority of one glucocorticoid regimen over another. Regarding treatment choices in case of severe or refractory JDM, there is a strong preference for IVIG, similar what is outlined in the CARRA treatment plans. Finally, the group agrees that patients with JDM should be managed in centers with an expertise in JDM. Furthermore, it is of course assumed that treatment decisions should always be shared between patients, families and providers. Since centers participating in the final consensus meeting manage more than half of all registered patients with JDM in Germany, it can be assumed that the consensus reached here is broadly generalizable in Germany. We have carefully worded the statements so that they are not confused with treatment guidelines or strict treatment recommendations.

There are several limitations to the PRO-KIND consensus strategies for JDM. First, the concepts outlined here may not represent the optimal way to manage JDM but rather represent current clinical practice among JDM experts in Germany and are based on a low level of evidence. Second, the statements and resulting strategies do not represent treatment protocols or "To Do"-lists. Management of patients with JDM will remain highly variable. Third, the field is constantly evolving: Some MSAs that were only recently reported in children, for example, anti-3-hydroxy-3-methylglutaryl-coenzyme A reductase (HMGCR) antibodies, are not included in our list but may be useful to determine in some patients, especially in case of refractory myositis [37, 46–48]. Fourth, some of the statements are rather vague, for example tapering of

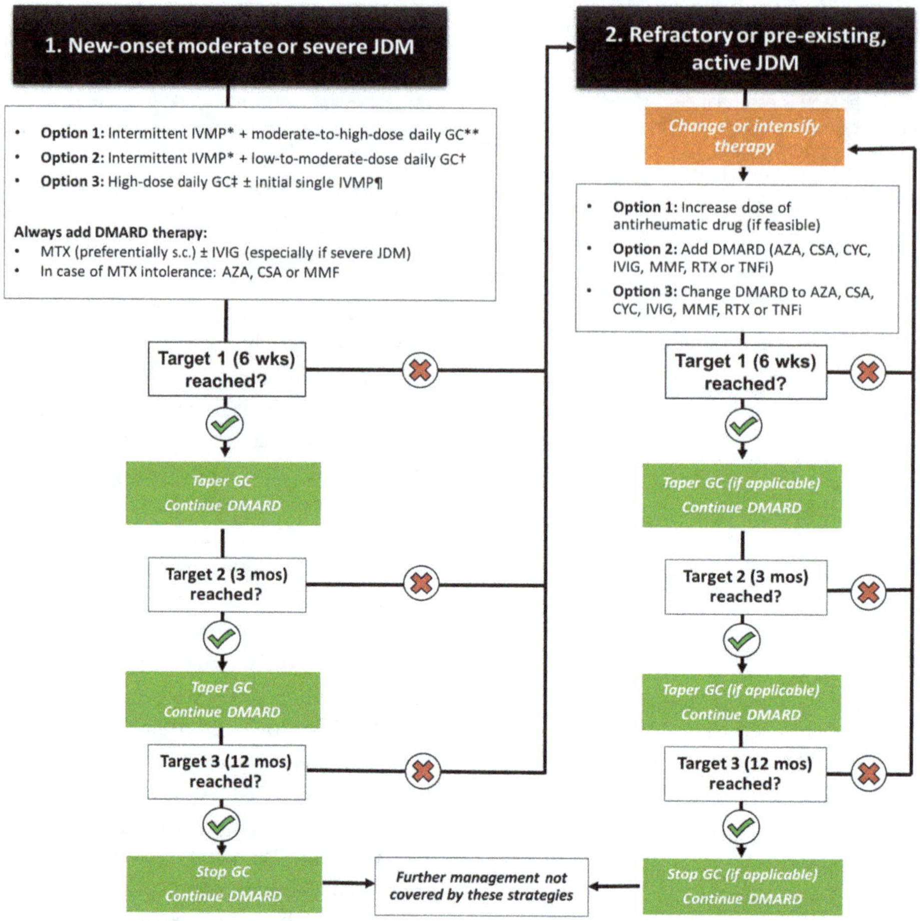

Fig. 1 Treatment strategies in juvenile dermatomyositis (JDM). Patients with new-onset active JDM are treated with 1 of 3 glucocorticoid regimens and always receive an additional disease-modifying antirheumatic drug, preferably methotrexate with or without intravenous immune globulins. If the predefined treatment targets are achieved, glucocorticoids are tapered according to a scheduled outlined in Table 3. If treatment targets are not reached, a modification in therapy is needed, i.e. either addition of a new therapy or switching therapy. There was no consensus as to a specific sequence of changes in therapy. Patients may also be treated according to these strategies if they have pre-existing, active JDM (see right side of this figure). *Repeated cycles of intravenous methylprednisolone 20–30 mg/kg (max. 1000 mg) daily for 3–5 days in a row. **Prednisone equivalent 0.5–2 mg/kg (max. 80 mg) daily. †Prednisone equivalent 0.2–0.5 mg/kg daily. ‡Prednisone equivalent 2 mg/kg (max. 80 mg) daily. ¶Single cycle of intravenous methylprednisolone 20–30 mg/kg (max. 1000 mg) daily for 3–5 days. Abbreviations: AZA, azathioprin; CSA, cyclosporin A; CYC, cyclophosphamide; DMARD, disease-modifying antirheumatic drug; GC, glucocorticoids; IVIG, intravenous immune globulins; IVMP, intravenous methylprednisolone pulse; JDM, juvenile dermatomyositis; MTX, methotrexate; MMF, mycophenolate mofetil; RTX, rituximab; s.c., subcutaneously; TNFi, tumor necrosis factor inhibitor

glucocorticoids, the choice of DMARD therapy beyond MTX, DMARD dosing regimens and the definitions of clinical inactive disease or disease flare. This is in part due to the difficulties achieving consensus on more precise statements which, in turn, results from the lack of convincing evidence for the preference of one option over another. We attempt to circumnavigate these issues by the implementation of a stringent treat-to-target strategy as outlined above. Fifth, many of the treatment options outlined in our strategies are not legally approved for the treatment of JDM, including the standard treatment with MTX. Therefore, treatment choices for individual patients may need to be adjusted based on local regulations for the off-label use of certain drugs. Sixth, some of the treatment options may not be widely available, again either due to regulation or due to cost.

Conclusions

In summary, we have developed consensus-based strategies for the diagnosis, monitoring and treatment of JDM by the harmonization of current clinical practice with the overarching goal is to improve the outcome of patients with JDM. Concerning therapy, we are placing an emphasis on a treat-to-target strategy using internationally accepted improvement criteria rather than on individual medications, fitting well into existing frameworks. As others have done previously, we define a minimal dataset to regularly collect in patients with JDM in order to allow comparative effectiveness research. We conclude that, due to the rarity of the condition, international collaboration will be critical in order to improve the outcome of patients with JDM. We believe that this work will add to the armamentarium of providers managing patients with JDM worldwide.

Acknowledgements
The authors thank Dipl.-Psych. Dr. Lea Höfel for her valuable support as a moderator at the consensus meeting. We are also grateful for the help of Jana Hörstermann with surveys and Nils Geisemeyer with data analyses; both are from the German Rheumatism Research Centre Berlin (DRFZ). The authors thank member of the GKJR and the GNP for their participation in the survey that assessed the current clinical practice in Germany.

Funding
The national pediatric rheumatology database is funded by the German Children's Arthritis Foundation (Deutsche Kinderrheumastiftung). The publication fees were supported by the Initiative für das rheumakranke Kind (www.irkk.de), a non-profit organization advocating for improved well-being of children with rheumatic diseases and their families, and a directed donation by the U can ride for arthritis (http://www.ucanr4a.eu/en/bicycle/) initiative.

Authors' contributions
CH participated in online surveys, the consensus meeting, analyzed data from the registries and survey and drafted the manuscript. FD, HF, JPH, AU and FWH developed the revised diagnostic criteria, participated in online surveys and the consensus meeting, and revised the manuscript critically. JB, FD, HF, DF, WMF, UN, CR and TS participated in the final consensus conference and revised the manuscript critically. EL and FS were members of the expert panel, participated in online surveys and revised the manuscript critically. All authors read and approved the final manuscript.

Consent for publication
Not applicable.

Competing interests
Dr. Hinze has received consulting fees, speaking fees, and/or honoraria from Novartis (less than $10,000 each). Dr. Oommen reports no potential competing interests. Dr. Dressler has received consulting fees, speaking fees, and/or honoraria from Novartis and Pfizer (less than $10,000 each). Dr. Weller-Heinemann has received honoraria from Abbvie, Novartis and Pfizer (less than $10,000 each). Dr. Lainka has received consulting fees, speaking fees, and/or honoraria from Novartis (less than $10,000 each) and research support from Sobi. Dr. Brunner has received consulting fees, speaking fees, and/or honoraria from Abbvie, MSD, Novartis, Pfizer and Roche (less than $10,000 each). Dr. Föll is a board member of the Society for Pediatric Rheumatoloy and has received honoraria from Novartis, Pfizer, Roche-Chugai and Sobi (less than $10,000 each) and research support from Novartis and Pfizer. Dr. Neudorf has received consulting fees, speaking fees, and/or honoraria from Chugai and Philips (less than $10,000 each), and research support from Novartis. Dr. Schwarz reports no potential competing interests. Dr. Schara is president of the Gesellschaft für Neuropädiatrie (GNP; Society for Pediatric Neurology in Germany) and has received consulting fees, speaking fees, and/or honoraria from PTC Therapeutics, Deutsche Myasthenie Gesellschaft (German Myasthenia Society) and benni &co (a non-profit organization benifitting patients with muscular dystrophy). Dr. Haas is the president of the Society for Pediatric Rheumatology has received research support from Novartis and Pfizer.

Author details
[1]Department of Pediatric Rheumatology and Immunology, University Hospital Münster, Albert-Schweitzer-Campus 1, Building D3, 48149 Münster, Germany. [2]Department of Pediatric Oncology, Hematology and Clinical Immunology, University Hospital Düsseldorf, Düsseldorf, Germany. [3]Department of Pediatric Pulmonology, Allergy and Neonatology, Hanover Medical School, Hanover, Germany. [4]Department of Pediatrics, St. Mary's Hospital, Amberg, Germany. [5]Division of Pediatric Rheumatology, Prof. Hess Children's Hospital, Bremen, Germany. [6]Division of Pediatric Rheumatology, University Medicine, Rostock, Germany. [7]Division of Immunology, Bone Marrow Transplantation and Rheumatology, University Hospital Ulm, Ulm, Germany. [8]Department of Pediatrics, University Hospital Essen, Essen, Germany. [9]Department of Pediatrics, Medical University Innsbruck, Innsbruck, Austria. [10]German Center for Pediatric and Adolescent Rheumatology, Garmisch-Partenkirchen Department of Dermatology, Oberammergau Center for Rheumatic Diseases, Oberammergau, Germany. [11]Department of Pediatric Neurology, University Hospital Munich, Munich, Germany. [12]Department of Pediatrics, Clementine Children's Hospital, Frankfurt, Germany. [13]Department of Pediatric Rheumatology, St. Josef Hospital, Sendenhorst, Germany. [14]Department of Pediatric Neurology, University Hospital Essen, Essen, Germany.

References
1. Feldman BM, Rider LG, Reed AM, Pachman LM. Juvenile dermatomyositis and other idiopathic inflammatory myopathies of childhood. Lancet. 2008; 371(9631):2201–12.
2. Brown VE, Pilkington CA, Feldman BM, Davidson JE, Network for Juvenile Dermatomyositis PRES. An international consensus survey of the diagnostic criteria for juvenile dermatomyositis (JDM). Rheumatology (Oxford). 2006; 45(8):990–3.
3. Stringer E, Bohnsack J, Bowyer SL, Griffin TA, Huber AM, Lang B, Lindsley CB, Ota S, Pilkington C, Reed AM, et al. Treatment approaches to juvenile dermatomyositis (JDM) across North America: the childhood arthritis and rheumatology research alliance (CARRA) JDM treatment survey. J Rheumatol. 2010;37(9):1953–61.
4. Oddis CV, Reed AM, Aggarwal R, Rider LG, Ascherman DP, Levesque MC, Barohn RJ, Feldman BM, Harris-Love MO, Koontz DC, et al. Rituximab in the treatment of refractory adult and juvenile dermatomyositis and adult polymyositis: a randomized, placebo-phase trial. Arthritis Rheum. 2013;65(2):314–24.
5. Ruperto N, Pistorio A, Oliveira S, Zulian F, Cuttica R, Ravelli A, Fischbach M, Magnusson B, Sterba G, Avcin T, et al. Prednisone versus prednisone plus ciclosporin versus prednisone plus methotrexate in new-onset juvenile dermatomyositis: a randomised trial. Lancet. 2016;387(10019):671–8.
6. Dressler F, Huppertz HI. Juvenile dermatomyositis. Z Rheumatol. 2006;65(7): 587–90. 592-584
7. Huppertz HI, Frosch M, Kuhn C, Christen HJ. Treatment of juvenile dermatomyositis (JDM) with highdose oral steroids or with steroid pulse therapy. Arthritis Rheum. 1998;41(9 Suppl):S264.
8. Kim S, El-Hallak M, Dedeoglu F, Zurakowski D, Fuhlbrigge RC, Sundel RP. Complete and sustained remission of juvenile dermatomyositis resulting from aggressive treatment. Arthritis Rheum. 2009;60(6):1825–30.
9. Lam CG, Manlhiot C, Pullenayegum EM, Feldman BM. Efficacy of intravenous Ig therapy in juvenile dermatomyositis. Ann Rheum Dis. 2011;70(12):2089–94.
10. Rouster-Stevens KA, Gursahaney A, Ngai KL, Daru JA, Pachman LM. Pharmacokinetic study of oral prednisolone compared with intravenous methylprednisolone in patients with juvenile dermatomyositis. Arthritis Rheum. 2008;59(2):222–6.
11. Rouster-Stevens KA, Ferguson L, Morgan G, Huang CC, Pachman LM. Pilot study of etanercept in patients with refractory juvenile dermatomyositis. Arthritis Care Res (Hoboken). 2014;66(5):783–7.
12. Rouster-Stevens KA, Morgan GA, Wang D, Pachman LM. Mycophenolate mofetil: a possible therapeutic agent for children with juvenile dermatomyositis. Arthritis Care Res (Hoboken). 2010;62(10):1446–51.
13. Riley P, Maillard SM, Wedderburn LR, Woo P, Murray KJ, Pilkington CA. Intravenous cyclophosphamide pulse therapy in juvenile dermatomyositis. A review of efficacy and safety. Rheumatology (Oxford). 2004;43(4):491–6.

14. Robinson AB, Reed AM. Clinical features, pathogenesis and treatment of juvenile and adult dermatomyositis. Nat Rev Rheumatol. 2011;7(11):664–75.
15. Bundesausschuss G. Arzneimittel-Richtlinie/ Anlage VI: Off-Label-Use Intravenöse Immunglobuline (IVIG) bei Polymyositis und bei Dermatomyositis. Bundesanzeiger. 2013. https://www.g-ba.de/informationen/beschluesse/1701/.
16. Enders FB, Bader-Meunier B, Baildam E, Constantin T, Dolezalova P, Feldman BM, Lahdenne P, Magnusson B, Nistala K, Ozen S, et al. Consensus-based recommendations for the management of juvenile dermatomyositis. Ann Rheum Dis. 2017;76(2):329–40.
17. Huber AM, Robinson AB, Reed AM, Abramson L, Bout-Tabaku S, Carrasco R, Curran M, Feldman BM, Gewanter H, Griffin T, et al. Consensus treatments for moderate juvenile dermatomyositis: beyond the first two months. Results of the second childhood arthritis and rheumatology research alliance consensus conference. Arthritis Care Res (Hoboken). 2012;64(4):546–53.
18. Spencer CH, Rouster-Stevens K, Gewanter H, Syverson G, Modica R, Schmidt K, Emery H, Wallace C, Grevich S, Nanda K, Zhao YD, Shenoi S, Tarvin S, Hong S, Lindsley C, Weiss JE, Passo M, Ede K, Brown A, Ardalan K, Bernal W, Stoll ML, Lang B, Carrasco R, Agaiar C, Feller L, Bukulmez H, Vehe R, Kim H, Schmeling H, Gerstbacher D, Hoeltzel M, Eberhard B, Sundel R, Kim S, Huber AM, Patwardhan A. Biologic therapies for refractory juvenile dermatomyositis: five years of experience of the Childhood Arthritis and Rheumatology Research Alliance in North America. Pediatr Rheumatol. 2017;15(1).
19. Hinze CH, Speth F, Oommen PT, Haas J-P: Current management of juvenile dermatomyositis in Germany: an online survey of pediatric rheumatologists and pediatric neurologists in Germany. 2018.
20. van Vollenhoven RF, Mosca M, Bertsias G, Isenberg D, Kuhn A, Lerstrom K, Aringer M, Bootsma H, Boumpas D, Bruce IN, et al. Treat-to-target in systemic lupus erythematosus: recommendations from an international task force. Ann Rheum Dis. 2014;73(6):958–67.
21. Kiltz U, Smolen J, Bardin T, Cohen Solal A, Dalbeth N, Doherty M, Engel B, Flader C, Kay J, Matsuoka M, et al. Treat-to-target (T2T) recommendations for gout. Ann Rheum Dis. 2017;76(4):632–8.
22. Smolen JS, Aletaha D, Bijlsma JW, Breedveld FC, Boumpas D, Burmester G, Combe B, Cutolo M, de Wit M, Dougados M, et al. Treating rheumatoid arthritis to target: recommendations of an international task force. Ann Rheum Dis. 2010;69(4):631–7.
23. Consolaro A, Negro G, Lanni S, Solari N, Martini A, Ravelli A. Toward a treat-to-target approach in the management of juvenile idiopathic arthritis. Clin Exp Rheumatol. 2012;30(4 Suppl 73):S157–62.
24. Hinze C, Gohar F, Foell D. Management of juvenile idiopathic arthritis: hitting the target. Nat Rev Rheumatol. 2015;11(5):290–300.
25. Hinze CH, Holzinger D, Lainka E, Haas JP, Speth F, Kallinich T, Rieber N, Hufnagel M, Jansson AF, Hedrich C, et al. Practice and consensus-based strategies in diagnosing and managing systemic juvenile idiopathic arthritis in Germany. Pediatr Rheumatol Online J. 2018;16(1):7.
26. Horneff G, Klein A, Ganser G, Sailer-Hock M, Gunther A, Foeldvari I, Weller-Heinemann F. Protocols on classification, monitoring and therapy in children's rheumatology (PRO-KIND): results of the working group Polyarticular juvenile idiopathic arthritis. Pediatr Rheumatol Online J. 2017;15(1):78.
27. Lilleker JB, Vencovsky J, Wang G, Wedderburn LR, Diederichsen LP, Schmidt J, Oakley P, Benveniste O, Danieli MG, Danko K, et al. The EuroMyositis registry: an international collaborative tool to facilitate myositis research. Ann Rheum Dis. 2018;77(1):30–9.
28. McCann LJ, Juggins AD, Maillard SM, Wedderburn LR, Davidson JE, Murray KJ, Pilkington CA, Juvenile Dermatomyositis Research G. The juvenile dermatomyositis National Registry and repository (UK and Ireland)–clinical characteristics of children recruited within the first 5 yr. Rheumatology (Oxford). 2006;45(10):1255–60.
29. McCann LJ, Kirkham JJ, Wedderburn LR, Pilkington C, Huber AM, Ravelli A, Appelbe D, Williamson PR, Beresford MW. Development of an internationally agreed minimal dataset for juvenile dermatomyositis (JDM) for clinical and research use. Trials. 2015;16:268.
30. Ruperto N, Ravelli A, Murray KJ, Lovell DJ, Andersson-Gare B, Feldman BM, Garay S, Kuis W, Machado C, Pachman L, et al. Preliminary core sets of measures for disease activity and damage assessment in juvenile systemic lupus erythematosus and juvenile dermatomyositis. Rheumatology (Oxford). 2003;42(12):1452–9.
31. Ravelli A, Trail L, Ferrari C, Ruperto N, Pistorio A, Pilkington C, Maillard S, Oliveira SK, Sztajnbok F, Cuttica R, et al. Long-term outcome and prognostic factors of juvenile dermatomyositis: a multinational, multicenter study of 490 patients. Arthritis Care Res (Hoboken). 2010;62(1):63–72.
32. Bitnum S, Daeschner CW Jr, Travis LB, Dodge WF, Hopps HC. Dermatomyositis. J Pediatr. 1964;64:101–31.
33. Bowyer SL, Blane CE, Sullivan DB, Cassidy JT. Childhood dermatomyositis: factors predicting functional outcome and development of dystrophic calcification. J Pediatr. 1983;103(6):882–8.
34. Crowe WE, Bove KE, Levinson JE, Hilton PK. Clinical and pathogenetic implications of histopathology in childhood polydermatomyositis. Arthritis Rheum. 1982;25(2):126–39.
35. Rider LG, Aggarwal R, Pistorio A, Bayat N, Erman B, Feldman BM, Huber AM, Cimaz R, Cuttica RJ, de Oliveira SK, et al. 2016 American College of Rheumatology/European league against rheumatism criteria for minimal, moderate, and major clinical response in juvenile dermatomyositis: an international myositis assessment and clinical studies group/Paediatric rheumatology international trials organisation collaborative initiative. Arthritis Rheumatol. 2017;69(5):911–23.
36. Gunawardena H, Wedderburn LR, North J, Betteridge Z, Dunphy J, Chinoy H, Davidson JE, Cooper RG, McHugh NJ. Clinical associations of autoantibodies to a p155/140 kDa doublet protein in juvenile dermatomyositis. Rheumatology (Oxford). 2008;47(3):324–8.
37. Kishi T, Rider LG, Pak K, Barillas-Arias L, Henrickson M, McCarthy PL, Shaham B, Weiss PF, Horkayne-Szakaly I, Targoff IN, et al. Association of Anti-3-Hydroxy-3-Methylglutaryl-coenzyme a reductase autoantibodies with DRB1*07:01 and severe myositis in juvenile myositis patients. Arthritis Care Res (Hoboken). 2017;69(7):1088–94.
38. Rider LG, Nistala K. The juvenile idiopathic inflammatory myopathies: pathogenesis, clinical and autoantibody phenotypes, and outcomes. J Intern Med. 2016;280(1):24–38.
39. Rider LG, Shah M, Mamyrova G, Huber AM, Rice MM, Targoff IN, Miller FW, Childhood Myositis Heterogeneity Collaborative Study G. The myositis autoantibody phenotypes of the juvenile idiopathic inflammatory myopathies. Medicine (Baltimore). 2013;92(4):223–43.
40. Stoffer MA, Schoels MM, Smolen JS, Aletaha D, Breedveld FC, Burmester G, Bykerk V, Dougados M, Emery P, Haraoui B, et al. Evidence for treating rheumatoid arthritis to target: results of a systematic literature search update. Ann Rheum Dis. 2016;75(1):16–22.
41. Lazarevic D, Pistorio A, Palmisani E, Miettunen P, Ravelli A, Pilkington C, Wulffraat NM, Malattia C, Garay SM, Hofer M, et al. The PRINTO criteria for clinically inactive disease in juvenile dermatomyositis. Ann Rheum Dis. 2013; 72(5):686–93.
42. Oddis CV, Rider LG, Reed AM, Ruperto N, Brunner HI, Koneru B, Feldman BM, Giannini EH, Miller FW, International Myositis A, et al. International consensus guidelines for trials of therapies in the idiopathic inflammatory myopathies. Arthritis Rheum. 2005;52(9):2607–15.
43. DeWitt EM, Brunner HI. The landscape of comparative effectiveness research in rheumatology. Nat Rev Rheumatol. 2014;10(1):57–62.
44. Lang B, Dooley J. Failure of pulse intravenous methylprednisolone treatment in juvenile dermatomyositis. J Pediatr. 1996;128(3):429–32.
45. Laxer RM, Stein LD, Petty RE. Intravenous pulse methylprednisolone treatment of juvenile dermatomyositis. Arthritis Rheum. 1987;30(3):328–34.
46. Tansley SL, Betteridge ZE, Simou S, Jacques TS, Pilkington C, Wood M, Warrier K, Wedderburn LR, McHugh NJ, Juvenile Dermatomyositis Research G. Anti-HMGCR autoantibodies in juvenile idiopathic inflammatory myopathies identify a rare but clinically important subset of patients. J Rheumatol. 2017;44(4):488–92.
47. Tiniakou E, Pinal-Fernandez I, Lloyd TE, Albayda J, Paik J, Werner JL, Parks CA, Casciola-Rosen L, Christopher-Stine L, Mammen AL. More severe disease and slower recovery in younger patients with anti-3-hydroxy-3-methylglutaryl-coenzyme a reductase-associated autoimmune myopathy. Rheumatology (Oxford). 2017;56(5):787–94.
48. Liang WC, Uruha A, Suzuki S, Murakami N, Takeshita E, Chen WZ, Jong YJ, Endo Y, Komaki H, Fujii T, et al. Pediatric necrotizing myopathy associated with anti-3-hydroxy-3-methylglutaryl-coenzyme A reductase antibodies. Rheumatology (Oxford). 2017;56(2):287–93.

22

Pediatric Rheumatology Collaborative Study Group – over four decades of pivotal clinical drug research in pediatric rheumatology

Hermine I. Brunner[1*], Lisa G. Rider[2], Daniel J. Kingsbury[3], Dominic Co[4], Rayfel Schneider[5], Ellen Goldmuntz[6], Karen B. Onel[7], Edward H. Giannini[1], Daniel J. Lovell[1] and for the PRCSG Advisory Council

Abstract

Importance: Specialized research networks are essential to achieve drug approvals for rare pediatric diseases. Such networks help realize the potential of global legislation enacted upon the recognition that most children are treated with drugs whose most beneficial dose and regimen have not been established in pediatric patients. The Pediatric Rheumatology Collaborative Study Group (PRCSG) is a North American clinical trials network that is specialized in the performance of clinical trials of new therapies for pediatric populations with rheumatic diseases. This review provides an overview of the strategies employed by this research network to achieve drug and biologic approvals for children with pediatric rheumatic diseases, particularly juvenile idiopathic arthritis.

Observations: Clinical trial conduct in rare pediatric diseases has required global recruitment. Supported or led by the PRCSG, highly responsive, validated, composite measures have been established to assess drug efficacy. For pediatric orphan diseases with high disease burdens, specialized investigative sites and study designs are needed to complete adequately powered trials at the high standard necessary to enable drug labeling by regulatory agencies. Novel trial designs have been utilized for more efficient testing of innovative drug candidates. All these have been developed or co-developed by the PRCSG research network.

Conclusions and relevance: Specialized research networks in pediatric rheumatology, such as the PRCSG, have changed the landscape of available therapies and improved overall disease outcomes for children with pediatric rheumatic diseases.

Keywords: Clinical trials, JIA, PRCSG, Drug approvals, Pediatrics, Networks

Background

There remains a profound unmet medical need for the effective and safe treatment of pediatric rheumatic diseases. As these diseases are rare, highly specialized and experienced research networks are best suited to support therapeutic trials of new drug compounds. The Pediatric Rheumatology Collaborative Study Group (PRCSG) has an over 40-year long track record of successfully supporting the design, conduct, analysis, and publication of such therapeutic trials in close collaboration with industry sponsors. The PRCSG has intensely focused on ensuring that clinical trial designs have scientific rigor, are practical for enrollment by pediatric rheumatologists, and acceptable to families of children with pediatric rheumatic diseases. Studies conducted in collaboration with the PRCSG changed the landscape of pediatric rheumatology care over the past decades. The objective of this review is to highlight the history of the PRCSG, including approaches developed and used by the research network that made effective therapies available to children with pediatric rheumatic diseases.

* Correspondence: Hermine.brunner@cchmc.org
[1]Division of Rheumatology, Cincinnati Children's Hospital Medical Center & Cincinnati Children's Research Foundation, MLC 4010, Cincinnati, OH 45229, USA
Full list of author information is available at the end of the article

Food and Drug Administration regulations for drugs for children with pediatric rheumatic diseases

The Food and Drug Administration (FDA) is the federal agency charged with overseeing drug manufacturing, labeling, advertisement, and safety of medications and biological products [1] in the United States (U.S.). The Food, Drug, and Cosmetic Act (FD&C Act) requires that there is "substantial evidence," resulting from "adequate and well controlled investigations" to demonstrate that a new drug "will have the effect it purports or is represented to have under the conditions of use prescribed, recommended, or suggested in the proposed labeling." New drug and biologic applications are submitted to and reviewed by the FDA for potential approval for marketing in the U.S [2].

Activism by professional organizations, families, and networks, such as the PRCSG, resulted in legislation that markedly changed the landscape of drug therapy for children. In the U.S., medication labeling and drug studies are governed largely by two sections of the FD&C Act: section 505A pertains to The Best Pharmaceuticals for Children Act (BPCA) [3] and section 505B to the Pediatric Research Equity Act (PREA) [4], respectively. Together these two laws encourage and/or require drug companies to study their products in children [5]. PREA necessitates new drugs and biologic therapies to be studied in children, if there is a pediatric disease that is similar to a non-orphan disease occurring in adults, and it is likely that the new agent will be used in children. The FDA considers juvenile idiopathic arthritis (JIA) with polyarticular joint involvement the pediatric correlate of adult rheumatoid arthritis (RA) [6]. BPCA provides pharmaceutical manufacturers with 6 months of additional market exclusivity after the completion of pediatric drug studies that have been done at request of the FDA. There is no exclusion for orphan diseases, but biologic therapies are not covered. The FDA Safety and Innovation Act (FDASIA) made PREA and BPCA permanent, which was important because, prior to 2012, PREA and BPCA were merely regulations intended to be in place for a limited time. Almost all stakeholders involved, including leaders of the PRCSG, asserted that permanence of PREA and BPCA was an important aspect for future drug development for children. Together, these laws resulted in the labeling of more than 600 products for pediatric indications, 149 of which occurred since the passage of FDASIA [7]. A recent review by the European Medicines Agency (EMA) and FDA confirmed that the existence of pediatric research networks, such as the PRCSG, is of utmost importance to realize the potential of this new pediatric legislation [2, 8].

Integration of pediatric planning and exclusivity requests are now a part of regular new drug and biologic product development programs at pharmaceutical companies. Key documents to be developed include the initial Pediatric Study Plan (iPSP) for submission to and approval by the Center for Drug Evaluation and Research (CDER) or the Center for Biologics Evaluation and Research (CBER) at FDA [9].

Importantly, the EMA passed similar legislation concerning pediatric drug testing and approval. Like the iPSP, a Pediatric Investigational Plan (PIP) must be submitted to the Paediatric Committee (PDCO), EMA's scientific committee that is responsible for activities concerning medicine testing in children. PDCO oversees the labeling of such medicines in the European Union. One difference between the U.S. and the European legislation is that PIP submission to PDCO takes place by the end of Phase I development in adults, while iPSP submission to FDA is expected to occur later around the end of Phase II development in adults.

It has been a long-term initiative of the FDA to facilitate international standardization in drug testing and drug approval ("harmonization"). Various FDA Centers coordinate regular conferences with colleagues in Europe, Japan, Canada, and Australia. The benefits of harmonization of drug and biologic DMARD testing in pediatric rheumatic diseases include a decrease of unnecessary exposure to placebo or potentially unsafe new medications. Harmonization efforts are especially evident in the context of pediatric drug trials. This is achieved by international agreement between the various regulatory agencies on the design and performance of only a single blinded controlled pediatric trial, rather than several studies.

Research network focused on promoting access to new medications for pediatric rheumatic disease therapy

Founded in 1973, the PRCSG is a research network of nearly 90 academic clinical pediatric rheumatology centers. At present, there are over 180 pediatric rheumatology investigators in North America and Puerto Rico who are members of the PRCSG. The mission of the PRCSG (http://www.prcsg.org) is to foster, facilitate, and conduct high quality clinical research in the field of pediatric rheumatology. The PRCSG Advisory Council provides oversight of the network's activities. Its members are established clinical investigators, a junior clinical investigator, and representatives of foundations, organizations, and government agencies pertinent to the mission of the network, such as the National Institutes of Health and FDA.

The impact of the PRCSG extends beyond North America. The PRCSG leadership was involved in the training of the leadership of the Paediatric Rheumatology International Trials Organisation (PRINTO; http://printo.it) [10], a research network that now includes centers in Europe, Latin America, Asia and Africa, and whose mission is aligned with that of the PRCSG. These two networks have been active collaborators for over 20 years, which ultimately supports licensure of new medicines in many countries throughout the world.

Studies in pediatric rheumatic diseases often require complex response measures; necessitate adjustment of background medications; and rules for early discontinuation of subjects for added safety. To ensure that study protocols are closely followed by the investigative sites, the PRCSG and PRINTO Coordinating Centers have developed standardized operating procedures, custom software, electronic data capture systems and databases, as well as data security and back-up systems. This robust infrastructure allows the Coordinating Centers to provide real-time feed-back to investigative sites throughout the world and across all time zones. Although focused on pharmaceutical supported trials, the PRCSG Coordinating Center also supports investigator-initiated studies [11, 12].

The scientific collaboration treaty between the U. S. and Union of Soviet Socialist Republics supported early clinical trials in JIA

During the Cold War era, and as part of a Scientific Collaboration Treaty between the State Departments of the U.S. and the Union of Soviet Socialist Republics (USSR), the PRCSG conducted trials of popular traditional Disease Modifying Anti-Rheumatic Drugs (DMARDs) with pediatric rheumatologists in the U.S. and the USSR. The motivation behind the Scientific Collaboration Treaty was that the fostering of scientific collaboration between the two countries was hoped to promote collaborations in other realms. Dr. Earl Brewer, the founder and first chairman of the PRCSG, considered the Scientific Collaboration Treaty a unique opportunity to obtain federal funding for clinical trials in JIA.

Facilitated by the Scientific Collaboration Treaty, three large, pivotal Phase III randomized, double-blind, placebo-controlled trials of DMARDs were successfully performed through the collaborative efforts of pediatric rheumatologists in the U.S. and the USSR. The first study compared the efficacy of D-penicillamine and hydroxychloroquine to placebo in polyarticular JIA [13]. Despite promising results in open-label clinical studies, the results of the controlled study proved that neither D-penicillamine nor hydroxychloroquine were superior to placebo in JIA. Thus, this PRCSG study spared other children with JIA treatment with these ineffective medications. A second clinical trial compared the efficacy and safety of oral gold to that of placebo in polyarticular JIA. Despite earlier positive clinical trials of oral gold in RA, this PRCSG study supported that oral gold was only marginally superior to placebo and had considerable toxicity when used in JIA [14]. Taken together, this PRCSG trial again prevented JIA patients from treatment with minimally effective yet potentially toxic oral gold therapy.

The third trial was of methotrexate versus placebo in active polyarticular JIA [15]. Only oral methotrexate at 10 mg/m^2 body surface area (BSA) once per week, but not the lower weekly dose of 5 mg/m^2 BSA, proved to be superior to placebo in JIA. The results of this study were specifically used for the subsequent labeled indication of methotrexate in reducing signs and symptoms of polyarticular JIA.

Other trials performed by the PRCSG were of various nonsteroidal anti-inflammatory drugs (NSAIDs), which were formerly the cornerstone of JIA treatments [16–23]. These studies led to FDA approval of five NSAIDs for JIA (Table 1).

Clinical trials of biological DMARDs result in markedly improved prognosis of JIA with polyarticular joint involvement

The first biologic DMARD studied in JIA was etanercept, a fusion protein targeting tumor necrosis factor alpha (TNFα) [24]. The efficacy of etanercept in JIA was tested and established using the then novel randomized

Table 1 Medications studied by the PRCSG Pediatric Rheumatology Collaborative Study Group for Juvenile Idiopathic Arthritis and other pediatric rheumatic diseases by route(s) of administration[a]

Medications studied but without approval/licensure by regulatory agencies	Medications studied with approval/licensure by regulatory agencies	Studies in Progress
Oral	Oral	Oral
D-penicillamine	Celecoxib	Baricitinib
Fenoprofen	Ibuprofen	Tofacitinib
Gold	Naproxen	Subcutaneous
Hydroxychloroquine	Rofecoxib[b]	*Certolizumab pegol*
Ketoprofen	Tolmetin	*Sarilumab*
Meclofenamate	Oral, subcutaneous or intramuscular	*Secukinumab*
Oxaprozin	Methotrexate	*Tocilizumab*
Pirprofen	Subcutaneous	Intravenous
Proquazone	*Adalimumab*	*Belimumab*[g]
Subcutaneous	*Canakinumab*[c]	*Golimumab*
Anakinra	*Etanercept*	*Rituximab*[h]
Intravenous	*Golimumab*[d]	
Intravenous immunoglobulin	Subcutaneous and/or intravenous	
Infliximab	*Abatacept*[e]	
Rilonacept	*Tocilizumab*[f]	

Biologic medications are printed in Italics
[b]Approval withdrawn by the U.S. Food and Drug Administration due to safety concerns in adults with rheumatoid arthritis
[c]Only for systemic juvenile idiopathic arthritis (JIA)
[d]Approved by European Medicines Agency only, but not by the U.S. Food and Drug Administration
[e]Both the intravenous and the subcutaneous form is approved for polyarticular JIA
[f]The intravenous forms are approved for systemic JIA and polyarticular JIA
[g]For systemic lupus erythematosus
[h]For antineutrophil cytoplasmic autoantibody (ANCA) associated vasculitis

withdrawal design (RWD). This RWD study ($n = 69$) was fully enrolled within 3 months from sites in North America because many children with JIA had failed all available medications. When the first JIA patient was dosed with etanercept, only about 300 adult patients with RA had been treated with this drug. Etanercept remains the first and presently only biologic DMARD that achieved regulatory approval by the FDA using the "fast track" approach. Eventually, world-wide approval of etanercept for polyarticular JIA was achieved based on the results of this PRCSG trial. However, given its small sample size and short duration of follow-up, the FDA required the Sponsor to establish a large post-marketing Phase IV JIA registry to document the continued effectiveness, benefits on quality of life, and longer-term safety of etanercept in routine clinical use, including usage in younger children [25]. These studies resulted in important additions to the label for etanercept pertaining to medication safety events, and broadened the approval to children as young as 2 years. Subsequent to the etanercept study, there have been a series of clinical trials managed by the PRCSG and PRINTO, which resulted in FDA approval of a total of six biologic DMARDs for polyarticular JIA [24, 26–30].

In the last decade, PRCSG investigators also participated in clinical trials in systemic JIA (SJIA) [31–33]. The trials of canakinumab, an interleukin (IL)-1β monoclonal antibody, and the anti-IL-6 monoclonal antibody, tocilizumab, in SJIA led to the regulatory approval of both biologic DMARDs in North America and Europe [32, 33]. A list of all medications studied by the PRCSG, including those that are now licensed for JIA, is provided in Table 1.

With the advent of designer drugs that target pathways only relevant to some rare JIA subsets, the corresponding clinical trials in children constitute an even larger challenge. Examples are drugs that inhibit the IL-17 or IL-12/23 pathways which are expected to only benefit children with juvenile psoriatic arthritis and /or enthesitis-related JIA. The PRCSG has also been involved in the planning and conduct of the pediatric clinical trials of the anti-B lymphocyte stimulator monoclonal antibody, belimumab, in systemic lupus erythematosus (SLE), and the anti-CD20 monoclonal antibody, rituximab, in anti-neutrophil cytoplasmic antibody associated vasculitis.

Global commitments and access to care

Since 2000, JIA medication trials generally involved pediatric rheumatology centers located all over the world, including in developing countries where access to affordable biologic DMARDs remains limited. The PRCSG and PRINTO have adopted the guiding principle that, irrespective of regulatory approval in the child's country, study participants must be provided long-term access to the study agent, as long as it is deemed medically beneficial to the child. The mechanism by which medication is provided to former study participants varies country by country. Despite the added cost, to date, all pharmaceutical companies have agreed to this request of the PRCSG and PRINTO.

Development of outcome and response measures for pediatric rheumatic diseases

The PRCSG published the first guidance papers concerning medication studies in JIA [34, 35]. Many of the recommendations from 1982 continue to be relevant: well validated outcome measures are deemed a *sine-qua-non* for the successful conduct of clinical trials. Members of the PRCSG Advisory Council have held the view that it is unethical and scientifically unacceptable to proceed with large scale trials, if validated response criteria [36] are unavailable. Often in collaboration with other pediatric rheumatic disease networks, the PRCSG has been an active participant in the development and validation of outcomes measures (see Table 2 for listing of developed measures). The most frequently used outcome measures and response criteria include those for

Table 2 Clinical trial outcome measures developed by the Pediatric Rheumatology Collaborative Study Group Leadership in collaboration with other pediatric rheumatology networks

PEDIATRIC RHEUMATIC DISEASE	Outcome measure	Reference
Juvenile Idiopathic Arthritis	Core set of Outcome Measures[a]	[35]
	Preliminary Definition of Improvement[a]	[36]
	Preliminary Flare Criteria[a]	[37]
	Provisional criteria for inactive disease & clinical remission[a]	[38]
	Macrophage Activation Syndrome[a]	[39]
Systemic Lupus Erythematosus	Disease activity	[40]
	Disease damage	[41]
	Core Set of Outcome Measures[a]	[42]
	Provisional Improvement Criteria[b]	[43]
	Preliminary Flare Criteria[b]	[44]
	Preliminary Inactive Disease Criteria[b]	[45]
Juvenile Dermatomyositis	Childhood Myositis Activity Assessment Scale[c]	[46]
	Core set measures of disease activity and damage[a]	[42]
	Provisional Criteria for Response to Therapy[a]	[47]

[a]Developed in collaboration with Pediatric Rheumatology International Trials Organization (PRINTO)
[b]Developed in collaboration with PRINTO and Childhood Arthritis and Rheumatology Research Alliance (CARRA)
[c]Developed in collaboration with Juvenile Dermatomyositis Disease Activity Collaborative Study Group (predecessor to International Myositis Assessment and Clinical Studies Group)

JIA [37–41]. The PRCSG leadership has also been involved in the delineation of core outcome measures and response criteria for SLE [42–47] and juvenile dermatomyositis [44, 48, 49].

Novel study designs to maximize study efficiency

Pediatric rheumatic diseases are uncommon, and almost all affect fewer than 200,000 individuals in the US, which is compared to 1.3 million adult patients diagnosed with RA [50]. Pediatric rheumatic diseases are considered orphan or rare diseases as defined by the Orphan Drug Act [51]. Although JIA is the most common pediatric rheumatic disease, its prevalence is only 44.7 (95% CI 39.1-50.2) per 100,000 persons in the U.S. [52]. Thus, children with pediatric rheumatic diseases are a precious resource, and adequately powered clinical trials require an international enrollment strategy. Considering the burden of active pediatric rheumatic diseases, it is also critical for controlled studies to minimize placebo exposure while maximizing the collection of safety data. Therefore, the PRCSG has developed and used a randomized withdrawal design (RWD) for many of the controlled trials [24, 27, 29]. Beyond pediatric rheumatology, the RWD is now also used for the studies in, among others, gastrointestinal and neuropsychiatric diseases [53, 54]. As shown in Fig. 1, RWD trials provide active study drug to all study participants during the open label lead-in period (Part 1). Only subjects who have experienced a protocol-defined improvement in disease signs and symptoms will be randomized to enter the blinded placebo-controlled of a RWD trial (Part 2), while non-responders are either discontinued from the study at the end of Part 1 or allowed enter an open-label extension phase with access to active study drug (Part 3). All subjects who complete the blinded Part 2 can continue to receive active drug during Part 3. Study participants remain in the blinded treatment phase until the last visit in Part 2 or until he/she experiences a 'disease flare', i.e., a protocol-defined disease worsening, whichever comes first. Therefore, study participants remain in Part 2 only as long as they continue to demonstrate at least a similar level of disease control as at the beginning of Part 2, which is better than at the beginning of Part 1. The primary endpoint of a RWD trial is either the proportion of patients with 'disease flare' compared to the time of randomization, or the time to 'disease flare' in Part 2. Advantages of the RWD include a high degree of efficiency in assessing drug efficacy, requiring fewer patients to be enrolled in the trial; an individualized duration of exposure to placebo with an option to restart open-label active drug upon experiencing a 'disease flare'. The disadvantages of the RWD trial are as follows: (1) there may exist a selection bias because only subjects who responded in the open lead-in phase are randomized into the double-blind phase, while children who failed to respond Part 1, and hence may have a lesser probability of favorable response to drug, are excluded from Part 2; (2) the primary outcome is not a direct comparison of response rates between treatment arms, but rather an indirect one (i.e., 'disease flare'); (3) given that patients receiving placebo in the blinded portion are more likely to have a 'disease flare' and exit Part 2 early, there is often only a small blinded placebo safety exposure dataset. Despite these limitations, the RWD has functioned well in numerous JIA trials [24, 27–29, 33].

Use of traditional double-blind placebo-controlled parallel design may be considered in pediatric rheumatic

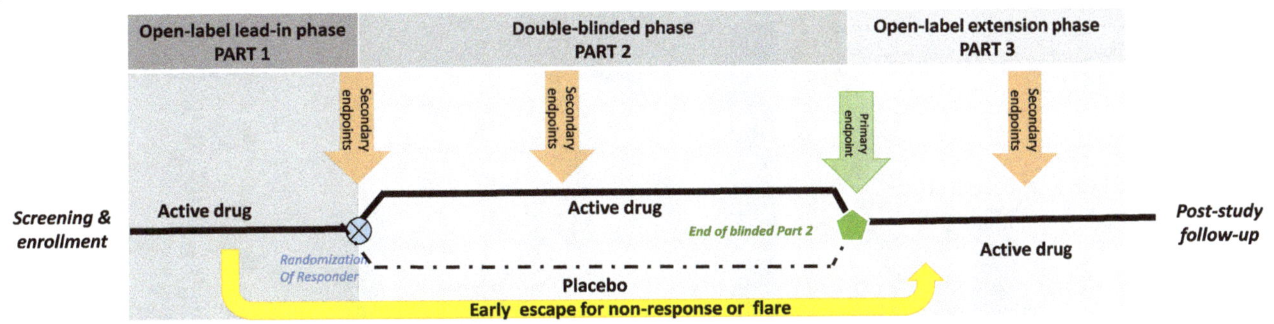

Fig. 1 Basic design of Randomized Withdrawal Design. A randomized withdrawal design (RWD) study consists of three parts. During Part 1 and Part 3 all study participants receive open-label active study drug. Participants who show a clinically meaningful response to study drug by the end of Part 1 are randomized to the double-blinded placebo-controlled Part 2. Participants move from Part 2 to Part 3 if there is a flare event during Part 2 or upon completion of all Part 2 visits, whichever comes first. Patients for whom study drug may be beneficial, but who did not meet criteria for a meaningful improvement during Part 1, may be allowed to enter Part 3. The primary endpoint of a RWD trial is 'the time to disease flare or the occurrence of a flare event during Part 2. The participant's disease status at the end of Part 1 is used as the baseline to assess whether disease worsening (flare) has occurred during Part 2. Secondary RWD study endpoints can be measured throughout the duration of the entire RWD trial (Part 1 through 3) and include achievement of inactive disease, success in tapering certain background medications and change in patient reported outcomes

diseases if (1) the new drug is fast-acting, hence the duration of placebo exposure is expected to be very short; (2) the new drug is not dosed continuously or has a very prolonged effect and therefore awaiting disease flare after therapy withdrawal would be impractical; or (3), there are safety concerns with sudden drug discontinuation of study drug in Part 2 of the RWD trials [32]. Whenever parallel designs are used, the PRCSG strongly advocates that there are liberal, early escape rules and an open label extension study. Such aspects of clinical development program ensure that patients with poor disease control have access to active drug early and over extended time periods.

In addition to placebo-controlled studies, the PRCSG uses open-label designs of studies for drug labeling purposes, provided the mechanism of action of a given drug is known to consistently result in improvement of a rheumatic disease in both children and adults, considering earlier controlled studies [55]. Open-label studies of "me-too" medications assume that the risk-benefit profile of a given drug is comparable to that of other drugs with a similar mechanism of action. The primary objective of such open-label studies in JIA is the identification of dosing regimens that result in drug exposures that have been found efficacious in RA. Regulatory agencies accepted an open-label study of certolizumab pegol in JIA (NCT01550003). This monoclonal antibody blocks TNFα-mediated inflammation in a similar manner to infliximab, adalimumab, and golimumab, i.e. biological DMARDs that have been found to be efficacious in controlled studies in RA and JIA. Other examples in JIA include intravenous golimumab (NCT02277444), and the study of subcutaneous abatacept.

Modification of the above-mentioned controlled and uncontrolled study designs include elements considered in adaptive trial designs. Examples are the reduction of sample size following planned interim analyses, the tapering of corticosteroids during the RWD trial of canakinumab in SJIA [33]; and protocolized discontinuation of methotrexate, NSAIDs, and even study drug, during the long-term phase of tocilizumab trial in SJIA [32].

Taken together, the PRCSG advocates study designs for new drugs that minimize placebo and background medication exposures. Nonetheless, any study by the PRCSG maintains sufficient scientific rigor needed for subsequent drug approval by regulatory agencies. Another prerequisite of PRCSG trials is that large-scale Phase III studies only proceed after the delineation of the dosing regimen that provides comparable drug exposure to those known to be efficacious in the related adult rheumatic disease. If the pathogenesis of the pediatric disease is distinct from the approved adult disease (e.g., RA and SJIA), dose-finding Phase II studies must be performed prior to the initiation of the Phase III trials used for achieving marketing approval [32]. Phase II dose finding studies were performed for both canakinumab and tocilizumab in SJIA [56, 57].

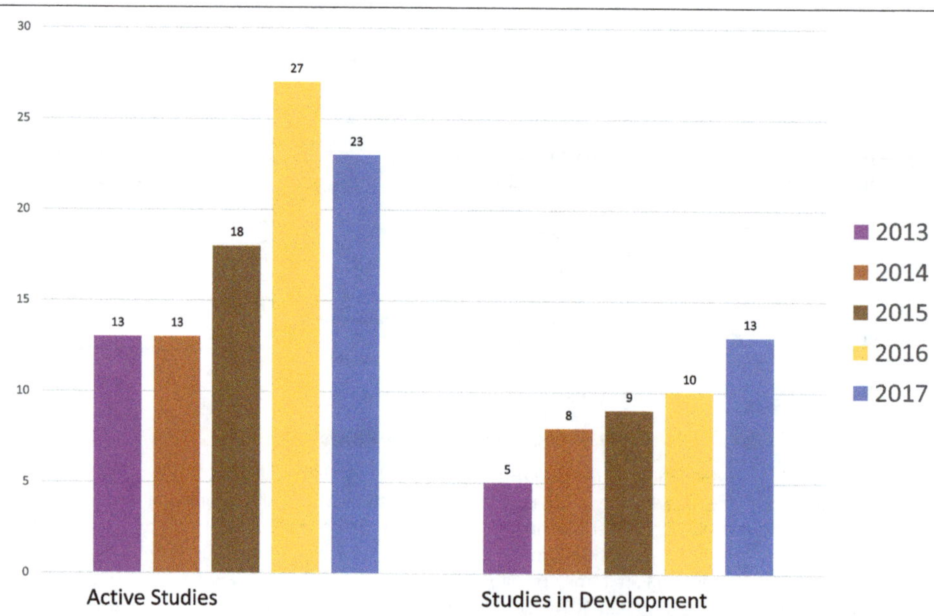

Fig. 2 The PRCSG is a productive collaborative research network with focus on medication studies in pediatric rheumatic diseases. The PRCSG network has been continuously active with the number of studies active or in development markedly increasing since the passage of FDA Safety and Innovation Act (FDASIA) in 2012

Other activities of the PRCSG

Besides optimizing study designs, the PRCSG is actively engaged in the training of pediatric rheumatology investigators. This includes formal training and certification of quantitated reporting of the joint evaluation in children (Joint Assessor Certification) [58] and the training in the completion of other outcome measures for clinical trials. The PRCSG also provides special mentoring and training to investigators or pediatric rheumatology sites new to drug trials. In recognition of the changing landscape of medical care, the PRCSG now actively invites membership applications from nurse practitioners, physician assistants, and pediatric rheumatology trainees involved in the care of children with rheumatic diseases.

It is the intent of the PRCSG to facilitate translational research studies in pediatric rheumatic diseases. This has proven to be difficult as pharmaceutical firms are determined to minimize trial costs and logistic demands. Generally, the collection of biological samples during studies paid for by biopharmaceutical companies focus on the demands of regulatory agencies and the pharmaceutical sponsor in-house research portfolio. To make matters worse, there were no internationally-accepted standard protocols for the collection, shipping, processing, and storage of pediatric rheumatology biological samples until recently. This short-coming has been addressed by the international consortium UCAN (Understanding Childhood Arthritis Network) [36, 59]. The PRCSG interacts with UCAN in supporting translational research by pediatric rheumatology investigators that make use of samples and data from drug trials. A recent example is the gene profiling study in SJIA patients treated with canakinumab [60].

Conclusions

Since the 1970's, the PRCSG has contributed to the methodology of performing trials in pediatric rheumatic diseases. Closely collaborating with PRINTO and industry sponsors, 25 drugs and biologic agents have been studied by the network, resulting in 13 drug and biologic therapies achieving labeling for JIA by the FDA and/or EMA as of 2018. These drugs have dramatically improved the outcomes of children with polyarticular and systemic forms of JIA, leading to improved growth, quality of life, and possibly reduced radiographic joint erosions [61–65]. Upcoming clinical studies undertaken by the PRCSG (see Fig. 2) are expected to yield the licensure of additional drugs for children with various subsets of JIA and other pediatric rheumatic diseases.

Abbreviations

BPCA: Best Pharmaceuticals for Children Act; BSA: Body surface area; CBER: Center for Biologics Evaluation and Research; CDER: Center for Drug Evaluation and Research; DMARDs: Disease Modifying Anti-Rheumatic Drugs; EMA: European Medicines Agency; FD&C Act: Food, Drug, and Cosmetic Act; FDA: Food and Drug Administration; FDASIA: FDA Safety and Innovation Act; IL: Interleukin; iPSP: Initial Pediatric Study Plan; JIA: Juvenile idiopathic arthritis; PDCO: Paediatric Committee; PIP: Paediatric Investigational Plan; PRCSG: Pediatric Rheumatology Collaborative Study Group; PREA: Pediatric Research Equity Act; PRINTO: Paediatric Rheumatology International Trial Organisation; RA: Rheumatoid arthritis; RWD: Randomized withdrawal design; U.S.: United States; UCAN: Understanding Childhood Arthritis Network; USSR: Union of Soviet Socialist Republics

Acknowledgements

We thank Drs. Robert Colbert and James McNamara for critical review of the manuscript. We would like to thank Drs. Suzette Peng and Sarah Yim for their service on the PRCSG Advisory Council.
Robert Colbert ColbertR@mail.nih.gov
James McNamara jmcnamara@niaid.nih.gov
Suzette Peng Suzette.Peng@fda.hhs.gov
Sarah Yim sarah.yim@fda.hhs.gov

Funding

This review was supported in part by the Intramural Research Program of the National Institute of Environmental Health Sciences (project ES101081, Lisa Rider) and National Institute of Allergy Immunology and Infectious Diseases (Ellen Goldmuntz), National Institutes of Health, Bethesda, MD. Salary support was provided for these two authors by NIH. Supervisors of Drs. Rider and Goldmuntz reviewed the manuscript and approved content and authorship of Drs. Rider and Goldmuntz.

Authors' contributions

First draft: HB. Critical feed-back, revisions and edits: HB; LGR; DJK; DC; RS; EG; KBO; EHG; DJL. Substantial contributions to conception and design, or acquisition of data, or analysis and interpretation of data. HB; LGR; DJK; DC; RS; EG; KBO; EHG; DJL. Final approval of submitted version: HB; LGR; DJK; DC; RS; EG; KBO; EHG; DJL. Agreed to be accountable for all aspects of the work in ensuring that questions related to the accuracy or integrity of any part of the work are appropriately investigated and resolved. HB; LGR; DJK; DC; RS; EG; KBO; EHG; DJL.

Consent for publication

Not applicable.

Competing interests

Dr. Lovell is Chairman of the PRCSG, Dr. Brunner is the Scientific Director of the PRCSG. All other named authors are members of the PRCSG Advisory Council. Drs. Yim and Peng are also members of the Advisory Council and reviewed the manuscript but deemed their contributions to the manuscript not significant enough to be included as named authors.

Author details

[1]Division of Rheumatology, Cincinnati Children's Hospital Medical Center & Cincinnati Children's Research Foundation, MLC 4010, Cincinnati, OH 45229, USA. [2]Environmental Autoimmunity Group, Clinical Research Branch, National Institute of Environmental Health Sciences, National Institutes of Health, Bethesda, MD, USA. [3]Randall Children's Hospital at Legacy Emanuel, Portland, OR, USA. [4]University of Wisconsin School of Medicine and Public Health, Madison, WI, USA. [5]The Hospital for Sick Children, University of Toronto, Toronto, Canada. [6]Division of Allergy, Immunology, and Transplantation, Rheumatologic Autoimmune Diseases Section, National Institutes of Health, Bethesda, MD, USA. [7]Hospital for Special Surgery, Weill Cornell Medicine, New York, NY, USA.

References

1. Neville KA, Frattarelli DA, Galinkin JL, et al. Off-label use of drugs in children. Pediatrics. 2014;133(3):563–7.
2. Rose AC, van't Hoff W, Beresford MW, Tansey SP. NIHR medicines for children research network: improving children's health through clinical research. Expert Rev Clin Pharmacol. 2013;6(5):581–7.
3. Best pharmaceuticals for children act of 2007. Food and Drug Administration Amendments Act (FDAAA), Title V Vol Public Law No. 110-85.
4. Pediatric Research Equity Act. Pub L; 2003. p. No. 108–55.
5. Field MJ, Boat TF, Institute of Medicine (U.S.), National Research Council (U.S.). Safe and effective medicines for children : pediatric studies conducted under the best Pharmaceuticals for Children act and the pediatric research equity act. Washington, D.C.: The National Academies Press; 2012.
6. U.S. Food and Drug Administration. Guidance for Industry: Clinical development programs for drugs, devices, and biological products for the treatment of rheumatoid arthritis (RA). 1999. https://www.fda.gov/downloads/Drugs/Guidances/ucm071579.pdf.
7. Califf R. Best Pharmaceuticals for Children act and Pediatric Research Equity act - July 2016 report to congress. 2016. https://www.fda.gov/downloads/ScienceResearch/SpecialTopics/PediatricTherapeuticsResearch/UCM509815.pdf.
8. Turner MA, Attar S, de Wildt SN, Vassal G, Mangiarini L, Giaquinto C. Roles of clinical research networks in pediatric drug development. Clin Ther. 2017; 39(10):1939–48.
9. U.S. Food and Drug Administration. Guidance for industry: pediatric study plans - content of and process for submitting initial pediatric study plans and amended initial pediatric study plans 2016. https://www.fda.gov/downloads/drugs/guidancecomplianceregulatoryinformation/guidances/ucm360507.pdf.
10. Ruperto N, Martini A. International research networks in pediatric rheumatology: the PRINTO perspective. Curr Opin Rheumatol. 2004;16(5): 566–70.
11. Wallace CA, Giannini EH, Spalding SJ, et al. Trial of early aggressive therapy in polyarticular juvenile idiopathic arthritis. Arthritis Rheum. 2012;64(6):2012–21.
12. Hashkes PJ, Spalding SJ, Giannini EH, et al. Rilonacept for colchicine-resistant or -intolerant familial Mediterranean fever: a randomized trial. Ann Intern Med. 2012;157(8):533–41.
13. Brewer EJ, Giannini EH, Kuzmina N, Alekseev L. Penicillamine and hydroxychloroquine in the treatment of severe juvenile rheumatoid arthritis. N Engl J Med. 1986;314(20):1269–76.
14. Brewer EJ Jr, Giannini EH, Barkley E. Gold therapy in the management of juvenile rheumatoid arthritis. Arthritis Rheum. 1980;23(4):404–11.
15. Giannini E, Brewer E, Kuzmina N, et al. Methotrexate in resistant juvenile rheumatoid arthritis: results of the USA-USSR double-blind, placebocontrolled trial. N Engl J Med. 1992;326(16):1043–9.
16. Bass J, Giannini E, Brewer E, et al. Pirprofen (Rengasil) in the treatment of juvenile rheumatoid arthritis. A segment I study. J Rheumatol. 1982; 9(1):140–3.
17. Brewer E, Giannini E, Baum J, et al. Aspirin and fenoprofen (Nalfon) in the treatment of juvenile rheumatoid arthritis results of the double blind-trial. A segment II study. J Rheumatol. 1982;9(1):123–8.
18. Brewer E, Giannini E, Baum J, et al. Sodium meclofenamate (Meclomen) in the treatment of juvenile rheumatoid arthritis. A segment I study. J Rheumatol. 1981;9(1):129–34.
19. Brewer E, Giannini E, Baum J, et al. Proquazone (Biarsan) in the treatment of juvenile rheumatoid arthritis. A segment I study. J Rheumatol. 1982;9(1):135–9.
20. Foeldvari I, Szer IS, Zemel LS, et al. A prospective study comparing celecoxib with naproxen in children with juvenile rheumatoid arthritis. J Rheumatol. 2009;36(1):174–82.
21. Levinson JE, Baum J, Brewer E, et al. Comparison of tolmetin sodium and aspirin in the treatment of juvenile rheumatoid arthritis. J Pediatr. 1977; 91(5):799–804.
22. Reiff A, Lovell DJ, Van Adelsberg J, et al. Evaluation of the comparative efficacy and tolerability of rofecoxib and naproxen in children and adolescents with juvenile rheumatoid arthritis: a 12-week randomized controlled clinical trial with a 52-week open-label extension. J Rheumatol. 2006;33(5):985–95.
23. Sobel RE, Lovell DJ, Brunner HI, et al. Safety of celecoxib and nonselective nonsteroidal anti-inflammatory drugs in juvenile idiopathic arthritis: results of the phase 4 registry. Pediatr Rheumatol. 2014;12(1):29.
24. Lovell DJ, Giannini EH, Reiff A, et al. Etanercept in children with polyarticular juvenile rheumatoid arthritis. Pediatric rheumatology collaborative study group. N Engl J Med. 2000;342(11):763–9.
25. Giannini EH, Ilowite NT, Lovell DJ, et al. Long-term safety and effectiveness of etanercept in children with selected categories of juvenile idiopathic arthritis. Arthritis Rheum. 2009;60(9):2794–804.
26. Ruperto N, Lovell DJ, Cuttica R, et al. A randomized, placebo-controlled trial of infliximab plus methotrexate for the treatment of polyarticular-course juvenile rheumatoid arthritis. Arthritis Rheum. 2007;56(9):3096–106.
27. Lovell DJ, Ruperto N, Goodman S, et al. Adalimumab with or without methotrexate in juvenile rheumatoid arthritis. N Engl J Med. 2008;359(8): 810–20.
28. Ruperto N, Lovell DJ, Quartier P, et al. Abatacept in children with juvenile idiopathic arthritis: a randomised, double-blind, placebo-controlled withdrawal trial. Lancet. 2008;372(9636):383–91.
29. Brunner HI, Ruperto N, Zuber Z, et al. Efficacy and safety of tocilizumab in patients with polyarticular-course juvenile idiopathic arthritis: results from a phase 3, randomised, double-blind withdrawal trial. Ann Rheum Dis. 2015; 74(6):1110–7.
30. Brunner HI, Ruperto N, Tzaribachev N, Horneff G, Chasnyk VG, Panaviene V, Abud-Mendoza C, Reiff A, Alexeeva E, Rubio-Pérez N, Keltsev V. Subcutaneous golimumab for children with active polyarticular-course juvenile idiopathic arthritis: results of a multicentre, double-blind, randomised-withdrawal trial. Ann Rheum Dis. 2017:annrheumdis-2016.
31. Lovell DJ, Giannini EH, Reiff AO, et al. Long-term safety and efficacy of rilonacept in patients with systemic juvenile idiopathic arthritis. Arthritis Rheum. 2013;65(9):2486–96.
32. De Benedetti F, Brunner HI, Ruperto N, et al. Randomized trial of tocilizumab in systemic juvenile idiopathic arthritis. N Engl J Med. 2012; 367(25):2385–95.
33. Ruperto N, Brunner HI, Quartier P, et al. Two randomized trials of canakinumab in systemic juvenile idiopathic arthritis. N Engl J Med. 2012; 367(25):2396–406.
34. Giannini EH, Brewer EJ Jr. Standard methodology for segment I, II, and III pediatric rheumatology collaborative study group studies. II. Analysis and presentation of data. J Rheumatol. 1982;9(1):114–22.
35. Brewer EJ Jr, Giannini EH. Standard methodology for segment I, II, and III pediatric rheumatology collaborative study group studies. I. Design. J Rheumatol. 1982;9(1):109–13.
36. Singh JA, Solomon DH, Dougados M, et al. Development of classification and response criteria for rheumatic diseases. Arthritis Rheum. 2006;55(3): 348–52.
37. Ruperto N, Giannini EH. Redundancy of conventional articular response variables used in juvenile chronic arthritis clinical trials. Ann Rheum Dis. 1996;55(1):73–5.
38. Giannini EH, Ruperto N, Ravelli A, Lovell DJ, Felson DT, Martini A. Preliminary definition of improvement in juvenile arthritis. Arthritis Rheum. 1997;40(7):1202–9.
39. Brunner HI, Lovell DJ, Finck BK, Giannini EH. Preliminary definition of disease flare in juvenile rheumatoid arthritis. J Rheumatol. 2002;29(5):1058–64.
40. Wallace CA, Giannini EH, Spalding SJ, et al. Clinically inactive disease in a cohort of children with new-onset polyarticular juvenile idiopathic arthritis treated with early aggressive therapy: time to achievement, total duration, and predictors. J Rheumatol. 2014;41(6):1163–70.
41. Ravelli A, Minoia F, Davì S, et al. 2016 classification criteria for macrophage activation syndrome complicating systemic juvenile idiopathic arthritis: a European league against rheumatism/American College of Rheumatology/Paediatric rheumatology international trials organisation collaborative initiative. Arthritis Rheumatol. 2016;68(3): 566–76.
42. Brunner HI, Feldman BM, Bombardier C, Silverman ED. Sensitivity of the systemic lupus erythematosus disease activity index, British isles lupus assessment group index, and systemic lupus activity measure in the evaluation of clinical change in childhood-onset systemic lupus erythematosus. Arthritis Rheum. 1999;42(7):1354–60.
43. Brunner HI, Silverman ED, To T, Bombardier C, Feldman BM. Risk factors for damage in childhood-onset systemic lupus erythematosus: cumulative disease activity and medication use predict disease damage. Arthritis Rheum. 2002;46(2):436–44.
44. Ruperto N, Ravelli A, Murray KJ, et al. Preliminary core sets of measures for disease activity and damage assessment in juvenile systemic lupus erythematosus and juvenile dermatomyositis. Rheumatology (Oxford). 2003; 42(12):1452–9.

45. Ruperto N, Ravelli A, Cuttica R, et al. The pediatric rheumatology international trials organization criteria for the evaluation of response to therapy in juvenile systemic lupus erythematosus: prospective validation of the disease activity core set. Arthritis Rheum. 2005;52(9): 2854–64.
46. Brunner HI, Mina R, Pilkington C, et al. Preliminary criteria for global flares in childhood-onset systemic lupus erythematosus. Arthritis Care Res (Hoboken). 2011;63(9):1213–23.
47. Mina R, Klein-Gitelman MS, Ravelli A, et al. Inactive disease and remission in childhood-onset systemic lupus erythematosus. Arthritis Care Res (Hoboken). 2012;64(5):683–93.
48. Lovell DJ, Lindsley CB, Rennebohm RM, et al. Development of validated disease activity and damage indices for the juvenile idiopathic inflammatory myopathies. II. The childhood myositis assessment scale (CMAS): a quantitative tool for the evaluation of muscle function. The juvenile dermatomyositis disease activity collaborative study group. Arthritis Rheum. 1999;42(10):2213–9.
49. Ruperto N, Pistorio A, Ravelli A, et al. The Paediatric rheumatology international trials organisation provisional criteria for the evaluation of response to therapy in juvenile dermatomyositis. Arthritis Care Res (Hoboken). 2010;62(11):1533–41.
50. Helmick CG, Felson DT, Lawrence RC, et al. Estimates of the prevalence of arthritis and other rheumatic conditions in the United States: part I. Arthritis Rheumatol. 2008;58(1):15–25.
51. Boat TF, Field MJ. Rare diseases and orphan products: accelerating research and development. Washington, DC: National Academies Press; 2011.
52. Harrold LR, Salman C, Shoor S, et al. Incidence and prevalence of juvenile idiopathic arthritis among children in a managed care population, 1996–2009. J Rheumatol. 2013;40(7):1218–25.
53. Biaggioni I, Freeman R, Mathias CJ, Low P, Hewitt LA, Kaufmann H. Randomized withdrawal study of patients with symptomatic neurogenic orthostatic hypotension responsive to droxidopa. Hypertension. 2014: HYPERTENSIONAHA. 114.04035.
54. Hibi T, Imai Y, Senoo A, Ohta K, Ukyo Y. Efficacy and safety of golimumab 52-week maintenance therapy in Japanese patients with moderate to severely active ulcerative colitis: a phase 3, double-blind, randomized, placebo-controlled study-(PURSUIT-J study). J Gastroenterol. 2017;52(10): 1101–11.
55. Ruperto N, Brunner HI, Lovell DJ, Martini A. Extrapolation or controlled trials in paediatrics: the current dilemma. Archives of disease in childhood. 2017: archdischild-2017.
56. Ruperto N, Quartier P, Wulffraat N, et al. A phase II, multicenter, open-label study evaluating dosing and preliminary safety and efficacy of canakinumab in systemic juvenile idiopathic arthritis with active systemic features. Arthritis Rheum. 2012;64(2):557–67.
57. Yokota S, Miyamae T, Imagawa T, et al. Therapeutic efficacy of humanized recombinant anti-interleukin-6 receptor antibody in children with systemic-onset juvenile idiopathic arthritis. Arthritis Rheumatol. 2005;52(3):818–25.
58. PRCSG / PRINTO. Joint Assessor certification. https://prcsg.org/index.php/prcsg-printo-joint-assessor-certification. Accessed 2 Jan 2018.
59. Yeung RS, Albani S, Feldman BM, Mellins E, Prakken B, Wedderburn LR. Enhancing translational research in paediatric rheumatology through standardization. Nat Rev Rheumatol. 2016;12(11):684–90.
60. Brachat AH, Grom AA, Wulffraat N, et al. Early changes in gene expression and inflammatory proteins in systemic juvenile idiopathic arthritis patients on canakinumab therapy. Arthritis Res Ther. 2017;19(1):13.
61. Nielsen S, Ruperto N, Gerloni V, et al. Preliminary evidence that etanercept may reduce radiographic progression in juvenile idiopathic arthritis. Clin Exp Rheumatol. 2008;26(4):688–92.
62. Simonini G, Giani T, Stagi S, de Martino M, Falcini F. Bone status over 1 yr of etanercept treatment in juvenile idiopathic arthritis. Rheumatology (Oxford). 2005;44(6):777–80.
63. Ruperto N, Lovell DJ, Li T, et al. Abatacept improves health-related quality of life, pain, sleep quality, and daily participation in subjects with juvenile idiopathic arthritis. Arthritis Care Res. 2010;62(11):1542–51.
64. Lovell DJ, Ruperto N, Mouy R, et al. Long-term safety, efficacy, and quality of life in patients with juvenile idiopathic arthritis treated with intravenous Abatacept for up to seven years. Arthritis Rheumatol. 2015; 67(10):2759–70.
65. De Benedetti F, Brunner H, Ruperto N, et al. Catch-up growth during tocilizumab therapy for systemic juvenile idiopathic arthritis: results from a phase III trial. Arthritis Rheumatol. 2015;67(3):840–8.

23

Unusual case of chronic recurrent multifocal osteomyelitis

Ausra Snipaitiene[1,2*], Rima Sileikiene[1,2], Justina Klimaite[2], Edita Jasinskiene[1,2], Rimantas Uktveris[1,2] and Lina Jankauskaite[1,2]

Abstract

Background: Chronic recurrent multifocal osteomyelitis (CRMO) is a rare auto-inflammatory bone disorder that primarily affects young girls, with a mean age of 10 years at onset. Generally, it is a self-limited disease. However, recent data indicate that more than 50% of patients have a chronic persistent disease and about 20% a recurring course of this condition. Also, there are more cases reported with associated auto-inflammatory and autoimmune diseases. In this case report, we present a rare case of sporadic CRMO in which the patient eventually developed C-ANCA (cytoplasmic anti-neutrophil cytoplasmic antibodies)-associated renal vasculitis and hyperparathyroidism.

Case presentation: A 14 year old female patient was brought to the emergency department with a sudden onset of left leg pain and oedema. After physical evaluation and initial investigation, she was diagnosed with femoral and pelvic deep vein thrombosis. While searching for possible thrombosis causes, osteomyelitis of the left leg was identified. Additional CT and MRI scans hinted at the CRMO diagnosis. Due to the multifocal lesions of CRMO, endocrinological evaluation of calcium metabolism was done. The results showed signs of hyperparathyroidism with severe hypocalcaemia. Moreover, when kidney damage occurred and progressed, a kidney biopsy was performed, revealing a C-ANCA associated renal vasculitis. Treatment was started with cyclophosphamide and prednisolone according to the renal vasculitis management protocol. Severe metabolic disturbances and hyperparathyroidism were treated with alfacalcidol, calcium and magnesium supplements. Secondary glomerulonephritis (GN) associated hypertension was treated with ACE (angiotenzine converting enzyme) inhibitors. Anticoagulants were prescribed for deep vein thrombosis. After 1.5 years of treatment, the patient is free of complaints. All microelement and parathormone levels are within normal range. Kidney function is now normal. To date, there are no clinical or diagnostic signs of deep vein thrombosis.

Conclusions: This case report presents a complex immunodysregulatory disorder with both auto-inflammatory and autoimmune processes. We hypothesize that the long lasting active inflammation of CRMO may induce an autoimmune response and result in concomitant diseases like C-ANCA-associated vasculitis in our patient. Any potential specific pathogenic relationships between these two rare pathologies may need to be further studied. Furthermore, there is a lack of specific biomarkers for CRMO and more studies are necessary to identify CRMO's characteristic patterns and how to best monitor disease progression.

Keywords: CRMO, C-ANCA, Renal vasculitis, GPA, Hyperparathyroidism, Paediatric, Auto-inflammation, Autoimmune

* Correspondence: a.snipaitiene@gmail.com
[1]The Lithuanian University of Health Sciences, A. Mickevičiaus g. 9, Kaunas, Lithuania
[2]The Hospital of Lithuanian University of Health Sciences Kauno Klinikos, Eiveniu g. 2, Kaunas, Lithuania

Background

Chronic recurrent multifocal osteomyelitis (CRMO) is a rare auto-inflammatory bone disorder that primarily affects young girls, with a mean age of 10 years at onset [1, 2]. The disease can cause multiple bone lesions, mostly affecting long bones of the lower extremities and vertebrae [3]. Generally, it is a self-limited disease; however, recent data show that more than 50% of patients have a chronic persistent and about 20% have a recurring course of this condition [1]. According to the Eurofever registry [4], there are only slightly more then 460 cases registered world-wide so far, with a prevalence of 1–9/million. [5]. As CRMO is the diagnosis of exclusion and can imitate other inflammatory bone conditions, it is thought to be underestimated [6]. Also, there are more cases emerging associated with other auto-inflammatory and autoimmune diseases, for example related to disorders with skin diseases [7, 8], peripheral arthritis [9–11], concomitant inflammatory bowel disease [12, 13], granulomatosis with polyangiitis (GPA, formerly known as Wegener granulomatosis) [14, 15] and others [16–19]. An association with several auto-inflammatory conditions can be detected in about one-third of CRMO patients [3]. Despite being well-known for about 50 years, CRMO still does not have approved treatment guidelines as the aetiology is unknown, and none of the therapies used currently have provided consistent outcomes. In this case report, we present a rare case of prolonged sporadic CRMO which eventually developed cytoplasmic anti-neutrophil cytoplasmic antibody (C-ANCA)-associated renal vasculitis and hyperparathyroidism.

Case presentation

A 14-year-old female patient presented to the emergency department with a sudden onset of left leg pain and oedema. She had a fever of 38 °C once a few days before. Physical evaluation revealed a swollen and painful left leg with reduced range of motion of the left hip and bumps palpated on the right tibia proximal metaphysis. No signs of arthritis, possible intestinal inflammation or skin changes were seen during physical evaluation. The patient's blood pressure and urinary output were normal. After the emergency ultrasound exam revealed a diagnosis of femoral and pelvic deep vein thrombosis, she was admitted to the hospital. According to her parents, the patient had had no chronic diseases to date. They indicated that she had a foot fracture at the age of 8 years. There were no autoimmune or auto-inflammatory disorders in the patient's family history.

Initial investigations revealed high levels of inflammatory markers (CRP and ESR), and a severe microcytic anaemia as well as thrombocytosis, hypoalbuminemia and elevated fibrinogen concentration and D-dimer values (Table 1). Suspecting an infectious cause, a urinalysis was performed, and haematuria and proteinuria

Table 1 Blood tests results

Test	Result	Reference value
CRP (mg/L)	249.19	0–7.5
ESR (mm/h)	125	0–11
Complete blood count:		
WBC ($X10^9/L$)	15.44	4.2–9.4
Neutrophil count ($X10^9/L$)	12.42	1.8–7.5
Hb (g/L)	45	108–133
Erythrocyte ($X10^{12}/L$)	2.81	3.9–4.9
MCV (fL)	62.6	77–91
MCH (pg)	17.1	24.8–30.2
Platelet count ($X10^9/L$)	676	194–345
Albumin (g/L)	21	31–48
Fibrinogen (g/L)	7.63	2–4
D-dimers (mg/L)	7.87	0–0.5
Creatinine (μmol/L)	185 → 307	26.5–88.4
eGFR ($ml/min/1,72m^2$)	33.5 → 20.2	90–120
BUN (mmol/L)	12.3	2.9–7.1
Feritine (μg/L)	448	15–150

CRP C-reactive protein, *ESR* erythrocyte sedimentation rate, *WBC* white blood cells *Hb* hemoglobin *MCV* mean corpuscular volume, *MCH* mean corpuscular hemoglobin, *eGFR* estimated glomerular filtration rate, *BUN* blood urea nitrogen

were detected. Both blood and urine cultures were sterile. X-rays of the legs were done (Fig. 1), showing sites of hyperostosis and sclerosis in the metaphysis of the right tibia along with a periosteal reaction, suggesting a possible osteomyelitis or oncological processes in the bones. As the diagnosis of acute osteomyelitis could not be disproved, broad-spectrum antibiotics were prescribed. However, the CRP level did not change significantly over the first few days, so other causes of acute thrombosis and inflammation were investigated. An abdominal ultrasound showed a giant, homogenous pelvic mass and hydronephrosis of the left kidney. Kidney function was quite abnormal as the creatinine level was 185 μmol/L and urinary protein excretion of 7 g over 24 h was detected. Within the next few days the patient's kidney function deteriorated further, with a creatinine value increasing to 307 μmol/L with poor urine output and high blood pressure. The patient had no prior history of kidney problems.

Due to the findings of the abdominal ultrasound and leg X-ray, the child underwent a whole-body computed tomography (CT) scan. Multiple bone lesions were observed, the most severe of which were located in the left scapula, the fifth rib projection near the spine and a large deformity of the left pelvic bone close to the acetabulum (Fig. 2). The left iliopsoas muscle also appeared to be abnormal. Moreover, renal parenchymal thickening and oedema were found. Investigations for possible

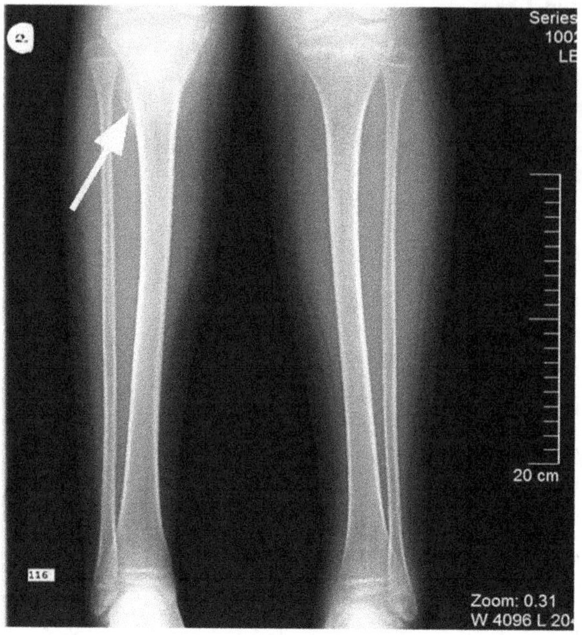

Fig. 1 X-ray of the legs.Hyperostosis on the left tibia metaphysis is indicated by a white arrow

endocrine disorders were performed (Table 2). Signs of hyperparathyroidism were present together with hypocalcaemia, hypomagnesaemia and a low vitamin D3 concentration, as well as hypocalciuria in the 24-h urine test and hyperphosphaturia based on phosphate fractional excretion (Table 3).

Bone and left kidney biopsies were performed. The bone biopsy from the affected site of the left pelvic bone demonstrated intertrabecular stromal fibrosis, several epithelioid granulomas with a central zone of necrosis and polymorphonuclear cells. Moreover, histological evaluation showed a few sites with plasma cell infiltration, including some cells positive for immunoglobulin G (IgG) and immunoglobulin G4 (IgG4). Histological examination of the surrounding connective tissue found mucoid oedema. The renal biopsy revealed an acute and active crescentic glomerulonephritis (GN) with ANCA-associated vasculitis (Fig. 3). Special staining was performed for the kidney sample, and no IgG subclasses were found.

Due to the results of left kidney biopsy together with thrombosis of the deep veins, additional screening for autoimmune diseases was carried out. The child tested positive for antinuclear antibodies (ANA 1:100), antibodies against centromere protein B (anti-CENP B), antibodies against proliferating cell nuclear antigens (anti-PCNA) and C-ANCA (Table 4). High levels of ferritin were also found (448 μg/L), indicating the possibility of both autoimmune and thrombotic causes of anaemia. However, antiphospholipid antibodies were not detected. Concerning the bone biopsy results, serum IgG levels were tested and only IgG4 was slightly increased (Table 4).

Since multiple bone lesions were detected, the fracture history was reviewed. At the age of 8 years our patient had not only a foot fracture, but also complained of pain in the left elbow and back. It appeared that she was diagnosed with CRMO at that time, based on the results of a biopsy from the fracture site as well as a CT of the left foot (Fig. 4) and a whole-body radionuclide scan. The radionuclide scan showed multiple sites of CRMO lesions, with three in the spine, one in the left hand, one in the left scapula, one in the left pelvic bone and two in the right leg. Surgery for the broken foot was performed and treatment with antibiotics and nonsteroidal anti-inflammatory drugs (NSAIDs) was prescribed for a month. When the patient's pain decreased over time, analgesics were discontinued due to the impression of a self-limiting disease

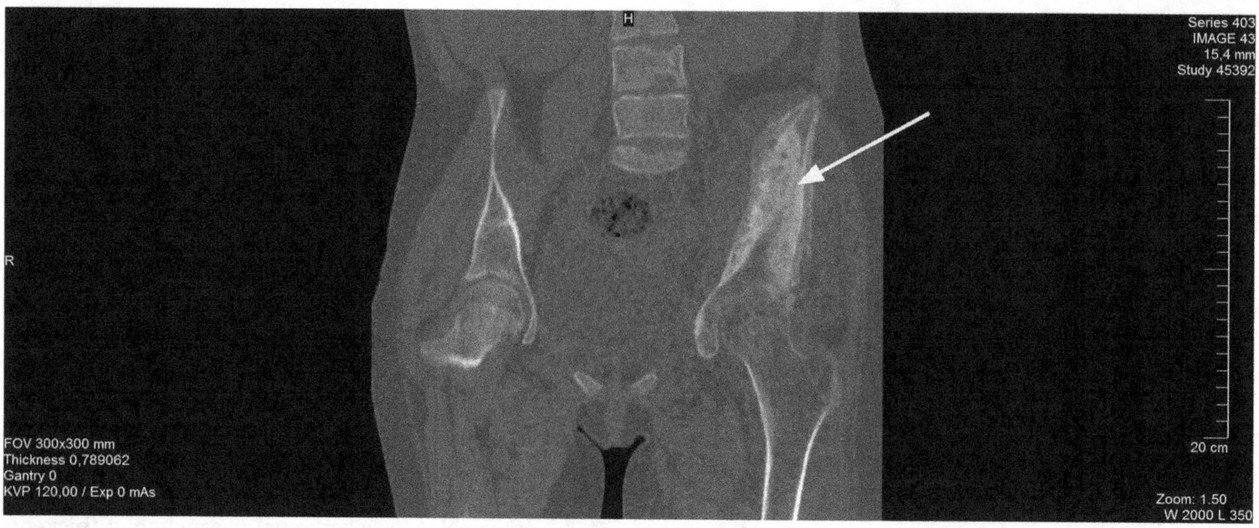

Fig. 2 Whole-body CT (pelvis region) showing destruction and sclerosis of the left hip bones

Table 2 Endocrine function tests results

Test	Result	Reference value
Ca (mmol/L)	1.9	2.23–2.58
Ionized Ca (mmol/L)	0.83	1.28–1.48
P (mmol/L)	1.34	1.07–2
Mg (mmol/L)	0.72	0,74-1,03
Vitamin D3 (25-OH) (nmol/L)	27.6	< 50 – deficiency, 51–69 – insufficiency, 70–250 – normal, > 250 – intoxication
PTH (pmol/L)	32.69	< 6.74
TSH (pmol/L)	2.6	0.4–3.6
FT4 (pmol/L)	19.03	10–19
FT3 (pmol/L)	3.39	3.34–5.14
Anti-TPO (kU/L)	< 3	0–3.2

Ca calcium, *P* phosphorus, *Mg* magnesium, *PTH* parathyroid hormone, *TSH* thyroid-stimulating hormone, *FT4* free thyroxine, *FT3* free triiodothyronine *Anti-TPO* anti-thyroid autoantibodies

course. For the next 6 years she was free from complaints except for painless unilateral right periorbital oedema appearing on and off for the last 2–3 years and observed without medical supervision. Due to this oedema and slight exophthalmos of the right eye during current episode, additional head and spine magnetic resonance imaging (MRI) was performed, and a new CRMO lesion in a right periorbital region was diagnosed (Fig. 5) together with deformation and lipoid degeneration of the seventh neck vertebrae (Fig. 6).

Treatment was started for the vasculitis with cyclophosphamide and prednisolone according to the renal-limited vasculitis management protocol. No pain reliever was necessary. Severe metabolic disturbances and hyperparathyroidism were treated with alfacalcidol, calcium and magnesium supplements. Kidney and ureter stents were placed for 1 month due to hydronephrosis. Secondary GN-associated hypertension was treated with ACE (angiotensin converting enzyme) inhibitors. Anticoagulants were prescribed for deep vein thrombosis for 6 months until full recanalisation of the left femoral vein had occurred.

Table 3 Urine test results

Test	Result	Reference value
Erythrocytes (/μL)	12,166	< 10
Leukocytes (/μL)	433	< 10
Protein (g/L)	3	< 0,1
Protein/24 h (g)	7	< 1
Creatinine (μmol/L)	3884	
Ca (mmol/24 h)	< 0.37	2.5–7.5
Fractional Ex of Ca (%)	1.54	1–2
P (mmol/24 h)	11.47	12.9–42
Fractional Ex of P (%)	38.59	10–20

Ca calcium, *Ex* excreation *P* phosphorus

After 1.5 years of treatment, the child is free of complaints. Her auto-inflammatory, metabolic and endocrinological conditions are being monitored by a multidisciplinary team of physicians. All microelements and parathormone levels are within the normal range. There are no signs of hypertension and the patient's kidney function has recovered. To date, there are no clinical or diagnostic signs of deep vein thrombosis. The patient is still on maintenance treatment with azathioprine according to the kidney vasculitis treatment protocol and receiving microelements supplementation.

Discussion

Chronic recurrent multifocal osteomyelitis has been recognized as a disease entity for several decades. It is a multi-faceted disease. The diagnosis is based on clinical signs, radiological findings and bone biopsy results. There are several diagnostic criteria suggested for this condition [3, 20], the latest ones are by Roderick et al. [20]. According to Zhao et al., these guidelines should be followed in clinical practice and their application in typical cases can prevent or minimise the need for bone biopsy [21]. Still, there is no unified protocol to identify and characterise this disease [22]. Regarding our case, biopsy results were essential, as various bone lesions and deformities were found together with highly elevated inflammation markers. Furthermore, possible oncological conditions such as osteoblastoma, osteosarcoma and others had to be ruled out [23]. Bone biopsy revealed all stages of bone inflammation, with fibrosis detected together with the presence of plasma cells (representing adaptive immunity) [24] and neutrophils (responsible for innate immune activation) [24]. These findings, together with symptomatic C-ANCA-associated kidney vasculitis and deep vein thrombosis, further illustrated the immune system disturbances.

Currently, there are an increasing number of CRMO cases associated with other auto-inflammatory and autoimmune conditions. According to different data, we found two more cases of CRMO that eventually developed GPA [14, 15]. However, both cases demonstrated typical signs of respiratory tract involvement. Our case presented with isolated C-ANCA-associated kidney vasculitis without respiratory tract injury by otorhinolaryngological examination or lung CT scans. Our case fulfils three criteria out of six for GPA diagnosis proposed by EULAR/PRINTO/PRES [25]. But the question remains if granulomatous lesions in bones are an expression of a separate skeletal inflammatory disorder which eventually caused kidney vasculitis (as a complication of persistent chronic inflammation) or if this sporadic CRMO could be the musculoskeletal expression of GPA [26]. The

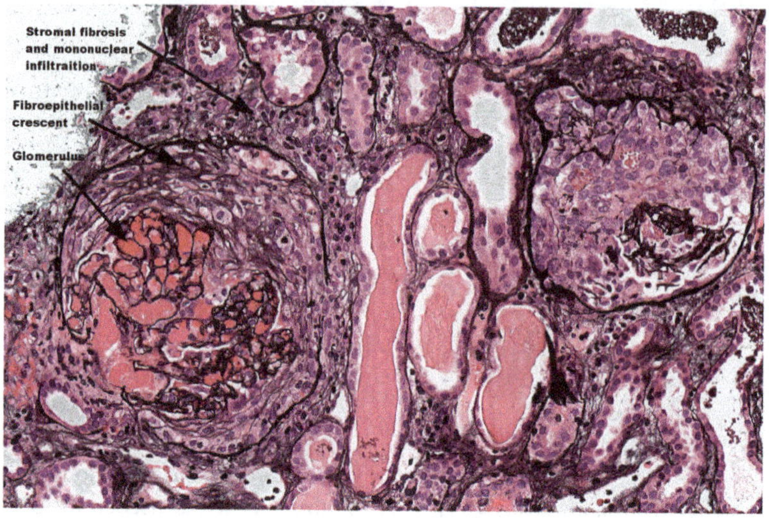

Fig. 3 Histological image of kidney tissue. PAS-stained sample, 400x magnification. The crescentic glomeruli, stromal fibrosis, normal mesangial region are indicated by arrows

recent studies of CRMO pathogenesis show a disturbed balance between pro- and anti-inflammatory cytokines such as interleukin 6 (IL-6), tumour necrosis factor alfa (TNFα) and interleukin 10 (IL-10) [24, 27]. Also, a reduced number of IL-10 producing cells in ANCA-associated vasculitis was shown in a study by Wilde et all. [28]. It may suggest a possible connection between these two conditions.

Moreover, it is reported that persistent inflammation and endothelial dysfunction associated with ANCA vasculitis increases the rate of thrombotic events and is linked to the active disease phase [29, 30]. Our patient's kidney biopsy results showed active vasculitis. Also, she had nephrotic proteinuria, which is known to increase the risk of thrombosis [31]. However, tests for protein C, protein S or antithrombin deficiencies, antiphospholipid antibodies and factor V Leiden mutation were negative in this case, indicating the possibility of other hypercoagulation mechanisms. Several hypotheses have also been proposed for activation of the coagulation cascade when well-known hypercoagulable risk factors remain undetected, including necrosis of endothelial cells and their circulation in the blood, wide-spread endothelial dysfunction, or thrombocyte activation [30].

Table 4 Autoimmune markers

Marker	Result	Reference value
ANA	1+ (1:100)	Negative < 1:40
Anti-CENP B	1+	Negative
Anti-PCNA	1+	Negative
C-ANCA	1+ (1:10)	Negative
P-ANCA	Negative	Negative
Anti-dsDNA (kU/L)	3.13	< 12
Complement C3 (g/L)	1.42	0.79–1.52
Complement C4 (g/L)	0.26	0.16–0.38
IgG (g/L)	24.09	7.9–16.4
IgG4 (g/L)	2.98	0.035–2.3

ANA antinuclear antibodies, *Anti-CENP B* antibodies against centromere protein B, *Anti-PCNA* antibodies against proliferating cell nuclear antigens, *C-ANCA* cytoplasmic anti-neutrophil cytoplasmic antibodies, *P-ANCA* perinuclear anti-neutrophil cytoplasmic antibodies, *Anti-dsDNA* anti-double stranded DNA antibodies, *IgG* immunoglobuline G, *IgG4* immunoglobuline G4

Interestingly, together with CRMO bone lesions, there were a few cells positive for IgG and IgG4 identified in the bone biopsy, pointing to another rare pathology, IgG4-related disease. To date, there are only 25 paediatric case reports of IgG-related disease identified and they usually involve ocular and parenchymal organs with positive histological results for IgG4 cells [32]. Although the IgG4 levels in the blood were slightly elevated compared to the reference values (Table 4), no other symptoms or signs of organ injury were detected in our patient. Also, the kidney histological examination was negative for IgG cells. A few studies have shown that increased IgG4 levels in serum can be found in a wide spectrum of diseases, including vasculitis [33, 34]. This could be the reason in our case too.

Our patient had several severe metabolic deficiencies including hypocalcaemia, hypomagnesemia and hyperparathyroidism leading to osteoporosis. In relation to these findings, the possibility of other metabolic bone diseases (like Camurati-Engelman syndrome and benign hyperostosis-pachydermoperiostosis) was considered. However, the lack of particular skin lesions and MRI results strongly supported CRMO diagnosis not the other two diagnoses. Information about the relationship between CRMO and calcium metabolism is still lacking.

We also considered a few possible conditions that could have caused hyperparathyroidism in our case.

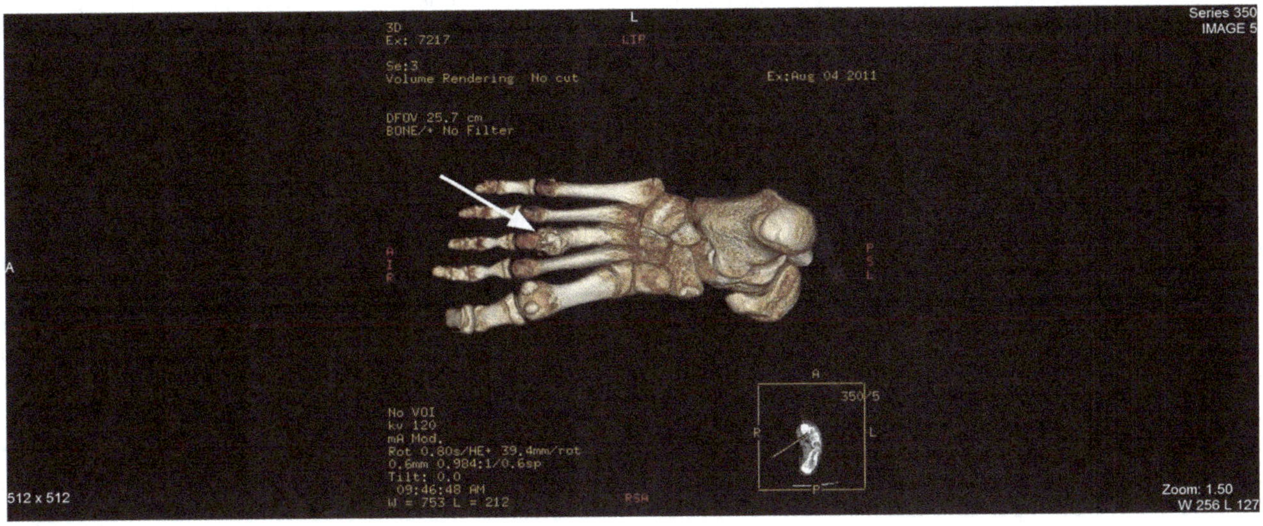

Fig. 4 Three-dimentional reconstruction CT of the left foot. The destruction and sclerosis of third metatarsus bone diaphysis and distal metaphysis parts are indicated by white arrows

First, we think that the hypocalcaemia may have developed due to the kidney damage and calcitriol production disturbances, which is well known in secondary hyperparathyroidism. This theory could be supported by the renal insufficiency and vitamin D3 hypovitaminosis that lasted for an unknown period. As our patient was free of complaints, her serum creatinine and vitamin D3 levels were not checked for several years. On the other hand, it is less likely that only renal insufficiency could have had influence on calcium metabolism as it was not severe on admission. Finally, as shown by Ata et al. [35], a high turnover rate of bone metabolism could be the most probable explanation for osteoporosis and hyperparathyroidism in this CRMO case. Closer follow-up of calcium metabolism might have provided an earlier hint of hyperparathyroidism and renal insufficiency due to the multiple bone lesions diagnosed after the first episode of CRMO 6 years ago.

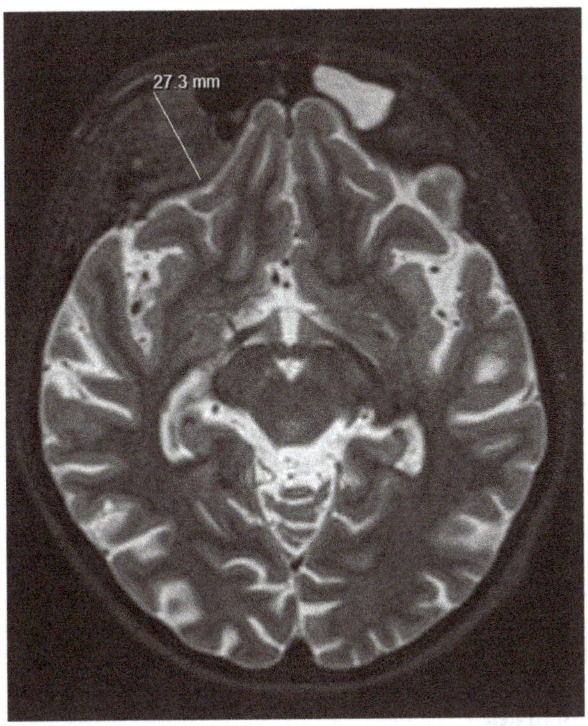

Fig. 5 MRI of the patient's head. Measuring of hyperostosis of frontal bone on the right is shown by a white line

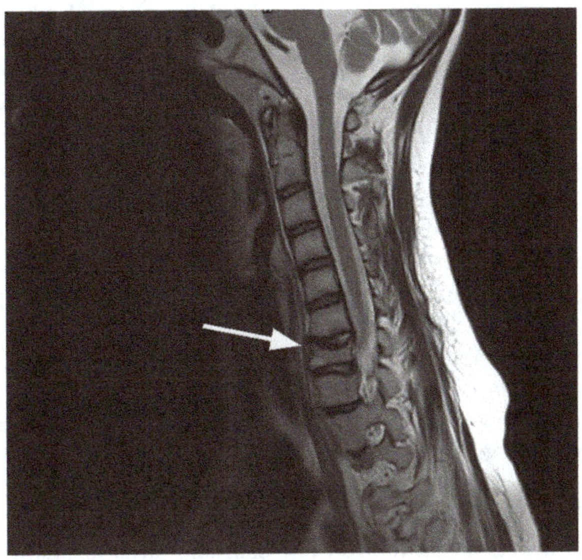

Fig. 6 MRI of the patient's neck. Destruction and lipoid degeneration in the seventh neck vertebrae is indicated by a white arrow

Chronic recurrent multifocal osteomyelitis is a very versatile disease. Several studies have been done to identify the possible connection between immunological defects and gene mutations. Different data show that genetic metabolism errors are responsible for some of CRMO syndromes [7, 16], for example, the *PSTPIP1* gene is associated with pyogenic arthritis, pyoderma gangrenosum and acne (PAPA) syndrome [7] as well as defects in *LPIN2* result in Majeed syndrome [16]. A few research groups suggested a link between sporadic CRMO and gene errors along the 18q chromosome [36]. However, more studies are needed. There is no data showing a specific genetic defects in most of the sporadic cases, especially those associated with other conditions like GPA, dermatomyositis and other auto-immune diseases. Genetic testing for the *PSTPIP1* gene mutation was performed for our patient and was negative.

Despite various attempts to understand CRMO pathogenesis and favour diagnostic processes, no auto-antibody production has been observed to date, thus supporting an auto-inflammatory pathogenic mechanism of this condition [24, 37, 38]. We did not observe high auto-antibody titres in our case too. However, several different auto-antibodies were found. Anti-PCNA antibodies are known to occur in Sjogren's syndrome [39], but no clinical signs of ocular or oral symptoms were present for this patient [40]. Also, we detected the presence of anti-CENP B antibodies, which are usually seen in systemic sclerosis [41]. Even so, our patient had no Raynaud's phenomenon, skin lesions or other signs of systemic sclerosis. Moreover, an inflammatory processes and not antibody production was predominant throughout the course of the disease.

Recent studies of CRMO have led to a better understanding of pathogenic mechanisms and contributed the treatment improvements as following. NSAID monotherapy is thought to influence osteoclast activation by inhibiting prostaglandins, and thus impacting bone remodelling [24]. Moreover, glucocorticoids were shown to be important in stopping the general inflammatory response, thus having a positive effect in some cases [2]. Considering recent studies about bone remodelling in CRMO [35] and previous reports about increased osteoclast activity in bone histology specimens [42, 43], bone resorption inhibitors may be an effective treatment option. Moreover, bisphosphonates are strong osteoclast activity inhibitors and they may reduce bone turnover. Furthermore, they have shown to be effective in recurrent cases and in cases unresponsive to first-line medication [44, 45]. In very severe cases, biological therapy, for instance IL-1 or TNF-α inhibitors, have had a beneficial effect and limited progress of the disease [24, 46].

Our patient did not feel any pain and physical disability close to the CRMO lesion sites. Moreover, no vertebral fractures were detected to date and no additional treatment for CRMO was prescribed. Only treatment for vasculitis with a continuous low dose of prednisone and high doses of calcium and alfacalcidol supplements for the osteoporotic changes were given.

According to clinical guidelines, pain relief of the affected area is thought to be one of the most important criteria for clinical improvement. Despite no specific treatment, our patient had no complaints for 6 years after the initial diagnosis. Still, the progression of CRMO was obvious with a new lesion present in the MRI and painless bone deformities as a complication of the chronic course of the disease. Interestingly, this phenomenon has been described before [47] showing that active CRMO can be found in MRI, both, in periods without complaints and after various treatment options, even more than 10 years after the initial bone injury. Regardless of this data, it is still unknown if these clinically undetectable and painless lesions have clinical relevance to the disease progression and how long the treatment should be administered, i.e. to a complete radiological remission or improvement of clinical and laboratory signs [47]. Having this in mind and seeking to monitor possible severe complications (like vertebral fractures in the absence of complaints) the whole-body MRI with short tau inversion recovery (STIR) images is currently preferred as it was shown to be of superior sensitivity for evaluating CRMO lesion activity [48]. Well-timed MRI could show bone oedema prior to the appearance of erosions and/or sclerosis [48, 49]. In our case, comparative bone scintigraphy was done in parallel to the one done 6 years ago. One new CRMO lesion site was found in the right orbital area. No negative progression was observed in the previously diagnosed lesions. The MRI of the right orbital area detected sclerotic changes without bone oedema, indicating a continuous inflammatory processes that had likely developed within months or even years when the patient was supposedly symptoms-free and in a benign course of the disease. Taking into account other cases in which the patients eventually developed C-ANCA-associated vasculitis, we suggest that patients with multiple CRMO lesions should be monitored closely regarding chronic inflammation despite no signs or symptoms of disease activity.

Recently, research on new biomarkers for CRMO diagnosis and monitoring CRMO progression has been done by Hofmann et al. It showed that some changes in interleukin levels (IL-6, IL-12, eotaxin and others) were significantly altered during the CRMO disease course, meaning they could potentially be used as CRMO activity markers [37]. In our opinion, these biomarkers would be especially useful in unusual cases with atypical clinical courses, when some monitoring tools, for instance the PedsCNO score [50], are difficult to apply objectively.

Conclusions

This case report presents a rare case of a complex immunodysregulatory disorder with both auto-inflammatory and autoimmune elements. We hypothesize that the long lasting active inflammation of CRMO may induce an autoimmune response, resulting in a concomitant disease such as the C-ANCA-associated vasculitis in our patient. Any potential specific pathogenic relationships between these two rare diseases may need to be further studied. Furthermore, there is still a lack of specific biomarkers for CRMO and more studies are necessary to identify CRMO's characteristic patterns and how to best monitor disease progression.

Abbreviations

ACF: Angiotenzine converting factor; ANA: Antinuclear antibodies; ANCA: Anti-neutrophil cytoplasmic antibodies; anti-CENP B: Antibodies against centromere protein B; anti-PCNA: Antibodies against proliferating cell nuclear antigens; C-ANCA: Cytoplasmic anti-neutrophil cytoplasmic antibodies; CRMO: Chronic recurrent multifocal osteomyelitis; CRP: C reactive protein; CT: Computed tomography; ESR: Erythrocyte sedimentation rate; EULAR: European League Against Rheumatism; GN: Glomerulonephritis; GPA: Granulomatosis with polyangiitis; IgG: Immunoglobulin G; IgG4: Immunoglobulin G4; IL-10: Interleukin 10; IL-12: Interleukin 12; IL-6: Interleukin 6; MRI: Magnetic resonance investigation; NSAIDs: Nonsteroidal anti-inflammatory drugs; PAPA: Pyogenic arthritis, pyoderma gangrenosum and acne syndrome; PedsCNO score: Paediatric chronic nonbacterial osteomyelitis score; PRES: Paediatric Rheumatology European Society; PRINTO: Paediatric Rheumatology INternational Trials Organization; STIR: Short tau inversion recovery; TNFα: Tumor necrosis factor alfa

Acknowledgements

We are grateful for the assistance of Professor Arvydas Laurinavicius from Vilnius University Hospital and the team at the Lithuanian National Center of Pathology for histological evaluation of the kidney biopsies.

Authors' contributions

AS was a major contributor in writing the manuscript. RS analysed and interpreted the patient's data regarding rheumatological diseases. JK analysed and interpreted the patient's data regarding oncological diseases and performed the bone biopsy. EJ analysed and interpreted the patient's data regarding endocrinological diseases. RU analysed and interpreted the patient's radiological scans. LJ designed and coordinated the writing of the manuscript, assisted in data interpretation and drafting of the manuscript. All authors read and approved the final manuscript.

Authors' information

AS is a paediatric rheumatology resident at The Lithuanian University of Health Sciences (LUHS) and the Hospital of Lithuanian University of Health Sciences Kauno Klinikos (HLUHS KK).
RS is an Associated Professor at the Paediatric Clinic of LUHS, and is Head of the Department of Paediatric Rheumatology and Cardiology at the HLUHS KK.
JK is a paediatric heamatology doctor at the Department of Paediatric Oncology at the HLUHS KK.
EJ is a lecturer at the Endocrinology Clinic of the LUHS and Head of the Department of Paediatric Endocrinology at the HLUHS KK.
RU is a lecturer at the Radiology Clinic of the LUHS and a radiologist in the Radiology Department at the HLUHS KK.
LJ is a lecturer at the Paediatric Clinic of the LUHS, post-doc at the Department of Physiology and Pharmacology of the LUHS, and a paediatric pulmonology doctor in the Paediatric department at the HLUHS KK.

Consent for publication

Written informed consent for publication of their clinical details and clinical images was obtained from the parent of the patient. A copy of the consent form is available for review by the Editor of this journal.

Competing interests

The authors declare that they have no competing interests.

References

1. Kaiser D, Bolt I, Hofer M, Relly C, Berthet G, Bolz D, Saurenmann T. Chronic nonbacterial osteomyelitis in children: a retrospective multicenter study. Pediatr Rheumatol Online J. 2015;13:25.
2. Wipff J, Costantino F, Lemelle I, Pajot C, Duquesne A, Lorrot M, et al. A Large National Cohort of French Patients With Chronic Recurrent Multifocal Osteitis. Arthritis and Rheumatology. 2015;67(4):1128–37.
3. Jansson A, Renner ED, Ramser J. Classification of non-bacterial osteitis: retrospective study of clinical, immunological and genetic aspects in 89 patients. Rheumatology (Oxford). 2007;46:154–60.
4. PRINTO. Eurofever registry. PRINTO web site. PRINTO. [Cited: June 12, 2017.] https://www.printo.it/eurofever/eurofever_registry.asp.
5. Orphanet. Orphanet Rare Disease Web site. [Cited: June 12, 2017] http://www.orpha.net.
6. Schnabel A, Range U, Hahn G, Siepmann T, Berner R, Hedrich CM. Unexpectedly high incidences of chronic non-bacterial as compared to bacterial osteomyelitis in children. Rheumatol Int. 2016;36(12):1737–45.
7. Wang D, Hoing S, Patterson HC, Ahmad UM, Rathinam VA, Rajewsky K, Fitzgerald KA, Golenbock DT. Inflammation in mice ectopically expressing human Pyogenic Arthritis, Pyoderma Gangrenosum, and Acne (PAPA) Syndrome-associated PSTPIP1 A230T mutant proteins. J Biol Chem. 2013; 288(7):4594–601.
8. Tlougan BE, Podjasek JO, O'Haver J, Cordova KB, Nguyen XH, Tee R, Pinckard-Hansen KC, Hansen RC. Chronic recurrent multifocal osteomyelitis (CRMO) and synovitis, acne, pustulosis, hyperostosis, and osteitis (SAPHO) syndrome with associated neutrophilic dermatoses: a report of seven cases and review of the literature. Pediatr Dermatol. 2009;26(5):497–505.
9. Walsh P, Manners PJ, Vercoe J, Burgner D, Murray KJ. Chronic recurrent multifocal osteomyelitis in children: nine years' experience at a statewide tertiary paediatric rheumatology referral centre. Rheumatology (Oxford). 2015;54(9):1688–91.
10. Tsitsami E, Dermentzoglou V, Moschovi M, Chrousos GP. Chronic recurrent multifocal osteomyelitis with concomitant features of juvenile idiopathic arthritis. Case Rep Rheumatol. 2011;2011:210795. https://doi.org/10.1155/2011/210795.
11. Zhao Y., Foster Shannon K., Murdock Todd J., Schlesinger M., Wallace Carol A. A rare case of chronic recurrent multifocal osteomyelitis with undifferentiated juvenile idiopathic arthritis, uveitis, and psoriasis. Case Rep Clin Med. 2016 5. DOI: https://doi.org/10.4236/crcm.2016.57041.
12. Girschick HJ, Zimmer C, Klaus G, Darge K, Dick A, Morbach H. Chronic recurrent multifocal osteomyelitis: what is it and how should it be treated? Nat Clin Pract Rheumatol. 2007;3(12):733–8.
13. Omidi CJ, Siegfried EC. Chronic recurrent multifocal osteomyelitis preceding pyoderma gangrenosum and occult ulcerative colitis in a pediatric patient. Pediatr Dermatol. 1998;15(6):435–8.
14. Pelkonen P, Ryoppy S, Jaaskelainen J, Rapola J, Repo H, Kaitila I. Chronic osteomyelitislike disease with negative bacterial cultures. Am J Dis Child. 1988;142(11):1167–73.
15. Brogan KS, Eleftheriou D, Biassoni L, Sebire N, Brogan PA. Multifocal noninfectious osteitis as a presentation of pediatric granulomatosis with polyangiitis (Wegener's). Arthritis Rheumatol. 2015;67(10):2748.
16. Ferguson PJ, Chen S, Tayeh MK, Ochoa L, Leal SM, Pelet A, Munnich A, Lyonnet S, Majeed HA, El-Shanti H. Homozygous mutations in LPIN2 are responsible for the syndrome of chronic recurrent multifocal osteomyelitis and congenital dyserythropoietic anaemia (Majeed syndrome). J Med Genet. 2005;42(7):551–7.
17. Dagan O, Barak Y, Metzker A. Pyoderma gangrenosum and sterile multifocal osteomyelitis preceding the appearance of Takayasu arteritis. Pediatr Dermatol. 1995;12(1):39–42.

18. Daniela SA, Dent PB, Ferguson PJ, Laxer RM. Chronic Non-bacterial Osteomyelitis in a Child with Previous Juvenile Dermatomyositis. J Rheumatol. 2013;40(3):339–40.
19. Vettiyil G, Punnen A, Kumar S. An Unusual Association of Chronic Recurrent Multifocal Osteomyelitis, Pyoderma Gangrenosum, and Takayasu Arteritis. J Rheumatol. 2017;44(1):127–8.
20. Roderick MR, Shah R, Rogers V, Finn A, Ramanan AV. Chronic recurrent multifocal osteomyelitis (CRMO) - advancing the diagnosis. Pediatric Rheumatology. 2016;14(1):47.
21. Y Zhao, RM Laxer, PJ Ferguson. Treatment Advances in Chronic Non-Bacterial Osteomyelitis and Other Autoinflammatory Bone Conditions. Curr Treat Opt Rheumatol. 2017;3(1)17–32.
22. Ferrari J, Pilkington C. Chronic recurrent multifocal osteomyelitis: the prevalence of lower-limb and foot involvement. J Am Podiatr Med Assoc. 2014;104(6):583–7.
23. Costa-Reis P, Sullivan KE. Chronic Recurrent Multifocal Osteomyelitis. J Clin Immunol. 2013;33:1043–56.
24. Hedrich C. M., Hofmann S.R., Pablik J., Morbach H., Girschick, H. J. Autoinflammatory bone disorders with special focus on chronic recurrent multifocal osteomyelitis (CRMO). Pediatr Rheumatol Online J. 2013 11.
25. Ozen S, Pistorio A, Iusan SM, Bakkaloglu A, Herlin T, Brik R, Buoncompagni A, Lazar C, Bilge I, Uziel Y, Rigante D, Cantarini L, Hilario MO, Silva CA, Alegria MA, Norambuena X, Belot A, Berkun Y, Ibanez Estrella A, Olivieri AN, Alpigiani MG, Rumba I, Sztainbok F. EULAR/PRINTO/PRES criteria for Henoch-Schönlein purpura, childhood polyarteritis nodosa, childhood Wegener granulomatosis, and childhood Takayasu arteritis: Ankara 2008. Part II: final classification criteria. Ann Rheum Dis. 2010;69(5):798–806.
26. Pangoux C. Joint and bone manifestations in GPA. Can Rheumatol Assoc J. 2011;21(2):25–7.
27. Hofmann SR, Schwarz T, Möller JC, Morbach H, Schnabel A, Rösen-Wolff A, et al. Chronic non-bacterial osteomyelitis is associated with impaired Sp1 signaling, reduced IL10 promoter phosphorylation, and reduced myeloid IL-10 expression. Clin Immunol. 2011;141(3):317–27.
28. Wilde B, Thewissen M, Damoiseaux J, et al. Regulatory B cells in ANCA-associated vasculitis. Annals of the Rheumatic Diseases. 2013;72(8):1416–9.
29. Von Scheven E, Lu TT, Emery HM, Elder ME, Wara DW. Thrombosis and pediatric Wegener's granulomatosis: Acquired and genetic risk factors for hypercoagulability. Arthr Rheum. 2003;49(6):862–5.
30. Tomasson G, Monach PA, Merkel PA. Thromboembolic disease in vasculitis. Curr Opin Rheumatol. 2009;21(1):41–6.
31. Singhal R, et al. Thromboembolic complications in the nephrotic syndrome: Pathophysiology and clinical management. Throm Res. 2006;118(3):397–407.
32. Karim F, Loeffen J, Bramer W, Westenberg L, Verdijk R, van Hagen M, et al. IgG4-related disease: a systematic review of this unrecognized disease in pediatrics. *Pediatric Rheumatology.* 2016;14:18.
33. Ryu JH, Horie R, Sekiguchi H, Peikert T, Yi ES. Spectrum of Disorders Associated with Elevated Serum IgG4 Levels Encountered in Clinical Practice. Int J Rheumatol. 2012;2012:232960. https://doi.org/10.1155/2012/232960.
34. Ebbo M, Grados A, Bernit E, et al. Pathologies Associated with Serum IgG4 Elevation. Int J Rheumatol. 2012;2012:602809. https://doi.org/10.1155/2012/602809.
35. Ata Y, Inaba Y, Choe H, Kobayashi N, Machida J, Nakamura N, et al. Bone metabolism and inflammatory characteristics in 14 cases of chronic nonbacterial osteomyelitis. Pediatr Rheumatol Online J. 2017;15(1):56.
36. Golla A, Jansson A, Ramser J, Hellebrand H, Zahn R, Meitinger T, et al. Chronic recurrent multifocal osteomyelitis (CRMO): evidence for a susceptibility gene located on chromosome 18q21.3-18q22. Eur J Hum Genet. 2002;10(3):217–21.
37. Hofmann SR, Kubasch AS, Range U, Laass MW, Morbach H, Girschick HJ, Hedrich CM. Serum biomarkers for the diagnosis and monitoring of chronic recurrent multifocal osteomyelitis (CRMO). Rheumatol Int. 2016;36(6):769–79.
38. Hofmann SR, Morbach H, Schwarz T, Rösen-Wolff A, Girschick HJ, Hedrich CM. Attenuated TLR4/MAPK signaling in monocytes from patients with CRMO resultsi n impaired IL-10 expression. Clin Immunol. 2012;145:69–76.
39. Mahler M, Silverman ED, Fritzler MJ. Novel diagnostic and clinical aspects of anti-PCNA antibodies detected by novel detection methods. Lupus. 2010; 19(13):1527–33.
40. Beckman KA, Luchs J, Milner MS. Making the diagnosis of Sjögren's syndrome in patients with dry eye. Clin Ophthalmol. 2015;2016(10):43–53.
41. Koenig M, Joyal F, Fritzler MJ, Roussin A, Abrahamowicz M, Boire G, Goulet J-R, Rich É, Grodzicky T, Raymond Y, Senécal J-L. Autoantibodies and microvascular damage are independent predictive factors for the progression of Raynaud's phenomenon to systemic sclerosis: A twenty-year prospective study of 586 patients, with validation of proposed criteria for early systemic sclerosi. Arthritis Rheum. 2008;58:3902–12.
42. Bjorksten B, Boquist L. Histopathological aspects of chronic recurrent multifocal osteomyelitis. J Bone Joint Surg. 1980;62(3):376–80.
43. Girschick HJ, Raab P, Surbaum S, Trusen A, Kirschner S, Schneider P, et al. Chronic non-bacterial osteomyelitis in children. Ann Rheum Dis. 2005;64(2): 279–85.
44. Pastore S, Ferrara G, Monasta L, Meini A, Cattalini M, Martino S, Alessio M, La Torre F, Teruzzi B, Gerloni V, Breda L, Taddio A, Lepore L. Chronic nonbacterial osteomyelitis may be associated with renal disease and bisphosphonates are a good option for the majority of patients. Acta Paediatr. 2016;105(7):328–33.
45. Roderick M, Shah R, Finn A, Ramanan AV. Efficacy of pamidronate therapy in children with chronic non-bacterial osteitis: disease activity assessment by whole body magnetic resonance imaging. Rheumatology (Oxford). 2014; 53(11):1973–6.
46. Eleftheriou D, Gerschman T, Sebire N, Woo P, Pilkington CA, Brogan PA. Biologic therapy in refractory chronic non-bacterial osteomyelitis of childhood. Rheumatology. 2010;49(8):1505–12.
47. Voit AM, Arnoldi AP, Douis H, Bleisteiner F, Jansson MK, Reiser MF, et al. Whole-body magnetic resonance imaging in chronic recurrent multifocal osteomyelitis: clinical longterm assessment may underestimate activity. J Rheumatol. 2015;42:1455–62.
48. Fritz J, Tzaribatchev N, Claussen CD, Carrino JA, Horger MS. Chronic recurrent multifocal osteomyelitis: comparison of whole-body MR imaging with radiography and correlation with clinical and laboratory data. Radiology. 2009;252(3):842–51.
49. Roderick M, Shah R, Finn A, Ramanan AV. Efficacy of pamidronate therapy in children with chronic non-bacterial osteitis: disease activity assessment by whole body magnetic resonance imagin. Rheumatology (Oxford). 2014;53: 1973–6.
50. Beck C, Morbach H, Beer M, Stenzel M, Tappe D, Gattenlöhner S, et al. Chronic nonbacterial osteomyelitis in childhood: prospective follow-up during the first year of anti-inflammatory treatment. Arthritis Res Ther. 2010; 12(2):R74.

24

Successful implementation of a clinical transition pathway for adolescents with juvenile-onset rheumatic and musculoskeletal diseases

Margot Walter[1*], Sylvia Kamphuis[2], Philomine van Pelt[1], Annemarie de Vroed[1] and Johanna M. W. Hazes[1]

Abstract

Background: In 2008 a clinical transition pathway for young people with juvenile-onset rheumatic and musculoskeletal diseases (jRMD) aiming at improving transitional care was instituted. Historical data on drop-out rate in our clinic was 35%, one year before the implementation of the transition pathway. This study aims to I) evaluate the effectiveness of the clinical transition pathway, II) evaluate the experiences and satisfaction of YP with the transitional process and evaluate their perceived self-management skills.

Methods: Young people with any jRMD transferred from the pediatric to the adult rheumatology department in our academic center were eligible to enroll in this quantitative cross-sectional observational study between 2009 and 2015. Notably in 2012, we created a dedicated adolescent JIA-clinic, located at the adult rheumatology department. Electronic patient records from all young people that were transferred between 2009 and 2015 were reviewed for drop-out of care. Young people were asked to rate a VAS for 'satisfaction with transition' and to complete the "on your own feet transfer experience scale" (OYOF-TES)-questionnaire regarding their experiences and satisfaction with transition. Self-management skills were measured with the "on your own feet self-efficacy scale" (OYOF-SES)-questionnaire.

Results: One hundred fifty-four young people were transferred to the adult department, of which 76 were transferred to the dedicated adolescent JIA-clinic. The mean age at transfer was 17.8 years for YP transferred to the adult clinic and 15.2 years for transfer to the adolescent clinic. Drop-out of care rate one year after transfer was 5.1% in the adult clinic and 1.3% in the adolescent JIA-clinic. Response rate of the returned questionnaires was 61% for the adolescent JIA clinic and 36% for the adult clinic. There was no difference between responders and non-responders in demographics and disease type besides age (non-responders were significantly younger). Young people transferred to the adult and adolescent JIA-clinic both had high scores on the satisfaction scale (7.7 and 7.5 on the VAS-scale and 72.0 and 74.5 on the OYOF-TES). Self-efficacy scores were high for both groups, with OYOF-SES 59.7 for those transferred to the adult clinic and 58.2 for those transferred to the adolescent JIA-clinic.

Conclusion: The implementation of the clinical transition pathway has led to a substantial improvement of patient care during the transitional process leading to low drop-out of care rate and high scores on satisfaction with transition. High scores on the self-reported self-efficacy scale suggests confidence of young people to have achieved sufficient skills to successfully manage their disease.

Keywords: Juvenile-onset rheumatic and musculoskeletal diseases, Young people, Transition, Clinical transition pathway, Outcome research

* Correspondence: m.walter@erasmusmc.nl
[1]Department of Rheumatology, Erasmus University Medical Centre, Postal box 2040, 3000, CA, Rotterdam, the Netherlands
Full list of author information is available at the end of the article

Background

It is generally accepted that young people (YP) with juvenile-onset rheumatic and musculoskeletal diseases (jRMD) need to be prepared well in advance, to achieve a successful transfer to adult rheumatology care [1–5]. Well-coordinated and effective management of the transitional process during adolescence is necessary to enable YP to acquire sufficient skills to independently manage their disease. Previously, we found that YP with jRMD who attended the pediatric rheumatology service before a dedicated transition program was established, were dissatisfied with the preparation for transfer to adult care [6]. The central points of YP in this study were that i) training self-management skills was neglected, ii) specific topics like education, vocation as well as the upcoming transfer to adult care were not discussed in clinic and iii) they didn't feel confident to attend the consultation without the support of their parents [6]. These findings are in line with results from other studies where ad hoc, unprepared transfer to adult care carried a high risk for lack of self-management skills and independence of YP, missed appointments and drop-out of care, non-compliance with medication and ultimately poor disease outcome [7–9].

Transition of care is a complex intervention, only few studies are available regarding the evaluation of the transitional process and there is a lack of clarity regarding which outcomes are relevant to determine the success of the transitional process. Drop-out of care rates are used as outcome measure for successful transition, being between 25 and 52% even after implementation of a transition program [10–13]. Other outcomes used are the satisfaction of YP with the transitional process and development of self-management skills [5, 14, 15]. Several studies also used physical, psychosocial and rheumatic specific health status as outcome measure for the success of implementing a transition program [11, 16–19]. However, there is no gold standard for successful transition [1, 5, 15, 18, 20]. Additionally, it is also unclear as to whose perception the success should be measured -success as perceived by the young person and/or parent and/or professional - and at which time point success of transition should be measured. These questions continue to be debated and are an area for further research.

Recently, EULAR/PReS endorsed recommendations for transitional care were published that include the definition of specific outcomes that can be used in future to measure successful transition to adult care [5]. Outcomes can be categorized in the area of health service outcomes (e.g attending medical appointments/drop-out, patients first visit no later than 3–6 months after transfer), individual outcomes (e.g self-management, adherence, quality of life, satisfaction with transition), social outcomes (having a social network) and alignment (assuring a good coordination and collaboration between pediatric and adult health care professionals) [1, 15].

The aims of the present study were I) to evaluate the effectiveness of a clinical transition pathway implemented in our institution since 2008 II) to evaluate the experiences and satisfaction of YP with jRMD with the transitional process III) to evaluate the perceived self-management skills of YP with jRMD.

Methods

Participants and study design

A quantitative cross-sectional observational study in a real life setting was conducted. All YP with any jRMD who were transferred from the pediatric to the adult rheumatology clinic between 2009 and 2015 in our academic hospital were eligible to enroll in this study. Notably, all patients preferred to continue care in our center after transfer, none transferred to another medical center due to 1) our active policy to advocate continuing care in the same center, 2) the expertise with adolescent care in our center and 3) the limited travel distances in our country. Patients with the subtype oligo-articular JIA with medication-free disease remission for ≥ one year before transfer, were not included as it is our policy to routinely discharge these patients from clinical care. All YP and their parents (if age < 18 years) gave written informed consent before inclusion.

Clinical transition pathway

The clinical transition pathway was described previously [6]. The most important points of this clinical transition pathway are an early start (12–14 years) with focus on development of self-management skills and independency using an individual transition plan (ITP) for each patient and his/her parents [6]. The ITP developed by McDonagh et al. (2006, 2015) was adjusted for this purpose [21, 22]. The ITP is an important tool for developing self-management skills and self-efficacy with attention for the entire transitional process (Additional file 1: Table S1).

During the study inclusion period (2009–2015), we created a dedicated adolescent JIA-clinic in 2012 at the adult rheumatology department. This was primarily developed for YP with JIA in the age of 12–23 years to optimally support the specific needs of adolescents and the transitional process (Additional file 2: Figure S1: clinical transition pathway, adjusted from [6]). In addition, patients with other (rare) diseases that were only seen by the rheumatologist were also transferred to the dedicated JIA-adolescent clinic. The adolescent JIA-clinic health care team consists of a mixture of paediatric and adult-care health professionals including (pediatric) rheumatologists, pediatric physiotherapists, specialized rheumatology nurses and nurse practitioners with certified training in pediatrics. The actual transfer to the adolescent JIA-clinic is between 12 and 14 years. The time of transfer is a joint decision by the patient and physician.

Clinical care for YP with systemic autoimmune diseases after 2012 continued to be delivered at the pediatric rheumatology department in the children's hospital, due to the necessity of involvement of other pediatric subspecialties (e.g.pediatric neurology, hematology, nephrology). Actual transfer to the adult clinic occurred around the age of 17–18 years, where timing of the transfer depends on the patient's achieved skills, personal wishes in discussion with health professionals (Additional file 3: Figure S2: clinical transition pathway as published previously [6]).

Data collection

To evaluate effectiveness, electronic patient records (n = 154) were reviewed on frequency of drop-out of care and the use of ITPs. YP were asked at study inclusion to complete a questionnaire that inventoried their experiences and satisfaction with the transitional process. They received the questionnaire once, a reminder by letter was sent after two weeks. The questionnaire included the following topics: demographic parameters, age, ethnicity, education, vocation, self-efficacy, self-management and satisfaction with transition.

Outcome measurements

Primary outcomes

The primary outcomes in this study were drop-out of care at one, two and three years after transfer and satisfaction with the transitional process. Drop-out was defined as YP who did not attend any follow up appointment at the dedicated adolescent JIA/adult clinic one year after the last appointment in the pediatric clinic.

Satisfaction with transition was measured by the "on your own feet transfer experience scale" (OYOF-TES) and a visual analogue scale assessing satisfaction with transition [10]. The OYOF-TES is a validated eighteen item patient reported outcome that measures experiences in transition, rated on five-point Likert scales (1 = strongly disagree to 5 = strongly agree) [10]. Seven items reflect the preparation for transition and eleven items reflect the alignment and collaboration between the pediatric and adult care [10]. A higher score on the OYOF-TES (score range 18–90) expresses higher experienced satisfaction of the YP with the transitional process, a specific cut-off point is not defined [10].

The VAS is a one-dimensional question asking: How satisfied were you with the overall process of transfer to the adolescent JIA/adult clinic on a Likert scale ranging from 1 to 10 (1 = completely unsatisfied to 10 = completely satisfied) [10].

Secondary outcomes

Secondary outcomes were independent visits of YP with the nurse and physicians defined as a visit without their parents being present for the whole visit, the number of ITP's present at transfer, self-management skills and the self-efficacy of the YP. To measure the efficacy of the implemented clinical transition pathway, the number of adolescents with an ITP were collected from the electronic patient records. Self-efficacy is measured with the on your own feet self-efficacy scale (OYOF-SES) [23]. This self-reported questionnaire consists of 17 items with a Likert scale from 1 to 4 (ranging from 1 = no, certainly not- 4 = yes, certainly). Four items reflect self-efficacy coping with the condition, six items reflect self-efficacy in disease-knowledge and six items reflect self-efficacy in skills for independent behavior. A higher score on the OYOF-SES (score range 10–64) expresses the perception of YP to have more self-reliance to manage the disease by themselves [23]. We asked YP an additional eight questions reflecting self-management skills. These questions were copied from a previous study [6] (Additional file 4: Table S2). Furthermore, we asked YP three additional questions regarding whether their disease had affected their educational achievements and whether the disease had affected their career choice.

Statistical analysis

We used descriptive statistics to describe the study sample by using STATA14. For continuous variables, the mean and standard deviation (SD) are shown, for categorical data percentages were presented. To compare the group of questionnaire responders and non-responders and the differences between YP transferred to the adolescents JIA clinic or adult clinic unpaired t-test or Wilcoxon's rank sum test, if data were not normally distributed, were used. Categorical variables were tested using Pear-son's chi-square test. P-value < 0.05 was considered statistically significant. Data from YP with JIA who were transferred to the dedicated adolescent JIA clinic and those transferred to the adult clinic, were separately analyzed.

Results

All electronic patient records of YP with jRMD who were transferred from the pediatric to the adult rheumatology department between 2009 and 2015 were reviewed (n = 154). In total 78 YP were transferred to the adult clinic and 76 to the dedicated adolescent JIA-clinic. Demographics and disease activity of all YP who were transferred are shown in Table 1. As expected the mean age at study inclusion of the YP transferred to the adult clinic was higher when compared with the YP

Table 1 Demographics of YP transferred from pediatric rheumatology to the adult rheumatology clinic and the adolescent JIA-clinic between 2009 and 2015

	YP transferred to the adult clinic (*n* = 78)	YP transferred to the adolescent JIA-clinic (*n* = 76)
Transfer period	2009–2015	2012–2015
Gender Female (%)	71%	56%
Mean age (SD) at time of study inclusion	22.2 (2.4)	18.6 (2.3)
Mean age (SD) at transfer	17.8 (1.5)	15.2 (2.1)
Diagnosis (*n* / %)		
• JIA – oligoarticular	• 21 / 27	• 26 / 37
• JIA – polyarticular	• 15 / 19	• 21 /30
• JIA – PSA	• 3 / 4	• 3 /4
• JIA – ERA	• 8 / 10	• 7 /10
• SLE	• 15 / 19	• 1 /2
• Other (e.g. GPA, FMF)	• 16 / 21	• 12 /17
Disease activity before transfer (median, IQR)		
• Number of tender joints	• 0 (0–0)	• 0 (0–0)
• Number of swollen joints	• 0 (0–0)	• 0 (0–0)
• ESR	• 8 (3–17)	• 8 (3–15)
Disease activity after transfer (median, IQR)		
• Number of tender joints	• 0.(0–0)	• 0 (0–1)
• Number of swollen joints	• 0.(0–0)	• 0 (0–1)
• ESR	• 9 (4–19)	• 8 (3–15)

Abbreviations: *JIA* Juvenile Idiopathic Arthritis, *PsA* Psoriatic Arthritis, *ERA* Enthesitis Related Arthritis, *SLE* Systemic Lupus Erythematosus, *GPA* Granulomatosis with Polyangiitis, *FMF* Familial Mediterranean Fever

transferred to the dedicated adolescent JIA-clinic. The majority of all study patients had oligo-articular or poly-articular JIA.

Results electronic patient records

The overall frequency of 'drop-out of care' one year after transfer to the adult clinic was low, with only 5.1% of YP that did not attend any clinical appointment within the first year after transfer. The drop-out of care frequency remained stable in the next two years after transfer to the adult rheumatology team (Table 2).

This percentage of drop-out of care was 1.3% for YP who were transferred to the dedicated adolescent-JIA clinic one year after transfer. The drop-out of care frequency of YP transferred to the adolescent JIA-clinic decreased to zero after three years (Table 2).

Almost all YP (94%) were transferred to the dedicated adolescent JIA-clinic with an ITP. This was in contrast to 55% ITPs in the group of YP who had been transferred to the adult clinic. This reflects the 'real life study' setting of this study, the frequency of not only discussing the ITP but also filing the results in the ITP became more and more incorporated in clinical care during the inclusion period of the study. This is reflected by the higher number of ITPs in the adolescent JIA clinic, as this study group primarily includes patients in a later time period of inclusion (2012–2015).

Table 2 Drop-out rate of YP and the presence ITP after transfer to adult rheumatology clinic and adolescent JIA clinic

	YP transferred to the adult clinic *N* = 78	YP transferred to the adolescent JIA clinic *N* = 76	*p*-value
Drop-out rate after 1 year (% / *N*)	5.1% (4 of 78)	1.3% (1 of 76)	0.18
Drop-out rate after 2 years (% / *N*)	6.7% (5 of 74) #	2.7% (2 of 75)	0.51
Drop-out rate after 3 years (% / *N*)	5.7% (4 of 69) #	0% (0 of 73)	0.10
Total drop-out rate (1–3 years after transfer)	16.6% (13 of 78)	3.9% (3 of 76)	
Presence of ITP at transfer (%)	55%	94%	< 0.01*

Abbreviations: *YP* Young People, *JIA* Juvenile Idiopathic Arthritis *: *P*-value < 0.05 was considered statically significant #: drop-out rate for *year 2 and year 3: the number of remaining patients in care were taken as the total number of patients in that year of follow up*

Results questionnaires

In total 46/76 YP transferred to the adolescent JIA-clinic and 28/78 YP transferred to the adult clinic returned questionnaires, leading to a response rate of respectively 61 and 36%. There were no differences between questionnaire-responders and non-responders regarding demographics or disease-type besides age (non-responders were younger 19.7 versus 21.4 years, $p = < 0.001$). Not surprisingly, the drop-out of care in the non-responders was higher (total number of drop-outs in non-responders $n = 5/80$ and in responders $n = 0/74$, $p = 0.02$). The mean age of the responders at the time of study inclusion was 18.4 years (SD 2.8) for the dedicated adolescent JIA-clinic and 21.46 years (SD 2.5) for the YP transferred to the adult clinic.

The satisfaction with the transitional process for both scales (OYOF-TES and VAS transition) of YP who either transferred to the adult clinic or to the dedicated adolescent JIA-clinic was high (Table 3). The questions regarding the alignment and collaboration between pediatric and adult health care resulted in high scores for both groups [10]; about 80% thought their new care provider was well informed about the condition of the YP and their treatment. Furthermore, 78.6% of the YP transferred to the adult clinic and 80% transferred to the adolescent JIA-clinic were convinced that there was a good collaboration between pediatric and adult care.

Self-management, measured with the OYOF-SES, was high in both groups (Table 3). More positive responses to the eight self-reported questions measuring self-management skills (e.g. independently visiting the nurse or physicians, ordering medication and making appointments independently) were seen in the group transferred to the adult clinic (Table 3). Furthermore, almost all YP in both transfer groups agreed that all important topics were discussed during the consultations. The transfer was discussed on time according to the YP in more than three quarters for both groups.

The answers to the three questions regarding education and vocation showed that the majority of all YP

Table 3 Questionnaire results of YP transferred to the adult or adolescent JIA-clinic

Questionnaires	Responders transferred to the adult clinic $N = 28$	Responders transferred to the adolescent JIA clinic $N = 46$	*p*-value
VAS satisfaction with transition ± (mean, SD)	7.7 (0.8)	7.5 (1.9)	0.79
OYOF-TES ± ± (mean, SD)	72.0 (14.7)	74.5 (12.1)	0.44
Treatment recommendations in the adult care setting are similar to those I used to receive in pediatric care (agreed,%)	85.7	79.5	0.51
There was good collaboration between pediatric and adult care (agreed,%)	78.6	80	0.88
OYOF-SES ± ± ± (mean, SD)	59.7 (2.9)	58.2 (5.0)	0.42
Independent visits physician (yes)	69%	47%	0.06
Independent visits nurse (yes)	75%	44%	0.01*
Important topics discussed (yes)	97%	96%	0.83
I order my medication at the pharmacy by myself (yes)	83%	52%	0.008*
Thinking about taking medication by myself (yes)	90%	80%	0.27
Forgetting medication (yes)	52%	80%	0.01*
Making appointments independently (yes)	86%	42%	< 0.01*
Transfer discussed on time (yes)	75%	79%	0.78
Education negatively influenced by the disease?			0.76
• No	• 30%	• 29%	
• Repeating a class	• 23%	• 19%	
• Lower level	• 12%	• 12%	
• More absenteeism	• 19%	• 29%	
• Other	• 15%	• 12%	
Taking the disease into account at choice for vocation (yes)	59%	42%	0.13
Restriction in career options by the disease (yes)	48%	25%	0.96

*: *p*-value * < 0.05 was considered statically significant
±: VAS satisfaction with transition: score range 1–10, higher score reflects higher satisfaction
±±: score-range of OYOF-TES 18–90, higher score reflects higher satisfaction of YP with transition
± ± ±: score-range of OYOF-SES 10–64, higher score reflects higher self-efficacy of YP
Abbreviations: *YP* Young People, *JIA* Juvenile Idiopathic Arthritis, *VAS* visual analogue scale, *OYOF-TES* on your own feet transfer experience scale, *OYOF-SES* on your own feet self-efficacy scale

thought that their education was negatively influenced by the disease (Table 3). This was seen in YP transferred to the adult clinic as well as in YP transferred to the adolescent JIA-clinic. In addition, around half of all YP had taken the disease into account when choosing their vocation. Almost half of the YP transferred to the adult clinic and a quarter of YP transferred to the adolescent clinic stated that they were restricted in career options by their disease.

Discussion

The implementation of the clinical transition pathway for YP with jRMD was successful: a low drop-out of care rate was seen and YP were satisfied with the transitional process in both groups. High levels on the self-efficacy scale were reported, suggesting confidence of all YP in this study to have achieved sufficient self-management skills and underlining the efficacy of the clinical transition pathway.

As a primary outcome of a successful transitional process, we evaluated the effectiveness of the clinical transition pathway by using the drop-out of care rate. Despite implementing transition programs, preventing drop-out of care is challenging. Previous studies showed drop-out frequencies between 25 and 52% after implementation of a transition program [10–13, 22]. In historical data from the electronic patient records in our hospital, we saw a drop-out rate of 35% after transfer to the adult clinic in 2007, one year before the implementation of our clinical transition pathway (unpublished data). At that time, there was no transition policy and preparation for transfer to adult care was not structurally given. Although these drop-out rates cannot be compared one-to-one, it gives an impression of the drop-out rates before implementation of the clinical transition pathway. The EULAR/PReS guidelines defined drop-out of care as a quality indicator to measure good transition [5]. We showed low frequencies of drop-out of care (5.1 and 1.3%) in the first year after transfer to the adult and adolescent JIA-clinic. This indicates that the implemented clinical transition pathway can improve attendance and adherence to follow up clinic visits and prevent drop-out of care. This low percentage might also be influenced by our active policy to continue care in the same academic hospital, the expertise with adolescent care and the limited travel distances in our country. Notably, the low drop-out of care rate of YP transferred to the adolescent JIA-clinic seems logical, as the mean age at transfer was lower (15.2 years) and we assume that parents are still making the clinic appointments and are more involved in the care process. However, three years later (mean age 18.0) years, the drop-out of care rate was even lower and decreased to zero. Additionally, when considering YP that transferred to the adolescent JIA-clinic at the age of 16 years and up to 21 years, we still found a low drop-out of care rate of 6%. Literature showed that the implementation of a dedicated adolescent clinic has shown to improve clinical outcome [23]. Our data of the adolescent JIA-clinic underline this conclusion.

Another quality indicator according to the EULAR/PReS recommendations on the individual outcome of the transitional process, is satisfaction of the YP with the transitional process [5]. In our study the overall satisfaction with the transitional process was high for both groups in our study. Another study with YP with jRMD resulted in almost similar scores of the VAS satisfaction after instituting a transition program [11]. Van Staa et al. investigated satisfaction with transition programs of YP with a broad range of chronic somatic conditions and showed lower percentages on both scales (respectively 61.8 and 6.6) [10].

Good alignment and collaboration between the pediatric and adult departments was seen as an important factor for higher satisfaction of YP with the transitional process [10]. The presence of good coordination between pediatric and adult health care professionals is also recommended as an outcome for successful transition [5, 15]. According to the EULAR/PReS recommendations this can be realized by direct communication before and after transfer by combining consultations [5]. We embedded this in the clinical transition pathway. Moreover, we evaluated the alignment between the pediatric and adult clinic from the perspective of the YP with the OYOF-TES. Almost all YP in both groups were convinced there was a good collaboration between both departments.

Self-management is an important individual outcome for successful transition. The high score on the self-reported self-efficacy scale assumes more responsibility in the self-management skills of the YP for both groups. Another important measured question regarding self-management skills, is independent visits, meaning visits of YP with care professionals without their parents [7, 14, 15, 24]. According to a study of Hilderson, many YP are not given the opportunity for independent visits with the physician [25]. Previous studies showed percentages between 46 and 59% of independent visits for YP between 15 and 23 years [26–28]. In our study, almost half of the YP transferred to the adolescent JIA-clinic had independent visits. More independent visits were reported in the group YP transferred to the adult clinic, which seemed logical because of the older age compared to those transferred to the adolescent JIA clinic. This was also observed in a study with YP with JIA, where frequency of independent visits increased with older age [17]. Notably, our historical data obtained before a clinical transition pathway was implemented, showed that 88% of YP between 14 and 20 years did not visit the physicians independently [6]. This suggests improved autonomy during clinic visits of the YP and may be contributed to the implementation of an ITP in the clinical transition pathway. Many items in the ITP are designed to help YP develop self-management skills and goals are set during the consultations. Indeed, the use of an ITP in the transitional process is strongly recommended by the EULAR/PReS recommendations for transitional care [5, 29, 30].

An important finding was that many YP perceived limitations in their education and vocation because of the disease. This was also found in other studies, where the time needed to finish studies tended to be longer and absenteeism was higher [31, 32]. These limitations might influence their future career as higher rates of unemployment were found in JIA patients [32–37]. These findings support the importance of vocational guidance and discussing vocation by health professionals [38] and should be a prominent subject in any transition plan.

This study has limitations. Paper-questionnaires were used with a mean response rate of 50%. Using electronic questionnaires might have led to higher response rates and therefore could have had an influence on the results. In addition, the number of YP discontent with the transitional process might be higher in the non-responders, leading to bias in the questionnaire results. Indeed, although the drop-out rate in the non-responder group was still relatively low, it was higher than the group that returned the questionnaires. The mean age of YP transferred to the dedicated adolescent JIA clinic was 15 years. These YP are still in the midst of the transition process and this has influenced the results of the study. Additionally, the success of this study is attributed in part to the fact that none of the patients transferred to another institution besides the Erasmus University MC. This is an exceptional situation and probably influences the external validity of this study. However, the transition process should start at an early age (12–14 years) and prepare young people to be ready for the actual transfer to adult rheumatology at age 17–18 and prevent drop-out even if transferred to another hospital. The transition pathway can be used to instruct the adult rheumatologist elsewhere regarding the follow up of care for this vulnerable patient group. The transition coordinator may play a role in this process as well and support the adult rheumatologist elsewhere.

Conclusion

The implementation of the clinical transition pathway for YP with jRMD has led to a substantial improvement of patient care during the transitional process leading to low drop-out rate, improved self-reported autonomy during the clinic visit, improved perceived self-management skills and high satisfaction of YP with the transitional process, which are all outcomes recently proposed in the EULAR/PreS recommendations for transitional care. This underlines the efficacy of the developed clinical transition pathway.

Abbreviations

ITP: Individual transition plan; jRMD: juvenile-onset rheumatic and musculoskeletal diseases; OYOF-SES: On your own feet self-efficacy scale; OYOF-TES: On your own feet transfer experience scale; VAS: Visual analogue scale; YP: Young people

Funding

Not obtained for this study.

Declarations

Not applicable.

Authors' contributions

Survey conception and design: MW, SK, MH. Acquisition of data: MW, AdV. Analysis and interpretation of data: MW, SK. All authors were involved in drafting the article and approved the final version of the manuscript to be published.

Consent for publication

Not applicable.

Competing interests

The authors declare that they have no competing interests.

Author details

[1]Department of Rheumatology, Erasmus University Medical Centre, Postal box 2040, 3000, CA, Rotterdam, the Netherlands. [2]Department of Pediatric Rheumatology, Sophia Children's Hospital – Erasmus University Medical Centre, Rotterdam, the Netherlands.

References

1. Fair C, Cuttance J, Sharma N, Maslow G, Wiener L, Betz C, et al. International and interdisciplinary identification of health care transition outcomes. JAMA Pediatr. 2016;170(3):205–11.
2. Sawyer S, Drew S, Yeo MS, Britto MT. Adolescents with a chronic condition: challenges living, challenges treating. Lancet. 2007;369(9571):1481–9.
3. Eleftheriou D, Isenberg D, Wedderburn L, Ioannou Y. The coming of age of adolescent rheumatology. Nat Rev Rheumatol. 2014;10(3):187–93.
4. Tattersall R, McDonagh J. Transition: a rheumatology perspective. Br J Hosp Med (Lond). 2010;71(6):315–9.
5. Foster H, Minden K, Clemente D, Leon L, McDonagh J, Kamphuis S, Berggren K, van Pelt P et al. EULAR/PReS standards and recommendations for the transitional care of young people with juvenile-onset rheumatic diseases. Ann Rheum Dis. 2017;76:639-46.
6. Walter M, Hazes J, Dolhain R, van Pelt P, Dijk A, Kamphuis S. Development of a clinical transition pathway for adolescents in the Netherlands. Nurs Child Young People. 2017;29(9):37–43.

7. Shaw K, Southwood T, McDonagh J, British Paediatric Rheumatology Group. User perspectives of transitional care for adolescents with juvenile idiopathic arthritis. Rheumatology (Oxford). 2004;43(6):770–8.
8. Fegran L, Hall E, Uhrenfeldt L, Aagaard H, Ludvigsen M. Adolescents' and young adults' transition experiences when transferring from paediatric to adult care: a qualitative metasynthesis. Int J Nurs Stud. 2014;51(1):123–35.
9. Lugasi T, Achille M, Stevenson M. Patients' perspective on factors that facilitate transition from child-centered to adult-centered health care: a theory integrated metasummary of quantitative and qualitative studies. J Adolesc Health. 2011;48(5):429–40.
10. van Staa A, Sattoe JN. Young adults' experiences and satisfaction with the transfer of care. J Adolesc Health. 2014;55(6):796–803.
11. Stringer E, Scott R, Mosher D, MacNeill I, Huber AM, Ramsey S, Lang B. Evaluation of a rheumatology transition clinic. Pediatr Rheumatol Online J. 2015;13:22.
12. Jensen PT, Karnes J, Jones K, Lehman A, Rennebohm R, Higgins J, et al. Quantitative evaluation of a pediatric rheumatology transition program. Pediatr Rheumatol Online J. 2015;13:17.
13. Hazel E, Zhang X, Duffy CM, Campillo S. High rates of unsuccessful transfer to adult care among young adults with juvenile idiopathic arthritis. Pediatr Rheumatol Online J. 2010;8:2.
14. Reid G, Irvine MJ, McCrindle BW, Sananes R, Ritvo PG, Siu SC, Webb GD. Prevalence and correlates of successful transfer from pediatric to adult health care among a cohort of young adults with complex congenital heart defects. Pediatrics. 2004;113(3 Pt 1):e197–205.
15. Suris JC, Akre Key C. Elements for, and indicators of, a successful transition: an international Delphi study. J Adolesc Health. 2015;56(6):612–8.
16. Shaw K, Watanabe A, Rankin E, McDonagh JE. Walking the talk. Implementation of transitional care guidance in a UK paediatric and a neighbouring adult facility. Child Care Health Dev. 2014;40(5):663–70.
17. McDonagh J, Southwood T, Shaw K. British Paediatric rheumatology group the impact of a coordinated transitional care programme on adolescents with juvenile idiopathic arthritis. Rheumatology (Oxford). 2007;46(1):161–8.
18. Castrejon I. Transitional care programs for patients with rheumatic diseases: review of the literature. Reumatol Clin. 2012;8(1):20–6.
19. Hilderson D, Moons P, Van der Elst K, Luyckx K, Wouters C, Westhovens RD, et al. The clinical impact of a brief transition programme for young people with juvenile idiopathic arthritis: results of the DON'T RETARD project. Rheumatology (Oxford). 2016;55(1):133–42.
20. Hersh A. Growing up and moving on--transition of care for patients with childhood-onset rheumatic disease. J Rheumatol. 2014;41(5):829–31.
21. McDonagh JE, Shaw KL, Southwood TR. Growing up and moving on in rheumatology: development and preliminary evaluation of a transitional care programme for a multicentre cohort of adolescents with juvenile idiopathic arthritis. J Child Health Care. 2006;10(1):22–42.
22. McDonagh JE, Hackett J, McGee M et al (2015) The evidence base for transition is bigger than you might think. Archives of disease in childhood. Education and practice edition. 100, 6, 321–322.
23. van Staa A, van der Stege HA, Jedeloo S, Moll HA, Hilberink SR. Readiness to transfer to adult care of adolescents with chronic conditions: exploration of associated factors. J Adolesc Health, 2011. 48(3): p. 295c302.
24. Jordan A, McDonagh JE. Transition: getting it right for young people. Clin Med (Lond). 2006;6(5):497–500.
25. Hilderson D, Moons P, Westhovens R, Wouters C. Attitudes of rheumatology practitioners toward transition and transfer from pediatric to adult healthcare. Rheumatol Int. 2012;32(12):3887–96.
26. Shaw KL, Southwood TR, JE MD. British Society of Paediatric and Adolescent Growing up and moving on in rheumatology: a multicentre cohort of adolescents with juvenile idiopathic arthritis. Rheumatology (Oxford). 2005; 44(6):806–12.
27. Suris J, Akre C, Rutishauser C. How adult specialists deal with the principles of a successful transition. J Adolesc Health. 2009;45(6):551–5.
28. Jensen P, Paul G, LaCount S, Peng J, Spencer C, Higgins G, Boyle B, et al. Assessment of transition readiness in adolescents and young adults with chronic health conditions. Pediatric Rheumatology. 2017;15:70.
29. Shaw K, Southwood T, McDonagh J, British Paediatric rheumatology group L, et al. Developing a programme of transitional care for adolescents with juvenile idiopathic arthritis: results of a postal survey. Rheumatology (Oxford). 2004;43(2):211–9.
30. McDonagh JE, et al. Unmet education and training needs of rheumatology health professionals in adolescent health and transitional care. Rheumatology (Oxford). 2004;43(6):737–43.
31. Minden K, Niewerth M, Listing J, Biedermann T, Bollow M, Schöntube M. Zink a long-term outcome in patients with juvenile idiopathic arthritis. Arthritis Rheum. 2002;46(9):2392–401.
32. Diaz-Mendoza A, Modesto Caballero C, Navarro-Cendejas J. Analysis of employment rate and social status in young adults with childhood-onset rheumatic disease in Catalonia. Pediatr Rheumatol Online J. 2015;13:29.
33. Minden K. Adult outcomes of patients with juvenile idiopathic arthritis. Horm Res. 2009;72(Suppl 1):20–5.
34. Jetha A, Badley E, Beaton D, Fortin PR, Shiff NJ, Gignac. Unpacking early work experiences of young adults with rheumatic disease: an examination of absenteeism, job disruptions, and productivity loss. MA Arthritis Care Res (Hoboken). 2015 Sep;67(9):1246–54. https://doi.org/10.1002/acr.22601.
35. Jetha A. The impact of arthritis on the early employment experiences of young adults: A literature review. Disabil Health J. 2015 ;8(3):317–24. doi: https://doi.org/10.1016/j.dhjo.2014.12.001. Epub 2014 Dec 20. Review.PMID: 25600476
36. Schlichtiger J, Haas J, Barth S, Bisdorff B, Hager L, Michels H, Hügle B, Radon K. Education and employment in patients with juvenile idiopathic arthritis – a standardized comparison to the German general population. Pediatric Rheumatology. 2017;15:45.
37. Bingham C, Scalzi L, Groh B, Boehmer S, Banks S. An assessment of variables affecting transition readiness in pediatric rheumatology patients. Pediatric Rheumatology. 2015;13:42.
38. Hanson H, Hart RI, Thompson B, McDonagh JE, Tattersall R, Jordan A, Foster HE. Experiences of employment among young people with juvenile idiopathic arthritis: a qualitative study. Disabil Rehabil. 2018;40(16):1921–8. PMID: 2850395

25

Clinical phenotypes and biologic treatment use in juvenile dermatomyositis-associated calcinosis

Amir B. Orandi[1,2*], Vikas R. Dharnidharka[3], Noor Al-Hammadi[4], Kevin W. Baszis[2] and for the CARRA Legacy Registry Investigators

Abstract

Background: Few risk factors have been identified for the development of calcinosis among patients with Juvenile Dermatomyositis, and currently no clinical phenotype has been associated with its development. We analyzed a large database of patients to further elucidate any relationships among patients with and without calcinosis.

Method: The CARRA legacy registry recruited pediatric rheumatology patients from 55 centers across North America from 2010 through 2014, including over 650 subjects with Juvenile Dermatomyositis. We compared the demographic characteristics, clinical disease features and treatment histories of those with and without calcinosis using univariate and multivariate logistic regression.

Results: Of the 631 patients included in the analysis, 84 (13%) had a current or prior history of calcinosis. These patients were statistically more likely to have longer durations of disease prior to diagnosis and treatment, have lipodystrophy and joint contractures, and to have received intravenous immune globulin or rituximab as treatments.

Conclusions: Calcinosis is found more often in patients with prolonged active disease, severe disease, and certain clinical features such as lipodystrophy and joint contractures. When these factors are combined with other known associations and predictors, groups of at-risk patients can be more effectively identified, treated and studied to improve overall outcomes.

Keywords: Juvenile dermatomyositis, Calcinosis, Biologics, Pediatric rheumatology

Introduction

As the most common inflammatory myopathy of childhood, Juvenile Dermatomyositis (JDM) affects 3.2 per million children annually in the United States [1]. Before the widespread use of glucocorticoids, followed by disease-modifying anti-rheumatic drugs (DMARDs), JDM was fatal in one-third of cases [2–4]. More recent studies have shown mortality as low as 3.1% [5] while simultaneously highlighting persistent morbidity from active disease or its sequelae [6–8]. An enigmatic source of morbidity comes from calcinosis, the dystrophic deposition of the mineral calcium hydroxyapatite in the skin, soft tissues or muscle, which is reported to occur in approximately 40% of patients [9]. When surveyed in 2016 regarding their experience and approach to assessing and treating JDM calcinosis, less than 20% of pediatric rheumatologists have treated more than 10 cases. In addition, the majority who have such experience have practiced for more than 20 years. [10].

There have been many studies attempting to identify risk factors or associations of calcinosis in JDM patients in order to further define the at-risk patient population. Actionable risk factors previously identified include a delay to treatment and/or prolonged disease duration [5, 11, 12] and initial treatment intensity [13, 14]; prognostic factors included race [15–17], male sex [15], underlying cardiac disease [18, 19], presence of joint contractures [18], and presence of certain myositis-specific antibodies [20, 21]; genetic risks were also identified [22, 23]. However, in some large cohorts, no risk factors are identified [24].

* Correspondence: Orandi.Amir@mayo.edu
[1]Division of Pediatric Rheumatology, Department of Pediatric and Adolescent Medicine, Mayo Clinic, 200 First Street SW, Rochester, MN 55902, USA
[2]Division of Pediatric Rheumatology, Department of Pediatrics, St. Louis, MO, USA
Full list of author information is available at the end of the article

Due to the rarity of JDM as a whole, and with calcinosis occurring in less than half of patients, there have been few studies of large numbers of patients with calcinosis. Lacking among all of these studies is a clinical phenotype of patient disease features that might also be associated with the development of calcinosis, apart from prolonged or severe disease, which has many connotations depending on the publication. Further, regarding treatment, much attention has been paid to the amount and duration of glucocorticoid use [25–27], but there has been no assessment made of whether the use of biologic treatments, now widely used, are associated with calcinosis. Our aim was to address these questions by analyzing a large patient registry of JDM patients with assessments of clinical features and treatment histories, including those who developed calcinosis during the course of follow-up.

Methods

The Childhood Arthritis and Rheumatology Research Alliance (CARRA) developed a multicenter registry for pediatric rheumatologic diseases across North America. Patients were enrolled from May 30, 2010 through October 31, 2014 from 55 CARRA centers. JDM was among the diseases included in the registry, and any patients whose disease began before 18 years of age and were less than 21 years of age at the time of enrollment were eligible for inclusion. All JDM patients must have met the Bohan and Peter criteria for diagnosis, modified to allow magnetic resonance imaging as an acceptable diagnostic modality [28].

Data collection

All data were submitted by the enrolling physician at each site after collecting clinical data using report forms for general information, demographics, functional and quality-of-life measures and JDM-specific information at baseline and follow-up visits. At baseline (the time of registry enrollment), the presence of several disease manifestations was assessed (present, absent or not assessed), including proximal muscle weakness (designated mild, moderate or severe), characteristic disease rashes, lipodystrophy, skin ulceration, periungal telangiectasias and contractures (not specified as due to muscle or joint disease). There was also documentation of presence or absence of other disease features (current, past or never), including calcinosis, small or large joint arthritis, dysphagia or dysphonia and organ involvement (cardiac, gastrointestinal or lung). At follow-up visits, these same clinical features were documented if present or absent. At enrollment, the patient's history of biologic medication use was assessed by current or prior use, and at follow-up visits, it was assessed if any biologic medication had been used in the visit interval. Patient data were kept in a centralized database by CARRA and after study approval were transmitted as a coded, deidentified dataset under code access agreement to the study team. This study was exempt from the Washington University School of Medicine institutional review board by not constituting human subject research.

Statistical analyses

All analyses were performed using SAS version 9.4 (SAS Institute Inc) and R version 3.3.1 (R Project for Statistical Computing). Any patients lacking requisite data in calcinosis were excluded. A cross-sectional analysis of baseline data in all JDM patients was performed comparing those with any history (current or past) of calcinosis to those without (never) in respect to demographic characteristics, clinical and disease features, and treatment with biologic agents and glucocorticoids. To calculate the duration of symptoms prior to treatment, the difference between symptom onset date and first rheumatology visit date was used, measured in months. Due to small respective numbers of each form of organ involvement (i.e. cardiac arrhythmia), a composite measure combining all different forms of organ toxicity (i.e. cardiac, pulmonary and gastrointestinal) was also used. For similar reasons, different tumor necrosis factor (TNF)-alpha inhibitors and interleukin-1 inhibitors were grouped as single entities for the purpose of analysis. Information on glucocorticoid treatment was collected in the registry by documenting only current or prior receipt of intravenous pulse steroids and/or systemic daily long-term use of specified durations. No dosages or intervals were recorded. In order to study possible effect of high or low glucocorticoid exposure, selected patients were grouped for the purpose of analysis. A patient with high steroid exposure was defined as one with a current or prior history of intravenous pulse steroids *and* current or prior use of daily systemic corticosteroids of at least one-month duration. Differences between patients with and without calcinosis were analyzed with t-test or Mann-Whitney-U tests for continuous variables as appropriate, while comparisons for categorical variables used Chi-square or Fisher's exact tests as appropriate. Statistically significant measures at the alpha level of 0.05 on univariate analyses were included in multivariate logistic regression modeling. Stepwise selection method during multivariate logistic regression modeling was used to adjust for collinearity of certain clinical features, where a variable had to be significant at the 0.25 level to be entered into the model and significant at 0.15 to stay. At the following step, the final model included variables significant at 0.05. A Forest Plot using R program was performed to illustrate the odds ratio and associated 95% confidence interval that were significant in the logistic regression model.

Results

A total of 654 patients with JDM were enrolled in the CARRA legacy registry. Twenty-three patients were excluded who lacked information on calcinosis, including five patients with follow-up data but no information at baseline. The remaining 631 were included in analysis, with 84 patients (13.3%) having a current or prior history of calcinosis at the time of enrollment. The registry cohort included 454 females (72%) and 177 males (28%) with a median age at diagnosis of 5.6 years. Caucasian race comprised 82% of patients, while Hispanic ethnicity represented 15% of patients, and African-American, 13%. The majority of patients were categorized as 'probable' JDM, which was used to define 490 patients (78%), while 48 (7.6%) were categorized as definite. Only nine patients (1.4%) were designated as amyopathic, and the remaining 13% had no selected category. Across the entire cohort, 38% had current or prior treatment with a biologic medication (Table 1).

Table 1 Cohort characteristics, $n = 631$

Characteristics		
Age (years) at diagnosis (median, IQR)	Median	IQR
	5.6	3.6–9.3
	N	%
Gender		
Male	177	28.1
Female	454	71.9
Ethnicity		
Hispanic	95	15.1
Race		
Caucasian	519	82.3
African-American	82	13
JDM Category		
Amyopathic	9	1.4
Probable	490	77.7
Definite	48	7.6
Missing	84	13.3
History of Calcinosis	84	13.3
History of biologic use	242	38.4
IVIG	225	35.7
Rituximab	26	4.1
Anti-TNF[a]	*35*	*5.6*
Certolizumab	0	0
Etanercept	22	3.5
Golimumab	1	0.2
Adalimumab	7	1.1
Infliximab	13	2
Abatacept	3	0.48
Anti-IL1[b]	2	0.32
High glucocorticoid exposure[c] ($n = 572$)	316	50

[a]Composite which includes etanercept, infliximab, adalimumab, certolizumab, golimumab
[b]Composite which includes anakinra, canakinumab, rilonacept
[c]Composite defined as history of IV pulse steroids and daily corticosteroids for ≥ 1 month

Clinical disease features

When comparing those with a history of calcinosis to those without, there were statistically significant differences in the proportions of the two groups for several demographic and clinical features (Table 2). There was no difference between groups in regards to cardiac, lung or gastrointestinal involvement, but when these events were combined as a single composite feature, "any organ involvement", the differences were statistically significant. In univariate analysis, statistical significance was maintained for characteristics of male sex (OR 1.811, 95% CI 1.123–2.919), time to diagnosis (OR 1.029, 95% CI 1.016–1.043) and African-American race (OR 2.264, 95% CI 1.270–4.038). For other clinical disease features, lipodystrophy (OR 5.993, 95% CI 2.588–13.874), joint contractures (OR 5.343, 95% CI 2.964–9.635), cutaneous ulcerations (OR 3.748, 95% CI 1.787–7.862), Gottron's or heliotrope rashes (OR 1.754, 95% CI 1.099–2.800), V or shawl sign (OR 2.410, 95% CI 1.083–5.361) and organ involvement (OR 2.506, 95% CI 1.127–5.573) also maintained significance (Table 2) and were included in multivariate analysis.

Treatment with biologics

In the overall cohort, 242 (38.4%) patients experienced current or prior use with a biologic agent. Intravenous immune globulin (IVIG) was the most common with 225 (35.6%) patients exposed followed by anti-TNF-alpha therapy with 35 (5.5%) patients. Etanercept comprised the majority of anti-TNF-alpha therapy with 22 patients reporting use, representing 63% of all anti-TNF-alpha therapy. Rituximab was used in 26 (4.1%) patients. When comparing patients with a history of calcinosis to those without, statistical significance between groups was maintained on univariate analysis for all treatments, except anti-IL1 agents as follows: Rituximab (OR 6.345, 95% CI 2.825–14.245), IVIG (OR 2.353 95% CI 1.479–3.743), anti-TNF-alpha (OR 3.797, 95% CI 1.812–7.960) and abatacept (OR 13.317, 95% CI 1.194–148.514). All were included in multivariable analysis except abatacept, since it was only used in three patients overall, and despite positive odds ratio had an extremely wide confidence interval (Table 3).

In the multivariable analysis including clinical features and treatments, the only predictors of association with calcinosis were increased time to diagnosis (OR 1.029, 95% CI 1.013–1.045), lipodystrophy (OR 3.038, 95% CI 1.014–9.106), joint

Table 2 Clinical characteristics by history of calcinosis

Risk factor	Descriptive analysis			Univariable analysis	
	Calcinosis			OR [95% CI]	*p*-value
	Yes	No			
Gender	n (%)		0.0138		
Male	33 (39.3)	144 (26.3)		1.811 [1.123–2.919]	0.0148
Female	51 (60.7)	403 (73.7)			
Age (years)	median (IQR)				
At symptom onset	6 (4.2–9)	5.5 (3.6–9.3)			
At diagnosis	8 (5.4–10.6)	6.3 (4.2–9.8)	0.0424		
Time to diagnosis (months)	8.8 (2–23.6)	3.8 (1.9–8.9)	0.0011	1.029 [1.016–1.043]	< 0.0001
Ethnicity	n (%)				
Hispanic	12 (14.3)	83 (15.2)			
Race			0.0047		
Caucasian	61 (72.6)	458 (83.7)			
African-American	19 (22.6)	63 (11.5)		2.264 [1.270–4.038]	0.0056
Missing	4 (4.8)	26 (4.8)			
JDM Category	n (%)				
Amyopathic	2 (2.4)	7 (1.3)			
Probable	61 (72.6)	429 (78.4)			
Definite	8 (9.5)	40 (7.3)			
Missing	13 (15.5)	71 (13)			
Clinical features	n (%)				
Lipodystrophy	11 (13.1)	13 (2.4)	< 0.0001	5.993 [2.588–13.874]	< 0.0001
Joint contractures	23 (27.4)	35 (6.4)	< 0.0001	5.343 [2.964–9.635]	< 0.0001
Cutaneous ulceration	12 (13.5)	23 (4.2)	0.001	3.748 [1.787–7.862]	0.0005
Gottron's or Heliotrope	50 (59.5)	244 (44.6)	0.0176	1.754 [1.099–2.800]	0.0186
Dysphagia or dysphonia	26 (31)	107 (19.6)	0.0178		
Small joint arthritis	25 (29.8)	115 (21.0)	0.041		
Malar or facial erythema	31 (36.9)	182 (33.3)			
V or Shawl sign	9 (10.7)	25 (4.6)	0.0377	2.410 [1.083–5.361]	0.0311
Periungal Telangiectasia	40 (47.6)	225 (41.1)			
Cardiac involvement	4 (4.8)	10 (1.8)			
Gastrointestinal ulceration	3 (3.6)	7 (1.3)			
Interstitial lung disease	4 (4.8)	11 (2.0)			
Any organ involvement[a]	9 (10.7)	25 (4.6)	0.0333	2.506 [1.127–5.573]	0.0243
Large joint arthritis	26 (31)	147 (26.9)			
Muscle enzyme elevation	74 (88.1)	481 (87.9)			
Severe muscle weakness	2 (2.4)	14 (2.6)			

[a]Composite outcome: includes cardiac, GI or lung involvement

contractures (OR 4.499, 95% CI 2.106–9.609), rituximab use (OR 3.955, 95% CI 1.551–10.089), and IVIG use (OR 1.891, 95% CI 1.062–3.366), as shown in Fig. 1.

Outcomes of calcinosis

Of the 631 patients included in analysis, only 422 had at least one follow-up visit. We reviewed the history of calcinosis in these 422 patients through the first follow-up visit. At baseline enrollment, 356 (84%) patients never had calcinosis and did not develop it through the first follow-up visit. A total of 42 patients had calcinosis present at the time of registry enrollment, and in 11 (26%) of these patients, the calcinosis resolved by the first follow-up visit, while in 31 (74%) patients,

Table 3 Treatment exposure by history of calcinosis

Risk factor	Descriptive analysis			Univariable analysis	
	Calcinosis			OR [95% CI]	*p*-value
	Yes	No			
Biologic treatment (Ever)	n (%)				
Any biologic	48 (57.1)	194 (35.5)	0.0001	2.426 [1.522–3.867]	
Rituximab	12 (14.3)	14 (2.6)	< 0.0001	6.345 [2.825–14.254]	< 0.001
IV Immune Globulin	45 (53.6)	180 (32.9)	0.0002	2.353 [1.479–3.743]	0.0003
Anti-TNF	12 (14.3)	23 (4.2)	0.0009	3.797 [1.812–7.960]	0.0004
Abatacept	2 (2.4)	1 (0.2)	0.048	13.317 [1.194–148.514]	0.0354
Anti-IL1	1 (1.2)	1 (0.2)			
High steroid exposure	47 (56)	269 (54.3)			

the calcinosis persisted. There were 14 patients with a prior history of but no calcinosis present at the time of enrollment. Three of these patients would develop a recurrence by the first follow-up visit.

Ten patients (2.5%) who never had calcinosis at the time of baseline enrollment, developed calcinosis by the first follow-up. The median age of JDM disease onset in these patients was 7 (IQR 4.5–8.2) with a median age at first follow-up (development of calcinosis) of 10.6 years (IQR 9.8–12.4). It should be noted that age of JDM disease onset could be different from age of diagnosis, and age of baseline enrollment. Eight patients were female. Six patients were Caucasian, three patients African-American and one patient mixed Caucasian and Hispanic. At the time of baseline enrollment, one patient had lipodystrophy, while one patient had joint contractures. For patients with available data, most (7/9, 78%) had previously received IV pulse steroids, and 7/9 (78%) were actively receiving daily long-term glucocorticoids for at least 1 month's duration. Four patients (50%) had previously received IVIG and 4/8 (50%) were actively receiving it. One patient had previously received rituximab (and also previously received IVIG), while one patient was actively receiving rituximab but had never received IVIG. None of the 10 patients had ever received anti-TNF-alpha therapy, abatacept or interleukin-1 inhibitors.

Discussion

Previous studies have highlighted differences between patients with calcinosis and those without. Duration of active JDM disease has been studied and described in two ways: the duration of symptoms prior to initial diagnosis and treatment, and as chronically active disease despite treatment. These two scenarios are not mutually exclusive. When expressed as the time until diagnosis

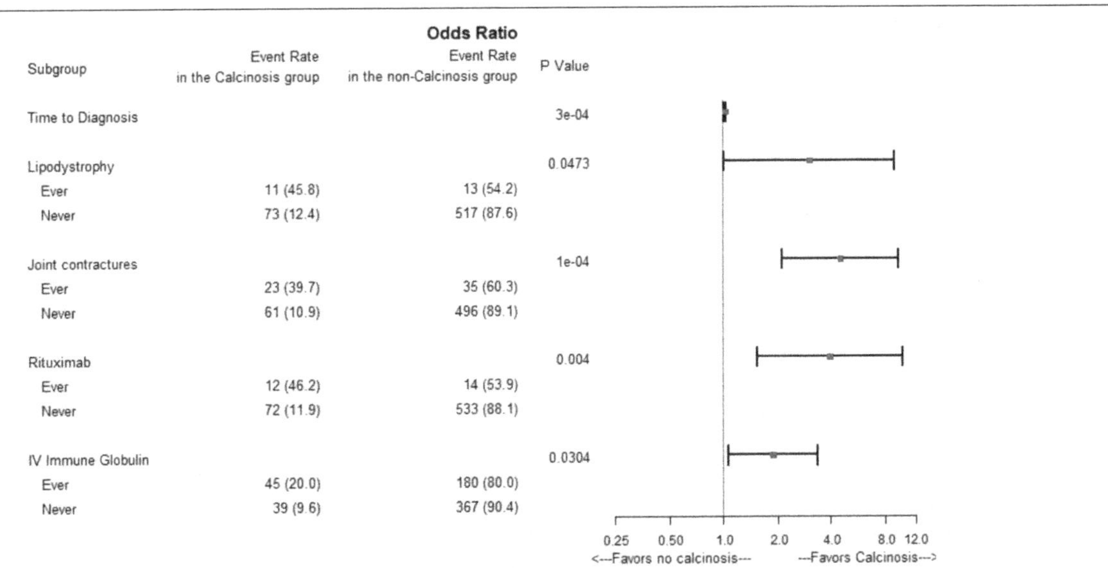

Fig. 1 Results of multivariate logistic regression analysis. Risk factors and event rates among patients with and without calcinosis are shown with *p*-values. Forest plot displays odds ratios and associated 95% confidence intervals of multivariate logistic regression

and treatment, increased symptom duration has been shown to be a risk factor for the development of calcinosis in some studies [5, 11, 18, 29, 30] but not in others [8, 19, 24], including a cohort with a high frequency of calcinosis. When the duration of active disease is expressed as chronically active disease despite treatment (i.e. cumulative disease duration), an association with calcinosis is also found in the studies that examined this feature [5, 6]. The combination of these assessments has led to the understanding that prolonged and/or severe disease activity is a risk factor for calcinosis. This understanding has subsequently been tested, with some evidence that early induction of remission can prevent calcinosis [13, 14]. Myositis antibodies are now widely used to guide prognosis and predict certain complications. In UK cohorts, calcinosis was associated with positive anti-MJ antibodies [20, 21], but this was not replicated in in a North American cohort, in which calcinosis occurred with equal frequency in patients with anti-p155/140, anti-MJ and negative serology [31]. African race, despite a low frequency of patients in all JDM cohorts, has been shown to be a risk factor for calcinosis [15–17]. Previously, the only non-demographic clinical features that were associated with calcinosis were cardiac disease [19] and joint contractures [18].

To our knowledge, our study includes the largest number of JDM patients with calcinosis collected and analyzed as a single cohort. Compared to other international series, our demographic characteristics of sex, age at onset, and JDM classification types are similar [5–8, 16, 24, 29]. We found no association that the age of JDM onset is associated with calcinosis. Male sex was associated with calcinosis on univariate analysis but did not hold significance on multivariable analysis. Our study demonstrated, as others have, that a delay in diagnosis and treatment is associated with the development of calcinosis; however, the effect in our study was small (OR 1.029, 95% CI 1.013–1.045). In addition, we showed that receiving IVIG or rituximab are more strongly associated with ever having calcinosis, and with higher odds ratios (OR 1.891, OR 3.955 respectively) than those with treatment delays. This effect was not seen with our variable of high steroid exposure. Given that IVIG and rituximab are typically reserved for those who fail standard treatment, we suspect those patients had more severe and/or prolonged active disease despite treatment. Clearly, untreated disease represents a risk for developing calcinosis, as was demonstrated in early studies with less effective treatments [2]. A delay in treatment imparts this same risk, and based on the intermittent association of this factor with calcinosis in various studies, this suggests that the effect may possibly be mitigated with *more* effective treatment, in addition to more timely treatment. Perhaps this implies that at even greater risk are the types of disease courses which are chronically active and difficult to control. Many studies, including those focusing on myositis antibodies are attempting to identify the pathophysiological mechanisms underlying these differences and therefore predict which patients might be at risk of calcinosis. If reliable, such predictions would encourage the development of screening techniques and potentially inform treatment approaches. In our study, we found that joint contractures (OR 4.499, 95% CI 2.106–9.609) and lipodystrophy (OR 3.038, 95% CI 1.014–9.106) were both independently associated with developing calcinosis, the latter of which to our knowledge has not been previously reported. Cutaneous ulcerations and any organ involvement (i.e. cardiac, pulmonary or gastrointestinal) were also associated with calcinosis on univariate analyses but did not hold significance in multivariate analysis. These associations may not have been identified in prior studies due to the small numbers of patients with calcinosis as a whole in those studies. Additionally, as collected in the legacy registry, the presence or absence of disease features were assessed simply as current, past or never without reference to chronology. Calcinosis, particularly across a joint may lead to joint contractures [9], which may partially explain this association. Previously, calcinosis was also identified as a predictor for lipodystrophy with affected areas often overlying areas of calcinosis or panniculitis [32]. By reviewing the limited follow-up data in the registry, we also describe that calcinosis occurs infrequently in this cohort over a short time period (2.5% of patients with one follow-up visit), but calcinosis tends to persist or recur once it has developed. It is also noted that in the 10 patients who developed calcinosis, most had received IVIG and/or rituximab suggesting they had either severe or refractory disease, but none of these patients had received anti-TNF-alpha therapy, since monoclonal antibody forms have been shown to be effective against JDM disease activity and calcinosis [33].

The limitations of our study include the retrospective methodology and that patients enrolled in this registry were a convenience sample with varying disease durations at the time of enrollment. Prior histories of treatment and/or complications are subject to recall bias by patients/parents and sufficient documentation at the many respective enrolling centers. Information on calcinosis itself was limited only to its presence or absence without further assessment of phenotype or complications such as infection. There was also no information on whether treatments received by patients were specifically intended for calcinosis or for other JDM disease activity. Additionally, information on testing of myositis-specific and myositis-associated antibodies was not collected. Further, there is inconsistent and relatively few follow-up dates, as the funding for this registry was limited to a short duration of data capture. Given these limitations, however, the CARRA legacy registry has provided important information about pediatric rheumatic diseases and JDM. Many of these limitations have been addressed in the newly created CARRA registry which began enrolling patients in 2015 with plans for several years of prospective follow-up. Apart from the full rationale and methodology already published [34], there are specific improvements in the data capture for JDM and calcinosis that address many of these limitations.

Conclusion

The pathogenesis and treatment approach for calcinosis remains a frontier of research in Juvenile Dermatomyositis. Identifying patients at risk for the complication is a critical step to improving treatment outcomes by focusing research efforts. From studying a large registry of patients, we confirm prior reports that a delayed time to diagnosis and treatment, joint contractures and organ disease are associated with calcinosis, and we also found that lipodystrophy is similarly associated. More aggressive therapy, namely IVIG and rituximab, in our study cohort is also associated with calcinosis which may reflect chronically active or refractory disease.

Abbreviations

CARRA: Childhood Arthritis and Rheumatology Research Alliance; CHAQ: Childhood health assessment questionnaire; DMARDs: Disease-modifying anti-rheumatic drugs; IVIG: Intravenous immune globulin; JDM: Juvenile Dermatomyositis; TNF: Tumor necrosis factor

Acknowledgements

We would also like to thank all participants and hospital sites that recruited patients for the CARRA Registry. The authors thank the following CARRA Registry site principal investigators and research coordinators: L. Abramson, E. Anderson, M. Andrew, N. Battle, M. Becker, H. Benham, T. Beukelman, J. Birmingham, P. Blier, A. Brown, H. Brunner, A. Cabrera, D. Canter, D. Carlton, B. Caruso, L. Ceracchio, E. Chalom, J. Chang, P. Charpentier, K. Clark, J. Dean, F. Dedeoglu, B. Feldman, P. Ferguson, M. Fox, K. Francis, M. Gervasini, D. Goldsmith, G. Gorton, B. Gottlieb, T. Graham, T. Griffin, H. Grosbein, S. Guppy, H. Haftel, D. Helfrich, G. Higgins, A. Hillard, J.R. Hollister, J. Hsu, A. Hudgins, C. Hung, A. Huttenlocher, N. Ilowite, A. Imlay, L. Imundo, C.J. Inman, J. Jaqith, R. Jerath, L. Jung, P. Kahn, A. Kapedani, D. Kingsbury, K. Klein, M. Klein-Gitelman, A. Kunkel, S. Lapidus, S. Layburn, T. Lehman, C. Lindsley, M. Macgregor-Hannah, M. Malloy, C. Mawhorter, D. McCurdy, K. Mims, N. Moorthy, D. Morus, E. Muscal, M. Natter, J. Olson, K. O'Neil, K. Onel, M. Orlando, J. Palmquist, M. Phillips, L. Ponder, S. Prahalad, M. Punaro, D. Puplava, S. Quinn, A. Quintero, C. Rabinovich, A. Reed, C. Reed, S. Ringold, M. Riordan, S. Roberson, A. Robinson, J. Rossette, D. Rothman, D. Russo, N. Ruth, K. Schikler, A. Sestak, B. Shaham, Y. Sherman, M. Simmons, N. Singer, S. Spalding, H. Stapp, R. Syed, E. Thomas, K. Torok, D. Trejo, J. Tress, W. Upton, R. Vehe, E. von Scheven, L. Walters, J. Weiss, P. Weiss, N. Welnick, A. White, J. Woo, J. Wootton, A. Yalcindag, C. Zapp, L. Zemel, and A. Zhu.

Funding

1. Washington University, Institute of Clinical and Translational Sciences, Core Usage Funding, Just-in-Time Grant, PI: Dr. Vikas Dharnidharka, via NIH grant NCATS UL1TR000448
2. Eunice Kennedy Shriver National Institute of Child Health and Development, T32 HD043010101
3. Washington University, Institute of Clinical and Translational Sciences, Mentored Training Program in Clinical Investigation via NIH grant NCATS UL1TR000448
4. The CARRA Legacy Registry was supported by a grant from the National Institute of Arthritis and Musculoskeletal and Skin Diseases of the National Institutes of Health under award Number RC2AR058934. The content is solely the responsibility of the authors and does not necessarily represent the official views of the National Institutes of Health. The CARRA Legacy Registry was also supported by CARRA, Friends of CARRA, the Arthritis Foundation, and the Duke Clinical Research Institute.

Authors' contributions

AO authored the manuscript. AO and KB made substantial contributes to study design, acquisition data and interpretation of statistical analysis. VD made substantial contribution to study design, co-acquisition of funding, interpretation of data and analyses. NA performed statistical analysis and made substantial contributions to study design and interpretation of data. All authors provided critical edits and approved the manuscript for publication.

Consent for publication

Not applicable.

Competing interests

The authors declare that they have no competing interests.

Author details

Division of Pediatric Rheumatology, Department of Pediatric and Adolescent Medicine, Mayo Clinic, 200 First Street SW, Rochester, MN 55902, USA. [2]Division of Pediatric Rheumatology, Department of Pediatrics, St. Louis, MO, USA. [3]Division of Pediatric Nephrology, Department of Pediatrics, St. Louis, MO, USA. [4]Division of Biostatistics, Washington University School of Medicine, St. Louis, MO, USA.

References

1. Mendez EP, Lipton R, Ramsey-Goldman R, Roettcher P, Bowyer S, Dyer A, et al. US incidence of juvenile dermatomyositis, 1995-1998: results from the National Institute of Arthritis and Musculoskeletal and Skin Diseases registry. Arthritis Rheum. 2003;49(3):300–5.
2. Bitnum S, Daeschner CW Jr, Travis LB, Dodge WF, Hopps HC. Dermatomyositis. J Pediatr. 1964;64:101–31.
3. Sullivan DB, Cassidy JT, Petty RE. Dermatomyositis in the pediatric patient. Arthritis Rheum. 1977;20(2 Suppl):327–31.
4. Jacobs JC. Methotrexate and azathioprine treatment of childhood dermatomyositis. Pediatrics. 1977;59(2):212–8.
5. Ravelli A, Trail L, Ferrari C, Ruperto N, Pistorio A, Pilkington C, et al. Long-term outcome and prognostic factors of juvenile dermatomyositis: a multinational, multicenter study of 490 patients. Arthritis Care Res (Hoboken). 2010;62(1):63–72.
6. Mathiesen P, Hegaard H, Herlin T, Zak M, Pedersen FK, Nielsen S. Long-term outcome in patients with juvenile dermatomyositis: a cross-sectional follow-up study. Scand J Rheumatol. 2012;41(1):50–8.

7. Ramanan AV, Feldman BM. Clinical features and outcomes of juvenile dermatomyositis and other childhood onset myositis syndromes. Rheum Dis Clin N Am. 2002;28(4):833–57.
8. Huber AM, Lang B, LeBlanc CM, Birdi N, Bolaria RK, Malleson P, et al. Medium- and long-term functional outcomes in a multicenter cohort of children with juvenile dermatomyositis. Arthritis Rheum. 2000;43(3):541–9.
9. Hoeltzel MF, Oberle EJ, Robinson AB, Agarwal A, Rider LG. The presentation, assessment, pathogenesis, and treatment of calcinosis in juvenile dermatomyositis. Curr Rheumatol Rep. 2014;16(12):467.
10. Orandi AB, Baszis KW, Dharnidharka VR, Huber AM, Hoeltzel MF, subgroup CJM. Assessment, classification and treatment of calcinosis as a complication of juvenile dermatomyositis: a survey of pediatric rheumatologists by the childhood arthritis and rheumatology research alliance (CARRA). Pediatr Rheumatol Online J. 2017;15(1):71.
11. Pachman LM, Abbott K, Sinacore JM, Amoruso L, Dyer A, Lipton R, et al. Duration of illness is an important variable for untreated children with juvenile dermatomyositis. J Pediatr. 2006;148(2):247–53.
12. Mathiesen PR, Zak M, Herlin T, Nielsen SM. Clinical features and outcome in a Danish cohort of juvenile dermatomyositis patients. Clin Exp Rheumatol. 2010;28(5):782–9.
13. Fisler RE, Liang MG, Fuhlbrigge RC, Yalcindag A, Sundel RP. Aggressive management of juvenile dermatomyositis results in improved outcome and decreased incidence of calcinosis. J Am Acad Dermatol. 2002;47(4):505–11.
14. Kim S, El-Hallak M, Dedeoglu F, Zurakowski D, Fuhlbrigge RC, Sundel RP. Complete and sustained remission of juvenile dermatomyositis resulting from aggressive treatment. Arthritis Rheum. 2009;60(6):1825–30.
15. Hoeltzel MF. Race is a risk factor for calcinosis in patients with JD - early results from the CARRAnet registry study. Pediatr Rheumatol. 2012;10(Suppl 1):A65.
16. Faller G, Mistry BJ, Tikly M. Juvenile dermatomyositis in south African children is characterised by frequent dystropic calcification: a cross sectional study. Pediatr Rheumatol Online J. 2014;12:2.
17. Phillippi K, Hoeltzel M, Byun Robinson A, Kim S, Childhood A. Rheumatology research Alliance legacy registry I. race, income, and disease outcomes in juvenile dermatomyositis. J Pediatr. 2017;184:38–44 e1.
18. Saini I, Kalaivani M, Kabra SK. Calcinosis in juvenile dermatomyositis: frequency, risk factors and outcome. Rheumatol Int. 2016;36(7):961–5.
19. Sallum AM, Pivato FC, Doria-Filho U, Aikawa NE, Liphaus BL, Marie SK, et al. Risk factors associated with calcinosis of juvenile dermatomyositis. J Pediatr. 2008;84(1):68–74.
20. Gunawardena H, Wedderburn LR, Chinoy H, Betteridge ZE, North J, Ollier WE, et al. Autoantibodies to a 140-kd protein in juvenile dermatomyositis are associated with calcinosis. Arthritis Rheum. 2009;60(6):1807–14.
21. Tansley SL, Betteridge ZE, Shaddick G, Gunawardena H, Arnold K, Wedderburn LR, et al. Calcinosis in juvenile dermatomyositis is influenced by both anti-NXP2 autoantibody status and age at disease onset. Rheumatology (Oxford). 2014;53(12):2204–8.
22. Pachman LM, Liotta-Davis MR, Hong DK, Kinsella TR, Mendez EP, Kinder JM, et al. TNFalpha-308A allele in juvenile dermatomyositis: association with increased production of tumor necrosis factor alpha, disease duration, and pathologic calcifications. Arthritis Rheum. 2000;43(10):2368–77.
23. Mamyrova G, O'Hanlon TP, Sillers L, Malley K, James-Newton L, Parks CG, et al. Cytokine gene polymorphisms as risk and severity factors for juvenile dermatomyositis. Arthritis Rheum. 2008;58(12):3941–50.
24. Clemente G, Piotto DG, Barbosa C, Peracchi OA, Len CA, Hilario MO, et al. High frequency of calcinosis in juvenile dermatomyositis: a risk factor study. Rev Bras Reumatol. 2012;52(4):549–53.
25. Callen AM, Pachman LM, Hayford J, Chung A, Ramseygoldman R. Intermittent high-dose intravenous methylprednisolone (iv pulse) therapy prevents calcinosis and shortens disease course in juvenile dermatomyositis (Jdms). Arthritis Rheum. 1994;37(6):R10-R.
26. Levy DM, Bingham CA, Kahn PJ, Eichenfield AH, Imundo LF. Favorable outcome of juvenile dermatomyositis treated without systemic corticosteroids. J Pediatr. 2010;156(2):302–7.
27. Tabarki B, Ponsot G, Prieur AM, Tardieu M. Childhood dermatomyositis: clinical course of 36 patients treated with low doses of corticosteroids. Eur J Paediatr Neurol. 1998;2(4):205–11.
28. Robinson AB, Hoeltzel MF, Wahezi DM, Becker ML, Kessler EA, Schmeling H, et al. Clinical characteristics of children with juvenile dermatomyositis: the Childhood arthritis and rheumatology research Alliance registry. Arthritis Care Res (Hoboken). 2014;66(3):404–10.
29. Pachman LM, Hayford JR, Chung A, Daugherty CA, Pallansch MA, Fink CW, et al. Juvenile dermatomyositis at diagnosis: clinical characteristics of 79 children. J Rheumatol. 1998;25(6):1198–204.
30. Malek A, Raeeskarami SR, Ziaee V, Aghighi Y, Moradinejad MH. Clinical course and outcomes of Iranian children with juvenile dermatomyositis and polymyositis. Clin Rheumatol. 2014;33(8):1113–8.
31. Rider LG, Shah M, Mamyrova G, Huber AM, Rice MM, Targoff IN, et al. The myositis autoantibody phenotypes of the juvenile idiopathic inflammatory myopathies. Medicine (Baltimore). 2013;92(4):223–43.
32. Bingham A, Mamyrova G, Rother KI, Oral E, Cochran E, Premkumar A, et al. Predictors of acquired lipodystrophy in juvenile-onset dermatomyositis and a gradient of severity. Medicine (Baltimore). 2008;87(2):70–86.
33. Riley P, McCann LJ, Maillard SM, Woo P, Murray KJ, Pilkington CA. Effectiveness of infliximab in the treatment of refractory juvenile dermatomyositis with calcinosis. Rheumatology (Oxford). 2008;47(6):877–80.
34. Beukelman T, Kimura Y, Ilowite NT, Mieszkalski K, Natter MD, Burrell G, et al. The new Childhood arthritis and rheumatology research Alliance (CARRA) registry: design, rationale, and characteristics of patients enrolled in the first 12 months. Pediatr Rheumatol Online J. 2017;15(1):30.

Clinical practice variation and need for pediatric-specific treatment guidelines among rheumatologists caring for children with ANCA-associated vasculitis

Clara Westwell-Roper[1], Joanna M. Lubieniecka[2], Kelly L. Brown[1], Kimberly A. Morishita[1], Cherry Mammen[1], Linda Wagner-Weiner[3], Eric Yen[4], Suzanne C. Li[5], Kathleen M. O'Neil[6], Sivia K. Lapidus[7], Paul Brogan[8], Rolando Cimaz[9], David A. Cabral[1*] and for ARChiVe Investigators Network within the PedVas initiative

Abstract

Background: Because pediatric antineutrophil cytoplasmic antibody-associated vasculitis is rare, management generally relies on adult data. We assessed treatment practices, uptake of existing clinical assessment tools, and interest in pediatric treatment protocols among rheumatologists caring for children with granulomatosis with polyangiitis (GPA) and microscopic polyangiitis (MPA).

Methods: A needs-assessment survey developed by an international working group of pediatric rheumatologists and two nephrologists was circulated internationally. Data were summarized with descriptive statistics. Pearson's chi-square tests were used in inferential univariate analyses.

Results: The 209 respondents from 36 countries had collectively seen ~1600 children with GPA/MPA; 144 had seen more than two in the preceding 5 years. Standardized and validated clinical assessment tools to score disease severity, activity, and damage were used by 59, 63, and 36%, respectively; barriers to use included lack of knowledge and limited perceived utility. Therapy varied significantly: use of rituximab rather than cyclophosphamide was more common among respondents from the USA (OR = 2.7 [1.3-5.5], $p = 0.0190$, $n = 139$), those with >5 years of independent practice experience (OR = 3.8 [1.3-12.5], $p = 0.0279$, $n = 137$), and those who had seen >10 children with GPA/MPA in their careers (OR = 4.39 [2.1-9.1], $p = 0.0011$, $n = 133$). Respondents who had treated >10 patients were also more likely to continue maintenance therapy for at least 24 months (OR = 3.0 [1.4-6.4], $p = 0.0161$, $n = 127$). Ninety six percent of respondents believed in a need for pediatric-specific treatment guidelines; 46% supported adaptation of adult guidelines while 69% favoured guidelines providing a limited range of treatment options to allow comparison of effectiveness through a registry.

Conclusions: These data provide a rationale for developing pediatric-specific consensus treatment guidelines for GPA/MPA. While pediatric rheumatologist uptake of existing clinical tools has been limited, guideline uptake may be enhanced if outcomes of consensus-derived treatment options are evaluated within the framework of an international registry.

Keywords: Pediatric rheumatology, Anti-neutrophil cytoplasmic antibody-associated vasculitis, Granulomatosis with polyangiitis, Microscopic polyangiitis, Physician practice patterns, Clinical practice guidelines, Disease classification, Vasculitis treatment, Outcome assessment

* Correspondence: dcabral@cw.bc.ca
[1]Clinical Professor, Division of Rheumatology, Department of Pediatrics, University of British Columbia, BC Children's Hospital, Room K4-119 4480 Oak Street Vancouver, Vancouver, BC V6H 3V4, Canada
Full list of author information is available at the end of the article

Background

Antineutrophil cytoplasmic antibody- (ANCA-) associated vasculitis (AAV) describes the subset of vasculitides primarily involving small vessels: granulomatosis with polyangiitis (GPA, formerly Wegener's granulomatosis), microscopic polyangiitis (MPA), eosinophilic granulomatosis with polyangiitis (EGPA, formerly Churg-Strauss syndrome), and renal-limited pauci-immune glomerulonephritis [1]. Although rare in childhood, AAV carries a high burden of morbidity. With the use of high-dose corticosteroids and cyclophosphamide, AAV is no longer rapidly fatal in the majority of affected children; however, these treatments have significant adverse effects. Balancing the risks associated with existing therapies against the damage associated with under- or overtreatment remains a challenge. In adult populations, this balance has been incrementally fine-tuned through clinical trials that rely on accurate disease sub-classification and scoring tools to stage disease severity, activity, and damage (Table 1). The rarity of pediatric AAV has limited opportunities for pediatric clinical trials such that management decisions are largely informed by adult data [2], with potential for significant practice variation.

A 2005 survey of Childhood Arthritis and Rheumatology Research Alliance (CARRA) members elicited overwhelming consensus on the need to study childhood-onset vasculitis independently from adult disease [3]. ARChiVe (A Registry for Childhood Vasculitis) was established in 2007 based on this imperative for pediatric-specific data collection. A concurrent initiative of the Pediatric Rheumatology European Society (PRES) also helped generate time-of-diagnosis data to support the development of pediatric-specific classification criteria and assessment tools. More recently, PedVas (Pediatric Vasculitis Initiative [4]; https://clinicaltrials.gov/ct2/show/NCT02006134) has allowed collection of clinical data and biological samples to ARChiVe. While pediatric clinical trials remain difficult, an international

Table 1 Definitions of clinical tools included in survey questions

Clinical tool	Description
Birmingham Vasculitis Activity Score (BVAS)	Scoring tool designed to document new or worseningfeatures of clinically active AAV. Items are categorized into 9 groups by organ system [11].
BVAS Version 3	2009 update to BVAS [11, 39].
BVAS for Wegener's Granulomatosis (WG)	Modification of BVAS that removes features unlikely to occur in GPA [13, 40].
Pediatric Vasculitis Activity Score (PVAS)	Pediatric version of BVAS preliminarily validated in children [12].
EUVAS Severity Score	Classification system for AAV based on disease extent and severity. Subgroups include localized, early systemic, generalized, severe renal, and refractory disease [41].
Five Factor Score	Scoring tool based on factors associated with poor prognosis: cardiac symptoms, gastrointestinal involvement, renal insufficiency, proteinuria, and central nervous system involvement [42].
Wegener's Granulomatosis Etanercept Trial (WGET) Severity Score	Sub-classification based on modified ACR criteria for limited versus extensive disease [43].
Disease Extent Index (DEI)	Tool for scoring disease activity based on organ system, with distinct domains from those included in BVAS [44].
Physician's Global Assessment (PGA)	Physician's global assessment of disease activity on a 10 cm visual analogue scale.
Vasculitis Damage Index (VDI)	Scoring tool used to record damage due to disease or treatment. Items are categorized into 11 groups by organ system with binary scoring [14].
Pediatric VDI (PVDI)	Pediatric modification of the adult VDI; not yet formally validated in children [14, 15].
AAV Index of Damage (AVID)	Tool for grading disease- or treatment-associated damage, with weighting of items based on potential morbidity and mortality [45].
Combined Damage Assessment Index	Combination of items from AVID and VDI, divided into 17 organ-based categories [46].

registry such as ARChiVe might provide the opportunity to compare effectiveness of a limited range of standardized treatment options and ultimately generate evidence-based guidelines. This strategy has been pursued for uvenile dermatomyositis, another rare pediatric rheumatic disease [5].

As a first step toward developing treatment guidelines for pediatric AAV, we sought to better understand the diversity of beliefs and practices associated with current care. We conducted an international needs assessment survey of physicians involved in the diagnosis and management of children with GPA and MPA, with the following aims: (1) to assess the level of community experience with pediatric AAV; (2) to assess uptake of existing classification criteria, clinical scoring tools, and treatment guidelines; (3) to assess the extent of variation in current treatment practices; and (4) to determine interest in and capacity for use of pediatric treatment protocols.

Methods

A survey draft developed by the Pediatric Rheumatology group and a nephrologist at British Columbia Children's Hospital was finalized with input from the Vasculitis Working Groups of CARRA and PRES. The survey comprised 47 predominantly categorical multi-choice questions in three sections (Additional file 1). The first section addressed practice type and experience with pediatric GPA and MPA (EGPA was excluded given its rarity in pediatrics). Respondents caring for fewer than two children with GPA and/or MPA over the past 5 years were then given the option to exit. The second section queried use and knowledge of classification criteria and formal scoring tools for disease severity, activity and damage (Table 1). Practitioners were also asked about their use of adult treatment guidelines and perceived need for pediatric-specific guidelines. The third section queried motivations for and barriers to participation in clinical registries. Levels of assigned value were requested using a five-point Likert scale from 1 (not important) to 5 (extremely important).

Members of CARRA, the Canadian Alliance of Pediatric Rheumatology Investigators (CAPRI), the Australian Pediatric Rheumatology Group, the PRES-CARRA Vasculitis Working Group, and the Pediatric Rheumatology Bulletin Board (ped-rhe-list@mcmaster.ca) were invited by email to complete the web-based survey (estimated 500 personal email invitations). The survey was administered using REDCap electronic data capture tools [6] hosted at the University of British Columbia (UBC) from July 24 to September 29, 2015. The survey was conducted as a quality assurance initiative for PedVas, which was approved by the Children's and Women's Research Ethics Board of UBC (H12-00894). Under Article 2.5 of the Tri Council Policy Statement, quality assurance/improvement activities are not subject to further institutional review.

Descriptive statistics were used to quantify response frequencies and means. Unless otherwise specified, frequencies are reported relative to the total number of respondents completing each question. Odds ratios (OR) were determined as measures of association. Limits of 95% confidence intervals of OR are reported in square brackets. Inferential univariate analysis with two-sided Pearson's chi-square tests and Benjamini-Hochberg correction for multiple comparisons was used to test 11 hypotheses with a false discovery rate of 5% [7]. Corrected p-values are reported. Analysis was performed using Microsoft Excel Version 14.6.7 and Prism Version 5.0a (GraphPad Software Inc., La Jolla, CA).

Results

Respondent characteristics

Of 216 respondents opening the survey, 209 completed it, yielding an estimated response rate of approximately 40%. Sixty-five (31%) chose to exit as they had not cared for two or more patients with GPA/MPA in the preceding 5 years. The 144 respondents completing the full survey practiced in 36 countries, predominantly the USA (48%), with others from Canada (13%), Italy (4%), Australia (3%), Germany (4%), Turkey (4%), United Kingdom (4%), Brazil (2%), and Sweden (2%). Most respondents (92%) belonged to one or more national or international rheumatology organizations, including CARRA (56%), PRES (32%), CAPRI (10%), the PRES-CARRA Vasculitis Working Group (10%), and others (18%). Approximately half of respondents had practiced for less than 10 years after formal training (21% for less than 5 years and 26% for 5-10 years); among the rest, 20% each had practiced for 10-20 and 20-30 years and 10% for 30-40 years. The combined lifetime experience of respondents was at least 1600 patients with GPA/MPA (some shared): 47% had seen fewer than ten patients, 39% had seen 10-20, and only 14% had seen more than 20. The majority of respondents (61%) had seen five or fewer patients with a new diagnosis of GPA or MPA within the past 5 years (mode 3, median 5, IQR 3-8 patients).

Most respondents belonged to group practices, sharing diagnostic and treatment decisions for all patients (46%) or managing patients independently while sharing on-call responsibilities (41%). A minority worked in a solo practice (7%) or in another practice arrangement (6%), predominantly hospital-based. For patients who had also been assessed by a nephrologist, the majority of respondents reported making collaborative treatment decisions, 30% in a combined nephrology/rheumatology clinic and 37% in separate clinic settings. Some reported variation in the responsible subspecialty depending on factors such as who had seen the patient first (18%), while 13 and 2% of respondents reported independent management by rheumatology or nephrology, respectively.

Classification criteria

There were between 129 and 144 responses (89-100%) to subsequent individual questions regarding diagnosis and management. While the majority (73%) reported that they always sub-classify AAV as either GPA or MPA, 26% endorsed only sometimes sub-classifying. Table 2 shows the number of respondents familiar with – and using – existing criteria for defining or classifying AAV. Most were familiar with ACR1990 [8] and EULAR/PRINTO/PRES 2008 [9] classification criteria for GPA, and with CHCC 1994 disease definitions [10]. Serology (cANCA/PR3 versus pANCA/MPO) and EULAR/PRINTO/PRES 2008 criteria [9] were most frequently used for distinguishing between GPA and MPA in clinical practice. Notably, 66% of all respondents reported using more than one set of criteria, and those using informal methods considered histopathology, antibody status, and specific organ involvement. The rationale for sub-classification was predominantly prognostication (73%), influence on treatment choice (48%), involvement in clinical studies/trials (39%), and access to treatments (29%). All respondents felt that distinguishing between GPA and MPA was at least somewhat important for research (mode 4, median 4, IQR 3-4).

Disease severity, activity, and damage

The proportions of respondents using formal tools to assess disease severity, activity, and damage are shown in Table 3. While most respondents used formal assessment tools for severity (59%) and activity (63%), only 36% had ever formally assessed disease damage. The Birmingham Vasculitis Activity Score (BVAS) [11], the Pediatric Vasculitis Activity Score (PVAS) [12], and BVAS for Wegener's Granulomatosis [13] – tools designed primarily for assessment of disease activity – were frequently used to stage severity, but tools such as the Five Factor Score and the EUVAS and WGET severity scores were used by a minority. PVAS, BVAS, and physician's global assessment on a 10 cm visual analogue scale (PGA) were the primary tools used by respondents for scoring disease activity, typically at the time of diagnosis: 39% at only some follow-up visits, 33% at all visits, 16% at prescribed times according to research protocols, and 7% at the time of diagnosis only. Most respondents felt formal assessment of disease activity was somewhat important to clinical management (mode 3, median 5, IQR 3-4), and more important to research (mode 5, median 5, IQR 4-5). Most commonly used tools for scoring disease damage include the Vasculitis Damage Index (VDI) [14] or its pediatric adaptation, PVDI [15]. Similar to scoring of disease activity, respondents assessed disease damage primarily at the time of diagnosis: 35% at only some follow-up visits, 23% at prescribed times only, and 31% at every visit. Respondent rationales for not

Table 2 Familiarity with and use of vasculitis classification criteria and disease definitions to differentiate GPA from MPA in children[a]

Criteria	Familiar (%)	Using (%)
EULAR/PRINTO/PRES 2008 criteria [9]	78	57
ANCA (PR3/MPO)	ND[b]	57
ACR 1990 criteria [8, 19]	72	29
CHCC 1994 [10]	62	32
CHCC 2012 [1]	47	
EMA classification algorithm (2007) [22]	18	5
Pediatric Modification of EMA classification algorithm (2012) [21]		
Informal criteria	ND[b]	19
Other formal criteria	ND[b]	1

[a]Data represent percentage of respondents out of $n = 144$ (familiar) or $n = 143$ (using)
[b]No data

Table 3 Use of formal disease severity, activity, and damage scoring tools by survey respondents in the assessment of children with GPA or MPA[a]

Parameter	Scoring tool	Respondents (%)
Severity[b]	PVAS [12]	41
	BVAS [11]	20
	BVAS for WG [13]	19
	EUVAS Severity Score [41]	11
	Five Factor Score [42]	8
	WGET Severity Score [43]	7
	Disease Extent Index [44]	1
	Other	1
	Never formally assess	41
Activity[c]	PVAS [12]	38
	Physician's Global Assessment	29
	BVAS [11]	19
	BVAS for WG [13]	13
	BVAS version 3 [39]	6
	Other tool	0
	Never formally assess	37
Damage[c]	Pediatric VDI [15]	31
	VDI [14]	10
	AAV Index of Damage [45]	3
	Combined Damage Assessment Index [46]	1
	Other	0
	Never formally assess	64

[a]Data represent percentage of respondents out of [b]$n = 142$, [c]$n = 141$

using formal assessment tools are shown in Table 4 and included use of histopathology, lack of effect on management, lack of familiarity, and inconvenience.

Treatment guidelines

A majority of respondents (53%) reported using a combination of resources to guide treatment decisions, most commonly EULAR/EUVAS recommendations (24%). A minority used site-specific standardized protocols (7%); others used pediatric textbook recommendations (4%), individualized approaches according to personal interpretation (4%), or advice from colleagues (6%). The majority of respondents (96%) believed in a need for pediatric treatment guidelines for GPA/MPA. Over half (58%) were interested in being involved in the process of consensus guideline development – 43% through an iterative survey – while others felt they did not have the time (13%) or relevant expertise (19%), or were unsure (9%). There was no association between group membership and the desire to participate in guideline development (OR = 1.4 [0.4, 5.1], $p = 0.7206$, $n = 131$), although respondents practicing outside the USA and Canada were more likely to want to participate than those within (OR = 4.2 [1.9, 9.0], $p = 0.0011$, $n = 135$). Most respondents supported consensus guidelines drafted by an expert group (69%) and believed in the need for a limited range of options to allow for comparative outcome assessment through a clinical registry (63%). Slightly less than half (46%) felt modification of recommendations for adult disease was an acceptable method for generating pediatric treatment guidelines.

Table 4 Reported rationales against use of formal assessment tools for scoring disease severity, activity, and damage in the assessment of children with GPA or MPA[a]

Parameter	Rationale against use of tool	Respondents (%)
Severity[b]	Use of histopathological findings	53
	No effect on management	34
	Lack of familiarity with tools	26
	No value added beyond clinical judgment	24
	Inconvenience	16
	Other	5.3
Activity[c]	Lack of familiarity with tools	47
	Inconvenience	43
	No effect on management	22
	Lack of applicability of tools for adults	20
	No value added beyond clinical judgment	18
Damage[d]	Lack of familiarity with tools	58
	Inconvenience	32
	Lack of applicability of tools for adults	20
	No effect on management	18
	No value added beyond clinical judgment	12

[a]Data represent percentage of respondents out of [b]$n = 38$, [c]$n = 51$, [d]$n = 91$

Treatment practices

All respondents followed a remission-induction and remission-maintenance model, switching from induction to maintenance therapy within 3-6 months. In adult studies, choice of induction agent may be adjusted based on measures of disease severity, primarily to limit use of aggressive life-saving treatment – specifically cyclophosphamide – that also has significant toxicity and may be unwarranted in milder disease. Two-thirds (67%) of respondents endorsed always using more aggressive treatment for patients with severe disease, while 32% reported only sometimes choosing induction therapy based on disease severity. Table 5 shows first-line induction and maintenance therapies preferred by respondents for treatment of AAV; respondents were not asked to distinguish between GPA- and MPA-specific regimens. In patients with severe disease not requiring intensive care, cyclophosphamide (CYC) was the first choice of remission-induction agent by 66% of respondents, while 31% stated they would choose rituximab (RTX). Use of RTX rather than CYC as an induction agent was more frequently reported by respondents from the USA (OR = 2.7 [1.3, 5.5], $p = 0.0190$, $n = 139$), those with greater than 5 years of experience (OR = 3.8 [1.3, 12.5], $p = 0.0279$, $n = 137$), and those who had seen more than 10 patients with GPA/MPA in their careers (OR = 4.39 [2.1, 9.1], $p = 0.0011$, $n = 133$).

Figure 1 shows the heterogeneity among prescribing practices for both CYC and RTX. Most respondents used CYC for induction until clinically inactive disease up to a maximum of 6 months (69%), while 16% treated

Table 5 Induction and maintenance agents used by respondents[a]

Indication	Agent	Respondents (%)
Induction agent in severe disease[b]	Cyclophosphamide	66
	Rituximab	31
	Other	2
Induction agent if not using CYC or RTX (e.g. for less severe disease)[c]	Methotrexate	40
	Azathioprine	30
	Mycophenolate	25
	Other	4
Maintenance therapy[d]	Azathioprine	45
	Methotrexate	23
	Mycophenolate	18
	Rituximab	11
	Other	3

[a]Data represent percentage of respondents out of [b]$n = 140$, [c]$n = 138$, [d]$n = 141$

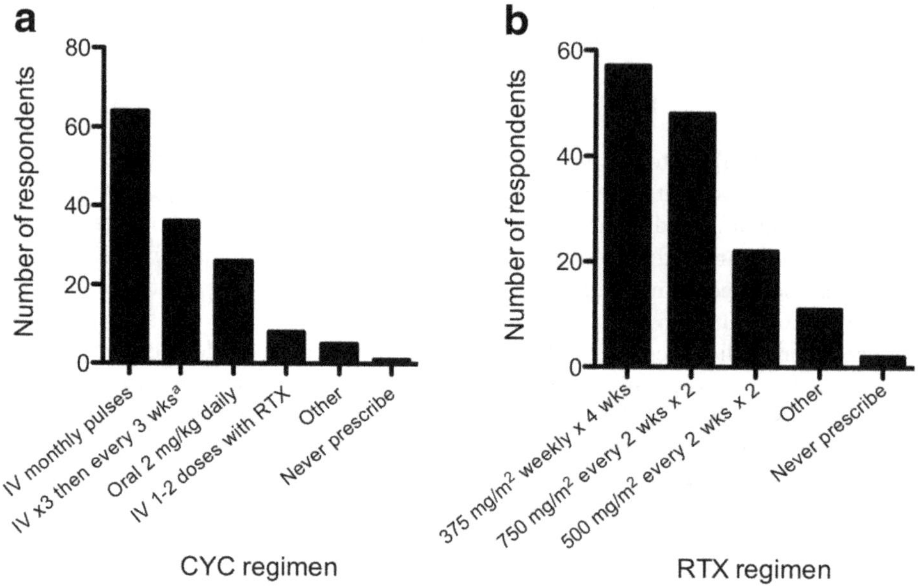

Fig. 1 Typical dosing regimens prescribed for cyclophosphamide (CYC) and rituximab (RTX) induction therapy. Data represent number of respondents out of n = 140 for both agents. [a]EUVAS protocol

for a defined duration between 3 and 7 months, 7% gave only 1-2 IV doses in conjunction with RTX, 5% continued induction therapy until clinical inactivity regardless of duration, and 2% employed some other regimen. The most common first choice of induction therapy in children not receiving CYC or RTX was methotrexate (MTX), followed by azathioprine (AZA) and mycophenolate mofetil (MMF) (Table 5).

The most commonly used remission-maintenance treatment was AZA, followed by MTX, MMF, and RTX (Table 5). There was no association between maintenance therapy and practice location (Canada vs. USA vs. other; p = 0.2009, n = 139), years of practice (<5 vs. 5 or more; p = 0.3042, n = 141), or total number of patients seen with GPA/MPA (<10 vs. 10 patients or more; p = 0.8328, n = 141). The provisional choice for maintenance therapy duration of 24 (46%), 18 (19%), 36 (14%), or 12 (13%) months was associated with total patient experience: 75% of respondents who had seen more than 10 GPA/MPA patients in their careers planned for at least 24 months of therapy, compared to 52% of those who had seen fewer than 10 patients (OR = 3.0 [1.4, 6.4], p = 0.0161, n = 127). Duration of maintenance therapy was not associated with practice location (Canada vs. USA vs. other; p = 0.3110, n = 130) or years of practice (<5 vs. 5 or more; OR = 1.6 [0.70, 3.89], p = 0.3109, n = 127). Concurrent corticosteroid duration initiated at induction was typically six (39%) or 12 (40%) months, with some respondents continuing for 18 (6%), 24 (4%), or 36 (0.7%) months and 11% chose variable periods according to disease severity. 93% of respondents routinely recommended plasma exchange in certain situations: severe pulmonary hemorrhage and/or rapidly progressive renal disease (76%), rapidly progressive renal disease only (8%), pulmonary hemorrhage only (5%), and with co-existent conditions (10%).

Interest in clinical registries

All respondents felt that an international collaborative registry was important for comparative outcome assessment of treatment strategies for GPA/MPA, with 64% of respondents selecting "very important" (mode 5, median 5, IQR 4-5). Primary motivations for participation in clinical studies or collaborative registries included the potential to improve outcomes for children with AAV (91%), access to available tools and resources (58%), endorsement by a formal network of investigators (49%), potential publication authorship (46%), and association with specific research objectives (40%). Only 15% of respondents felt that a monetary stipend was a major motivation. Registry-associated resources believed to be of most value included an automated PVAS calculator (82%), an online algorithm to stage disease severity with links to corresponding treatment guidelines (68%), an automated PVDI calculator (66%), a classification tool based on entered patient data (54%), and a printable table to track patient data over multiple visits (54%). Most clinicians had resources available to assist with the use of registry data entry and clinical tools, including computer and internet access in the clinic (80% each) and a trainee or fellow (58%). Fewer had a research assistant (47%), support for review board applications (37%), technology support (33%), or a research nurse (23%). Major barriers to registry participation included insufficient support for data entry (59%), lack of time (43%), burden of ethics review board approval (32%), and lack of patients (24%).

Discussion

This survey emphasizes the limited individual experience among clinicians caring for children with GPA and MPA and reiterates clinicians' aspirations to study childhood-onset vasculitis independently from adult disease [3]. International collaborations within the last decade have facilitated the development of pediatric-specific classification criteria for GPA [9] and scoring tools for disease activity and damage [12, 15]. They have also evaluated the pediatric utility of adult patient algorithms for classifying MPA [16] and staging disease severity [17]. Moreover, the recent revision of the CHCC definitions is relevant to both adults and children [1]. These newly developed criteria, definitions, and clinical tools are essential for systematic evaluation of drug efficacy. However, the present survey reveals limited uptake by pediatric caregivers and identifies several challenges in the development, implementation, and evaluation of pediatric treatment guidelines.

Distinguishing GPA from MPA

Most respondents believed that the distinction between GPA and MPA in patients with AAV was important for prognostication, consistent with meta-analyses of adult studies showing lower 5-year survival in MPA versus GPA [18] and of pediatric studies showing less frequent relapses [18] and more severe renal disease [16] in MPA. While respondents were familiar with both the ACR 1990 criteria for GPA [9] and its EULAR/PRINTO/PRES 2008 pediatric adaptation, neither organization includes criteria to define MPA [8, 19]. Not surprisingly, respondents often used multiple methods to differentiate (subclassify) GPA and MPA phenotypes, and 25% reported sometimes not differentiating. Frequently, ANCA specificity to PR3 or MPO was used "erroneously" as the primary differentiating criterion to define GPA and MPA, respectively. Adult studies suggest that genetics, pathophysiology, and clinical outcomes may be more strongly associated with antibody status than with the clinical syndromes [20]; although the populations defined by PR3 or MPO antibodies overlap with GPA and MPA, respectively, they are not the same. Indeed, most respondents were not aware of the recently revised CHCC 2012 definitions that do not incorporate ANCA specificity but arguably provide the clearest discriminating definitions of GPA and MPA [1]. Moreover, less than 20% of respondents were familiar with the European Medicines Agency (EMA) classification algorithm or its pediatric modification [21, 22]. However, this is a complicated tool primarily used in the research setting.

Clinical scoring tools

Multiple national and international rheumatology organizations have published treatment guidelines for management of AAV in adults [23–31]. Many require formal clinical measurement tools to assess disease "severity" (to stratify appropriate therapy) and "activity" (to determine when to start, stop, or modify therapy). These standardized measures also guide entry of adult patients into research studies and will inevitably guide research eligibility in children. However, one third of respondents reported only sometimes tailoring induction therapy to a formalized disease severity scale, suggesting that other factors – likely including informal assessment, histopathology [32], and specific organ involvement – influence management decisions. In children, PVAS [12] may show better correlation with treatment decisions than the BVAS v.3 [33]; nevertheless, equal proportions of respondents used BVAS or its variants. Furthermore, evaluation of permanent damage from disease or treatment is required for outcome assessment and may allow prediction of mortality [34]. The PVDI is a relatively recent pediatric modification of the adult VDI [14] yet to be validated [15]; however, few respondents used either tool. Lack of knowledge or familiarity – as well as perceived lack of utility – may account for some lack of uptake. Successful implementation of practice guidelines requiring standardized assessment tools will depend on improved clinician engagement, clear clinical utility, and feasibility of use.

Treatment practices

Consistent with guidelines for treatment of adults with AAV, all survey respondents employed a remission-induction and remission-maintenance model. Although 25% of respondents used EULAR/EUVAS recommendations to guide their treatment decisions, many employed a combination of resources. There was significant variation in medication and dosing regimens for childhood GPA/MPA, with variable use of evidence-based recommendations from existing adult guidelines.

Potential engagement in comparative effectiveness research

An overwhelming majority of respondents believed in the need for pediatric-specific treatment guidelines and supported guideline development by expert group consensus. It is not simple to reconcile these aspirations with the limited uptake of recent pediatric-specific research and consensus reports, although the described lack of knowledge or familiarity – as well as unclear added benefit beyond current practice – likely contribute. In view of the high frequency of renal disease (75%) among pediatric AAV patients [16] and the existing high level of cross-specialty collaboration, future efforts towards developing and implementing guidelines for managing patients with AAV must further engage pediatric nephrologists.

A recent European initiative to develop standards of care for pediatric rheumatic diseases, SHARE (Single Hub and Access point for Paediatric Rheumatology in Europe) [35], will soon provide consensus-based guidelines for management of pediatric vasculitides, including GPA [36]. While many of these recommendations will be based on adult data, most survey respondents favored longer-term comparative outcome assessment of a range of possible consensus approaches. Given barriers to uptake of existing pediatric-specific tools – many of which will be part of standardized guidelines – incentives for implementation are critical. A registry that provides treatment guidelines endorsed by national/international rheumatology organizations, access to clinical tools with automated scoring calculators, and individual patient summary progress reports might further improve engagement and uptake.

Limitations of this study include a sample population that likely underestimates true variability in practice given the selection bias associated with elective survey completion [37] and response rates below 50% [38]. Participants were reached through formal organizations and therefore may represent a particularly informed group, leading to overestimation of the use of clinical tools and guidelines. Moreover, the survey included few respondents outside Europe and North America, and therefore is limited in generalizability particularly with respect to practice variation in Asian and African countries.

Conclusions

Taken together, these data suggest a need for and interest in consensus treatment guidelines for pediatric GPA and MPA. They also point to potential challenges associated with guideline development and implementation. Understanding the barriers to uptake of existing classification criteria and formal assessment tools will inform efforts to improve standardization of classification and assessment to guide therapy. Physicians' aspirations for pediatric-specific, evidence-based treatments may motivate uptake of guidelines that evolve from this needs assessment survey and, imminently, from SHARE. Consensus-derived guidelines that include a range of specific treatment options – if provided together with mechanisms for comparative effectiveness research through an international registry – may facilitate clinician engagement and ultimately lead to improved outcomes for children with AAV.

Abbreviations

AAV: Antineutrophil cytoplasmic antibody-associated vasculitis; ANCA: Antineutrophil cytoplasmic antibody; ARChiVe: A registry for childhood vasculitis; AZA: Azathioprine; BVAS: Birmingham vasculitis activity score; CAPRI: Canadian alliance of pediatric rheumatology investigators; CARRA: Childhood arthritis and rheumatology research alliance; CHCC: Chapel hill consensus conference; CYC: Cyclophosphamide; EGPA: Eosinophilic granulomatosis with polyangiitis; EMA: European medicines agency; EULAR: European league against rheumatism; EUVAS: European vasculitis study group; GPA: Granulomatosis with polyangiitis; IQR: Interquartile range; MMF: Mycophenolate mofetil; MPA: Microscopic polyangiitis; MTX: Methotrexate; PedVas: Pediatric vasculitis initiative; PRES: Pediatric Rheumatology European Society; PRINTO: Paediatric rheumatology international trials organisation; PVAS: Pediatric vasculitis activity score; PVDI: Pediatric vasculitis damage index; RTX: Rituximab; SHARE: Single hub and access point for Paediatric Rheumatology in Europe; VDI: Vasculitis damage index; WGET: Wegener's granulomatosis etanercept trial

Acknowledgements

The authors thank CARRA, CAPRI, the Vasculitis Working Group of PRES, and the Australian Paediatric Rheumatology Group for input into survey design and/or distribution to their members. CARRA is supported by NIAMS, Friends of CARRA, and the Arthritis Foundation. We also thank Angelyne Sarmiento Rivera and Jayson Tan (British Columbia Children's Hospital) for assistance with REDCap and preliminary data analysis, respectively.

Funding

This work was supported by a Canadian Institutes of Health Research grant for the PedVas Initiative [TR2-119188 to DAC].

Authors' contributions

DAC conceived of the study. CW-R, KLB, KAM, CM, and DAC developed the pilot survey. LW-W, EY, SCL, KMO, SKB, PB, RC reviewed, pilot-tested, and modified the survey for the final draft. CW-R analyzed the data with input from JML and prepared the initial manuscript draft. All authors participated in the writing of the manuscript and also read and approved the final draft for submission.

Consent for publication

Not applicable

Competing interests

The authors declare that they have no competing interests.

Author details

[1]Clinical Professor, Division of Rheumatology, Department of Pediatrics, University of British Columbia, BC Children's Hospital, Room K4-119 4480 Oak Street Vancouver, Vancouver, BC V6H 3V4, Canada. [2]Simon Fraser University, Burnaby, BC, Canada. [3]University of Chicago Comer Children's Hospital, Chicago, USA. [4]University of California – Los Angeles, Los Angeles, CA, USA. [5]Joseph M. Sanzari Children's Hospital, Hackensack, NJ, USA. [6]Riley Hospital for Children at IU Health, Indianapolis, IN, USA. [7]Morristown Medical Center, Morristown, NJ, USA. [8]Great Ormond Street Hospital NHS Foundation Trust, London, UK. [9]Ospedale Pediatrico Meyer Firenze, Florence, Italy.

References

1. Jennette JC, Falk RJ, Bacon PA, Basu N, Cid MC, Ferrario F, Flores-Suarez LF, Gross WL, Guillevin L, Hagen EC, et al. Revised international Chapel Hill consensus conference nomenclature of Vasculitides. Arthritis Rheum. 2012;2013(65):1–11.
2. Morishita K, Brown K, Cabral D. Pediatric vasculitis: advances in treatment. Curr Opin Rheumatol. 2015;27:493–9.

3. Wilkinson NM, Page J, Uribe AG, Espinosa V, Cabral DA. Establishment of a pilot pediatric registry for chronic vasculitis is both essential and feasible: a childhood arthritis and rheumatology alliance (CARRA) survey. J Rheumatol. 2007;34:224–6.
4. Cabral D, Benseler S, Foell D, Hancock RE, Ross C, Graham J, Luqmani R. Chronic primary vasculitis in children: a new research opportunity. CRAJ. 2012;22:10–1.
5. Huber AM, Giannini EH, Bowyer SL, Kim S, Lang B, Lindsley CB, Pachman LM, Pilkington C, Reed AM, Rennebohm RM, et al. Protocols for the initial treatment of moderately severe juvenile dermatomyositis: results of a Children's arthritis and rheumatology research alliance consensus conference. Arthritis Care Res. 2010;62:219–25.
6. Harris PA, Taylor R, Thielke R, Payne J, Gonzalez N, Conde JG. Research electronic data capture (REDCap) - a metadata-driven methodology and workflow process for providing translational research informatics support. J Biomed Inform. 2009;42:377–81.
7. Benjamini Y, Hochberg Y. Controlling the false discovery rate - a practical and powerful approach to multiple testing. J R Stat Soc Series B Stat Methodol. 1995;57:289–300.
8. Leavitt RY, Fauci AS, Bloch DA, Michel BA, Hunder GG, Arend WP, Calabrese LH, Fries JF, Lie JT, Lightfoot RW Jr, et al. The American College of Rheumatology 1990 Criteria for the classification of Wegener's granulomatosis. Arthritis Rheum. 1990;33:1101–7.
9. Ozen S, Pistorio A, Iusan SM, Bakkaloglu A, Herlin T, Brik R, Buoncompagni A, Lazar C, Bilge I, Uziel Y, et al. EULAR/PRINTO/PRES criteria for Henoch-Schonlein purpura, childhood polyarteritis nodosa, childhood Wegener granulomatosis and childhood Takayasu arteritis: Ankara 2008. Part II: final classification criteria. Ann Rheum Dis. 2010;69:798–806.
10. Jennette JC, Falk RJ, Andrassy K, Bacon PA, Churg J, Gross WL, Hagen EC, Hoffman GS, Hunder GG, Kallenberg CG, et al. Nomenclature of systemic vasculitides. Proposal of an international consensus conference. Arthritis Rheum. 1994;37:187–92.
11. Luqmani RA, Bacon PA, Moots RJ, Janssen BA, Pall A, Emery P, Savage C, Adu D. Birmingham Vasculitis activity score (BVAS) in systemic necrotizing vasculitis. QJM. 1994;87:671–8.
12. Dolezalova P, Price-Kuehne FE, Ozen S, Benseler SM, Cabral DA, Anton J, Brunner J, Cimaz R, O'Neil KM, Wallace CA, et al. Disease activity assessment in childhood Vasculitis: development and preliminary validation of the paediatric Vasculitis activity score (PVAS). Ann Rheum Dis. 2013;72:1628–33.
13. Stone JH, Hoffman GS, Merkel PA, Min YI, Uhlfelder ML, Hellmann DB, Specks U, Allen NB, Davis JC, Spiera RF, et al. A disease-specific activity index for Wegener's granulomatosis: modification of the Birmingham Vasculitis activity score. International network for the study of the systemic Vasculitides (INSSYS). Arthritis Rheum. 2001;44:912–20.
14. Exley AR, Bacon PA, Luqmani RA, Kitas GD, Gordon C, Savage CO, Adu D. Development and initial validation of the Vasculitis damage index for the standardized clinical assessment of damage in the systemic vasculitides. Arthritis Rheum. 1997;40:371–80.
15. Dolezalova P, Wilkinson NW, Brogan PA, Anton J, Benseler SM, Brunner J, Cabral DA, Cimaz R, O'Neil KM, Özen S, Luqmani R. Paediatric Vasculitis damage index: a new tool for standardised disease assessment. Ann Rheum Dis. 2014;73:696–7.
16. Cabral DA, Canter DL, Muscal E, Nanda K, Wahezi DM, Spalding SJ, Twilt M, Benseler SM, Campillo S, Charuvanij S, et al. Comparing presenting clinical features of 48 children with microscopic polyangiitis (MPA) against 183 having granulomatosis with polyangiitis (GPA). An ARChiVe study. Arthritis Rheumatol. 2016;68:2514–26.
17. Morishita K, Guzman J, Chira P, Muscal E, Zeft A, Klein-Gitelman M, Uribe AG, Abramson L, Benseler SM, Eberhard A, et al. Do adult disease severity subclassifications predict use of cyclophosphamide in children with ANCA-associated vasculitis? An analysis of ARChiVe study treatment decisions. J Rheumatol. 2012;39:2012–20.
18. Iudici M, Quartier P, Terrier B, Mouthon L, Guillevin L, Puechal X. Childhood-onset granulomatosis with polyangiitis and microscopic polyangiitis: systematic review and meta-analysis. Orphanet J Rare Dis. 2016;11:141.
19. Fries JF, Hunder GG, Bloch DA, Michel BA, Arend WP, Calabrese LH, Fauci AS, Leavitt RY, Lie JT, Lightfoot RW, Jr., et al: The American College of Rheumatology 1990 criteria for the classification of vasculitis. Summary. Arthritis Rheum 1990, 33:1135-1136.
20. Pepper RJ, Salama AD. Classifying and predicting outcomes in ANCA-associated glomerulonephritis. Nephrol Dial Transplant. 2012;27:2135–7.
21. Uribe AG, Huber AM, Kim S, O'Neil KM, Wahezi DM, Abramson L, Baszis K, Benseler SM, Bowyer SL, Campillo S, et al. Increased sensitivity of the European medicines agency algorithm for classification of childhood granulomatosis with polyangiitis. J Rheumatol. 2012;39:1687–97.
22. Watts R, Lane S, Hanslik T, Hauser T, Hellmich B, Koldingsnes W, Mahr A, Segelmark M, Cohen-Tervaert JW, Scott D. Development and validation of a consensus methodology for the classification of the ANCA-associated vasculitides and polyarteritis nodosa for epidemiological studies. Ann Rheum Dis. 2007;66:222–7.
23. McGeoch L, Twilt M, Famorca L, Bakowsky V, Barra L, Benseler S, Cabral DA, Carette S, Cox GP, Dhindsa N, et al. CanVasc recommendations for the management of antineutrophil cytoplasm antibody (ANCA)-associated vasculitides - executive summary. Can J Kidney Health Dis. 2015;2:43.
24. Lapraik C, Watts R, Bacon P, Carruthers D, Chakravarty K, D'Cruz D, Guillevin L, Harper L, Jayne D, Luqmani R, et al. BSR and BHPR guidelines for the management of adults with ANCA associated vasculitis. Rheumatology. 2007;46:1615–6.
25. Ntatsaki E, Carruthers D, Chakravarty K, D'Cruz D, Harper L, Jayne D, Luqmani R, Mills J, Mooney J, Venning M, et al. BSR and BHPR guideline for the management of adults with ANCA-associated vasculitis. Rheumatology. 2014;53:2306–9.
26. French Vasculitis Study Group: Vascularites nécrosantes systémiques - Protocole national de diagnostic et de soins. L'Haute autorité de santé de France; 2009.
27. Charles P, Bienvenu B, Bonnotte B, Gobert P, Godmer P, Hachulla E, Hamidou M, Harle JR, Karras A, Lega JC, et al. Rituximab: recommendations of the French Vasculitis study group (FVSG) for induction and maintenance treatments of adult, antineutrophil cytoplasm antibody-associated necrotizing vasculitides. Presse Med. 2013;42:1317–30.
28. KDIGO Work Group. Kidney Disease: Improving Global Outcomes (KDIGO) Glomerulonephritis Work Group: KDIGO Clinical Practice Guideline for Glomerulonephritis. Kidney Int. 2012;2:139–274.
29. Mukhtyar C, Guillevin L, Cid MC, Dasgupta B, de Groot K, Gross W, Hauser T, Hellmich B, Jayne D, Kallenberg CG, et al. EULAR recommendations for the management of primary small and medium vessel vasculitis. Ann Rheum Dis. 2009;68:310–7.
30. Menahem S, Hiremagalur B, Mudge D, Toussaint N, Walters G. Caring for Australians with renal impairment: the CARI guidelines. Induction and maintenance therapy in ANCA-associated systemic vasculitis. Nephrology. 2008;13(Suppl 2):S24–36.
31. Japanese Circulation Society Joint Working Group: Guideline for management of vasculitis syndrome (JCS 2008). Japanese Circulation Society. Circ J. 2011(75):474–503.
32. Berden AE, Ferrario F, Hagen EC, Jayne DR, Jennette JC, Joh K, Neumann I, Noel LH, Pusey CD, Waldherr R, et al. Histopathologic classification of ANCA-associated glomerulonephritis. J Am Soc Nephrol. 2010;21:1628–36.
33. Morishita K, Li SC, Muscal E, Spalding S, Guzman J, Uribe A, Abramson L, Baszis K, Benseler S, Bowyer S, et al. Assessing the performance of the Birmingham Vasculitis activity score at diagnosis for children with antineutrophil cytoplasmic antibody-associated Vasculitis in a registry for childhood Vasculitis (ARChiVe). J Rheumatol. 2012;39:1088–94.
34. Bhamra K, Luqmani R. Damage assessment in ANCA-associated vasculitis. Curr Rheumatol Rep. 2012;14:494–500.
35. Wulffraat NM, Vastert B. SHARE consortium: time to share. Pediatr Rheumatol Online J. 2013;11:5.
36. de Graeff N, Groot N, Kamphuis S, Beresford M. FRI0271 final evidence-based recommendations for diagnosis and treatment of paediatric Vasculitides. Ann Rheum Dis. 2015;74:522–3.
37. Khazaal Y, van Singer M, Chatton A, Achab S, Zullino D, Rothen S, Khan R, Billieux J, Thorens G. Does self-selection affect samples' representativeness in online surveys? An investigation in online video game research. J Med Internet Res. 2014;16:e164.
38. Edwards PJ, Roberts I, Clarke MJ, DiGuiseppi C, Wentz R, Kwan I, Cooper R, Felix LM, Pratap S. Methods to increase response to postal and electronic questionnaires. Cochrane Database of Systematic Reviews. 2009. Issue 3. Art. No.: MR000008. doi:10.1002/14651858.MR000008.pub4.
39. Mukhtyar C, Lee R, Brown D, Carruthers D, Dasgupta B, Dubey S, Flossmann O, Hall C, Hollywood J, Jayne D, et al. Modification and validation of the Birmingham Vasculitis activity score (version 3). Ann Rheum Dis. 2009;68:1827–32.
40. Mahr AD, Neogi T, Lavalley MP, Davis JC, Hoffman GS, McCune WJ, Specks U, Spiera RF, St Clair EW, Stone JH, et al. Assessment of the item selection and weighting in the Birmingham vasculitis activity score for Wegener's granulomatosis. Arthritis Rheum. 2008;59:884–91.

41. European therapeutic trials in ANCA-associated systemic vasculitis: disease scoring, consensus regimens and proposed clinical trials. European Community study group on clinical trials in systemic Vasculitis ECSYSVASTRIAL. Clin Exp Immunol. 1995;101(Suppl 1):29–34.
42. Guillevin L, Pagnoux C, Seror R, Mahr A, Mouthon L, Le Toumelin P. French Vasculitis study G: the five-factor score revisited: assessment of prognoses of systemic necrotizing vasculitides based on the French Vasculitis study group (FVSG) cohort. Medicine. 2011;90:19–27.
43. Stone JH. Wegener's Granulomatosis Etanercept trial research group: limited versus severe Wegener's granulomatosis: baseline data on patients in the Wegener's granulomatosis etanercept trial. Arthritis Rheum. 2003;48:2299–309.
44. de Groot K, Gross WL, Herlyn K, Reinhold-Keller E. Development and validation of a disease extent index for Wegener's granulomatosis. Clin Nephrol. 2001;55:31–8.
45. Seo P, Luqmani RA, Flossmann O, Hellmich B, Herlyn K, Hoffman GS, Jayne D, Kallenberg CG, Langford CA, Mahr A, et al. The future of damage assessment in vasculitis. J Rheumatol. 2007;34:1357–71.
46. Suppiah R, Flossman O, Mukhtyar C, Alberici F, Baslund B, Brown D, Hasan N, Holle J, Hruskova Z, Jayne D, et al. Measurement of damage in systemic Vasculitis: a comparison of the Vasculitis damage index with the combined damage assessment index. Ann Rheum Dis. 2011;70:80–5.

Fecal calprotectin in juvenile idiopathic arthritis patients related to drug use

Kristiina Aalto*, Pekka Lahdenne and Kaija-Leena Kolho

Abstract

Background: Patients with juvenile idiopathic arthritis (JIA) on non-steroidal anti- inflammatory drugs (NSAIDs) may experience abdominal pain. In adults, NSAID use has been linked to an increase in fecal calprotectin (FC) levels, a surrogate marker for gut inflammation. In JIA, data on gut inflammation related to drug use is scarce.

Methods: JIA patients followed up at the outpatient pediatric rheumatology clinic in Children's Hospital, Helsinki University Hospital, Helsinki, Finland were routinely assessed for FC if they complained about abdominal pain, had an elevated erythrocyte sedimentation rate (ESR) or used NSAIDs on a daily basis. The FC levels were related to the presence of abdominal pain, to ESR, and to the presence of HLA-B27.

Results: Of the total group of 90 patients (median age 9.1 years; 45 JIA patients with disease modifying anti-rheumatic drugs (DMARDs), 25 without DMARD medication, and 20 arthralgia patients as controls), approximately 50% used NSAIDs, of whom 40% complained about abdominal pain. In patients with abdominal pain, one-third had elevated FC values (>100 μg/g). The FC values, for the most part, declined along with the discontinuation or reduction of NSAIDs and after intensifying the DMARD medication, where after the pain disappeared. In patients with an elevated ESR, the FC values and ESR normalized in parallel. The presence of HLA-B27 was not associated with FC levels.

Conclusion: In patients with JIA and abdominal pain, it may be useful to determine the FC when evaluating the need for further gastrointestinal examinations.

Keywords: Abdominal pain, Biological markers, Child, Diagnosis, Gut, IBD

Background

In patients with juvenile idiopathic arthritis (JIA), a chronic joint inflammation of childhood, non-steroidal anti-inflammatory drugs (NSAIDs) are frequently needed. When the disease activity is low, NSAIDs can be used as a monotherapy for up to two months [1]. However, it has been reported that JIA patients may experience abdominal pain related to NSAID use [2]. NSAIDs may cause intestinal damage in adults [3], but there are less data about children [4, 5]. The differential diagnosis of abdominal symptoms, however, is challenging. On the other hand, a considerable proportion of patients with inflammatory bowel disease (IBD) may have joint pains [6, 7].

To assess the presence of inflammation in the gut in detail, endoscopy is needed. However, especially in children this procedure is challenging; it is invasive and has to be performed under anesthesia. Thus, during recent years, the use of surrogate markers of gut inflammation, such as fecal calprotectin (FC), has emerged as a valuable screening tool [8–12]. In active IBD, the correlation between the endoscopy results and FC levels is good [9–11, 13]. Several reports have shown that NSAID use in adults may result in an increase in FC levels, reflecting intestinal inflammation, and furthermore, the FC levels decline when the drug is discontinued, suggesting healing of the gut mucosa [14].

Calprotectin, a major cytosolic protein released during the activation of neutrophils, is a relatively new marker for inflammatory processes in the endothelium [15]. An increase in the serum calprotectin level is seen in several inflammatory conditions, including JIA [16]. Calprotectin is stable in feces, and fecal concentrations reflect not only colonic inflammation, but the presence of small bowel

* Correspondence: kristiina.aalto@hus.fi
Helsinki University Central Hospital, Children's Hospital, University of Helsinki, Helsinki 00029 HUCH, Finland

involvement as well [9, 10]. FC levels are high among patients with active IBD, providing a diagnostic tool for differentiating between recurrent abdominal pain and chronic inflammatory disease in the intestine [11, 12, 17] and reducing the need of referrals for further investigations [18]. The significance of minor elevations in FC levels is poorly understood, but dysfunctional pain is not related to FC values [12]. Constipation may be associated with a slight elevation in FC values [19].

In patients with JIA, data on the performance of FC levels in the assessment of intestinal inflammation are limited. At our hospital, we have routinely used FC measurements for several years to screen for the presence of gut inflammation in paediatric patients with non-specific abdominal symptoms, e.g. abdominal pain. The aim of this study was to evaluate the usefulness of FC measurements in patients with JIA associated with NSAID use and abdominal pain.

Methods

A group of 90 patients followed up at the outpatient clinic of pediatric rheumatology in Children's Hospital, Helsinki University Hospital, Helsinki, Finland, a tertiary care hospital, were routinely assessed for FC when they complained about abdominal pain, had an elevated erythrocyte sedimentation rate (ESR) or used NSAIDs on a daily basis. Of the 90 patients, 50 had JIA for at least 6 months, 20 patients had newly diagnosed JIA (Table 1). As controls we had 20 patients with arthralgia who were referred to our hospital for evaluation of JIA (Table 1). No patients with systemic-onset JIA were included and there were no patients with psoriasis or undifferentiated arthritis.

Table 1 Clinical characteristics of the patients; 70 having the JIA diagnosis and 20 arthralgia

All patients *n* = 90	Oligo *n* = 33	Poly *n* = 29	JSpA *n* = 8	All JIA *n* = 70	Arthralgia *n* = 20
Age	10.2 ± 3.8	8.1 ± 3.5	11.8 ± 3.0	9.6 ± 3.9	8.7 ± 4.9
Female	25 (57%)	19 (43%)	0	44 (63%)	13 (65%)
ANA-Ab +	4 (12%)	6 (21%)	0	9 (13%)	1 (5%)
Anaemia	10 (30%)	9 (31%)	3 (38%)	22 (31%)	1 (5%)
HLA-B27 +	9 (27%)	6 (21%)	7 (88%)	22 (31%)	5 (25%)
Active disease	8 (24%)	9 (31%)	0	17 (24%)	0
NSAID +	15 (45%)	14 (48%)	5 (63%)	34 (49%)	12 (60%)
DMARD +	20 (61%)	20 (69%)	5 (63%)	45 (64%)	0
Biologicals +	3 (10%)	2 (7%)	0	5 (7%)	0

JIA juvenile idiopathic arthritis
Oligo juvenile oligoarthritis, *Poly* juvenile polyarthritis (RF-negative), *JSpA* juvenile spondyloarthritis (including enthesitis related arthritis)
ANA-Ab antinuclear antibodies
DMARD disease-modifying anti-rheumatic drug
mainly methotrexate (MTX), other DMARDS: leflunomide, sulphasalazine (SSZ), hydroxychloroquine, cyclosporine A (CyA)
- Ten patients had ≥1 DMARD (usually MTX + SSZ), one patient had CyA with SSZ
NSAID non-steroidal anti-inflammatory drug

JIA diagnosis was based on the criteria of the International League of Associations for Rheumatology (ILAR) [20]. At the time of JIA diagnosis, the presence of HLA-B27, serum antinuclear antibodies (S-ANA) and rheumatoid factor were routinely determined. The disease was considered active (Table 1) if there were active joints in the clinical examination and the doctor's global assessment of the disease using a visual analogue scale (VAS) was > 1 (range 0–10) or if the ESR was higher than 20 mm/h, which is comparable to a JIA disease activity score of JADAS10 > 2 [21].

Fecal calprotectin (FC)

The FC levels were analyzed using a quantitative, enzyme-linked immunoassay (PhiCal Test, Calpro AS, Oslo, Norway) in routine analyses of the central laboratory services of the Helsinki University Hospital. The fecal samples were stored at –20°C until analyzed. FC values <100 µg/g in the stools were considered normal and values <50 µg/g very low, whereas values >1000 mg/g were found to be exceedingly high [22–24]. Measurements of FC levels were made on clinical grounds, i.e. when the patient complained of abdominal pain or had an elevated ESR or was using NSAIDs on a daily basis. Elevated FC levels were controlled at regular follow-up visits until normal.

Endoscopies were performed when the FC value was > 200-300 µg/g. When the FC value was only mildly or moderately elevated with no major symptoms, NSAIDs were discontinued.

Statistical analyses

Data are presented as means (± standard deviation), or as ranges and medians, as appropriate. Correlations between the parameters were calculated using either a Spearman rank correlation, the Kruskall-Wallis test, or logistic regression (with a threshold of elevated FC value <100 µg/g or <50 µg/g), when appropriate and statistical comparisons between groups were performed using the Student's *t*-test (normal distribution) or the Mann-Whitney *U* test. Statistical analyses were performed using Microsoft® software Excel 2010 or with IBM® SPSS® Statistics 19 software. A *p*-value <0.05 was considered significant.

Results

FC values in the patients

Of the 70 patients with JIA, 45 (64%) were on DMARD medication (Table 1). In these 45 patients, FC values ranged from 1 to 1617 µg/g (Table 2): ten (22%) had elevated FC values (>100 µg/g), six had FC values between 50 and 100 µg/g, and 29 had FC values less

Table 2 Diagnoses of the patients and proportion of patients with abdominal pain, NSAID usage, and their ESR and FC values

All patients (*n* = 90)	Abdominal pain *n* (%)	NSAID usage *n* (%)	ESR mm/h range (median) elevated (*n*)	FC µg/g range (median) elevated (*n*)
JIA patients				
Oligoarthritis (33)	13 (39%)	15 (45%)	1–80 (12) *n* = 15	1–368 (17) *n* = 5
Polyarthritis (29)	11 (38%)	14 (48%)	1–94 (16) *n* = 15	2–1617 (34) *n* = 7
JSpA* (8)	1 (13%)	5 (63%)	10–35 (19) *n* = 4	11–184 (18) *n* = 1
All JIA (70)	27 (39%)	34 (70%)	1–94 (15) *n* = 34 (49%)	1–1617 (25) *n* = 13 (19%)
Arthralgia (20)	12 (60%)	12 (60%)	7–50 (10) *n* = 7 (35%)	0–113 (32) *n* = 1 (5%)

JIA juvenile idiopathic arthritis
**JSpA* juvenile spondylarthritis
NSAID non-steroidal anti-inflammatory drug
ESR erythrocyte sedimentation rate
FC fecal calprotectin, cut-off of 100 µg/g for elevated values [17–19]

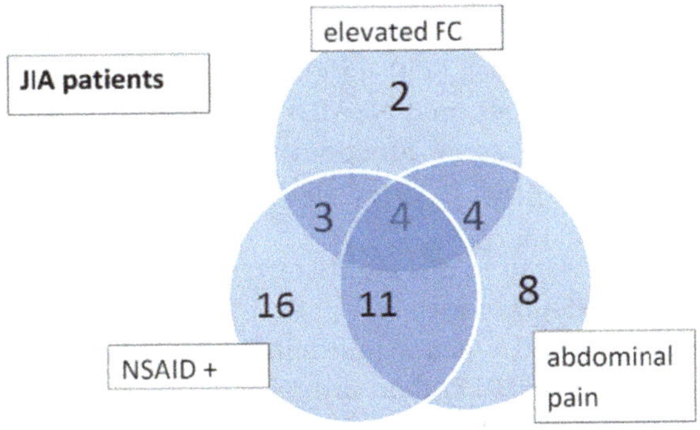

FC = fecal calprotectin, cut-off of 100 µg/g for elevated values (22 - 24)
JIA = juvenile idiopathic arthritis
NSAID = non-steroidal anti-inflammatory drug

Fig. 1 JIA patients with elevated FC-values and/or regular NSAID use and/or abdominal pain. Of the 70 patients with JIA 48 had elevated FC value and/or NSAID use and/or abdominal pain. The numbers in overlapping areas show the combinations e.g. JIA patients having both abdominal pain and elevated FC values (*n* = 8), and four of them used NSAIDs as regular bases. See the text for other details

than 50 µg/g. JIA patients with DMARDs had significantly more often a FC value > 50 µg/g than patients without DMARDs ($p = 0.029$). Of the 20 arthralgia patients (Table 2) one (5%) with abdominal pain had a mildly elevated FC value of 113 µg/g (Fig. 2) which returned to normal two months later. Twelve patients with arthralgia used NSAIDs on a daily basis.

Of the ten JIA patients on DMARDs and with elevated FC values, seven presented with abdominal pains (Tables 2 and 3, Fig. 1) and five used NSAIDs on a regular basis. Three patients underwent endoscopies. One of them had an exceedingly high FC value (1617 µg/g). This particular patient reported abdominal pain, and after medication for endoscopy-confirmed esophagitis with a proton pump inhibitor (PPI) and dietary adjustment, her pains disappeared and the FC value declined after three months. Two other patients underwent endoscopies because of abdominal pain and elevated FC values (both with values > 200 µg/g). In these two, biopsy findings revealed mild gastritis and irritation in the bowel but no pathological changes in the capsule endoscopy of the small intestine. Naproxen was discontinued, and abdominal pain subsequently disappeared in both patients. FC-values normalized in two to three months.

Table 3 FC-values of the JIA patients in relation to their abdominal pain, NSAID usage, and ESR values

All JIA patients (*n* = 70)	Abdominal pain	NSAID usage	elevated ESR >20 mm/h
FC 0–50 µg/g (*n* = 51)	38%	43%	41%
FC 50–100 µg/g (*n* = 6)	50%	83%	83%
FC 100–200 µg/g (*n* = 10)	50%	60%	70%
FC > 200 µg/g (*n* = 3)	100%	67%	67%

JIA juvenile idiopathic arthritis
NSAID non-steroidal anti-inflammatory drug
ESR erythrocyte sedimentation rate
FC fecal calprotectin

The remaining seven JIA patients using DMARDS and with FC values >100 µg/g (all with values less than 200 µg/g) did not undergo endoscopies (Tables 2 and 3). Of these patients, two suffered from constipation. After successful treatment of constipation, their FC values fell within normal ranges. The five other patients were advised to take NSAIDs only for short periods when they used NSAIDs on daily bases. Their FC values returned to normal after restricting NSAID use in all except one. In this particular patient, the FC values fluctuated between 89 and 181 µg/g during the follow-up even when he was not on NSAIDs. He also had a diagnosis of IgA deficiency and autoimmune (AI) hepatitis.

FC values were between 50 and 100 µg/g in six JIA patients with DMARDs, of whom three suffered from abdominal pain. These three had an active joint disease and used NSAIDs regularly. Several months later, one of them had an even higher FC value, 258 µg/g, but after reducing the amount of NSAIDs he was taking and increasing the dosage of DMARDs his abdominal pain disappeared, and the FC value declined to normal after two months. Similarly, when the joint disease of the other two patients was better controlled, the patients' need for NSAIDs decreased, and the FC values fell below 50 µg/g also after three to four months.

Twenty-five patients with JIA were not on DMARDS, and the majority (*n* = 20) of them had a disease duration of less than 6 months. The FC values ranged from 2 to

189 µg/g (Fig. 1, Table 3). Of the 25 patients three (12%) had elevated values (>100 µg/g), and the rest 88% had very low FC values (<50 µg/g). The three patients with elevated FC values used NSAIDs daily (Fig. 1). They also presented with some functional gastrointestinal symptoms, but only one reported abdominal pain.

FC values related to disease characteristics, abdominal pain, and NSAID usage

Patients with JIA had significantly more often elevated FC value (p = 0.017) than arthralgia patients. The presence of ANA antibodies or HLA-B27 was not associated with the elevation of FC, nor was the subtype of JIA.

In total, 27 (39%) of the 70 patients with JIA and 12 (60%) of the 20 with arthralgia experienced abdominal pain (Figs. 1 and 2, Table 2). There was a linked association between abdominal pain, elevated ESR values and elevated FC values (overall p = *0.001*). Of the 14 patients (13 with JIA and one with arthralgia) with elevated FC values (>100 µg/g, Tables 2 and 3), nine had abdominal pains and six of them had elevated ESR values. In patients with an elevated ESR, anti-rheumatic treatment was intensified which led to a decline of both the FC and ESR (data not shown).

Of the 29 JIA patients on DMARDs who had FC values of less than 50 µg/g, 11(38%) reported some abdominal pain. All except one were girls, aged 5 to 15 years, and they all had a tendency to experience other non-specific pains as well, such as limb pain and headaches.

About half of the JIA patients (n = 34) used NSAIDs regularly, and 15 (44%) of them reported abdominal pains. Among the patients taking NSAIDs daily and experiencing abdominal pain, one third had elevated FC values >100µg/g (Fig. 1, Table 2). In the whole group of 90 patients, the use of NSAIDs was associated with elevated FC levels (p = *0.03*). Even though there was no clear correlation between NSAID use and abdominal pain, in many cases, abdominal pains lessened after lowering the NSAID dosage. At the same time the DMARD medication of the JIA patients was intensified.

If the threshold of elevated FC value was lowered to 50 µg/g and a multivariate analysis made, the correlation of NSAID use came more evident. Logistic regression analysis showed that NSAID (OR = 3.96) and DMARD (OR = 3.78) use together with abdominal pain (OR = 3.96) were significantly (overall p = *0.046*) correlated to the FC elevation. Of these three parameters abdominal pain associated most strongly to the elevated FC-value.

In the JIA group, 24% had an active joint disease. Disease activity was not associated with abdominal pain or the elevated FC value (data not shown). None of the patients had celiac disease or food allergies; each child tolerated milk, except for two, one was lactose intolerant and one with a cow's milk allergy and Down's syndrome.

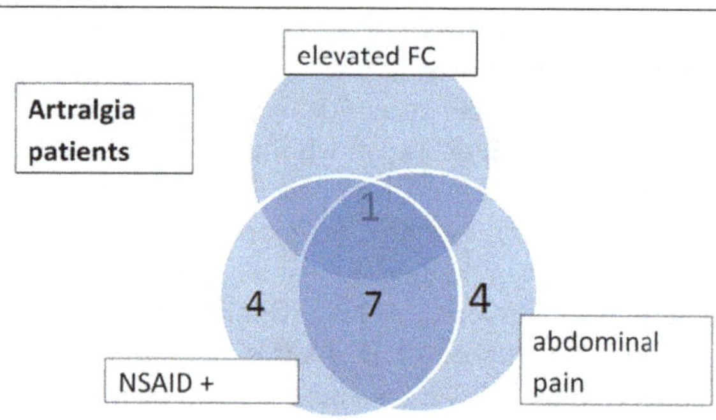

FC = fecal calprotectin, cut-off of 100 µg/g for elevated values (22 - 24)
JIA = juvenile idiopathic arthritis
NSAID = non-steroidal anti-inflammatory drug

Fig. 2 Arthralgia patients with elevated FC-values and/or regular NSAID use and/or abdominal pain. Of the 20 patients with arthralgia 12 had abdominal pain of which eight used NSAIDs (overlapping areas). See text for details

Discussion

JIA patients who were on DMARDs had significantly higher FC values than the other JIA patients, possibly suggesting intestinal inflammation. The difference, however, seemed to be associated with NSAID use, too. The higher FC values in those patients who used NSAIDs regularly returned to normal after tapering the NSAID dosage. Concurrently, in most JIA patients, DMARD medication was also intensified. Thus, it can be speculated that JIA patients may have some low activity also in the intestinal mucosa when their joint disease is not adequately controlled.

A recent comprehensive study in 44 adult spondyloarthritis (SpA) patients showed that FC can be elevated even without obvious GI symptoms [25]. There are no such studies of children. As reported in adults, the use of NSAIDs may induce a modest increase in the FC values, but rarely above 300 µg/g [26], which is in line with our findings. In a recent study [27] of adult rheumatoid arthritis (RA) and osteoarthritis (OA) patients using NSAIDs small intestinal lesions were identified significantly more often in RA (56.8%) patients compared to OA (31.9%) suggesting a possible influence of the underlying disease. They did not find any laboratory marker (hemoglobin, ESR, or fecal occult blood test) to be used as a diagnostic factor but they did not test FC. In our study the arthralgia patients had clearly lower FC values suggesting also that the underlying disease might have an explanatory role and not only the NSAID usage.

In our study most patients with higher FC values had abdominal pain, but the presence of pain varied among patients with lower FC values. The FC levels in patients without GI problems were comparable to those observed in healthy children [28]. However, our upper normal limit (<100 μg/g) is somewhat higher when compared to the manufacturer's instructions (50 μg/g) and several other studies with a different immunoassay [18, 28]. Since it has been suggested that pediatric patients having FC values greater than 50μg/g should be monitored for a possible flare-up of intestinal inflammation [28], we also stratified the patient groups according to a lower cut-off level for FC values (>50μg/g). With this lower cut-off level, the JIA patients on NSAIDs showed significantly more elevated values than other patients. These patients with elevated FC values had significantly more often also abdominal pain and DMARD medication.

When the joint disease was active patients took NSAIDs more regularly, but as such, the presence of active joint inflammation was not associated with an increase in FC values. When the joint disease was appropriately controlled and NSAIDs less often needed, the patients did not report abdominal pain. Their FC values were not elevated anymore in the control samples taken approximately two months afterwards. The fact that only five JIA patients in our study group were taking biological DMARDs indirectly shows that patients using biologics have such a low disease activity that they did not fulfill the criteria of this study (elevated ESR, NSAID usage or abdominal pain). Also, in Finland, we apply an aggressive step-down treating model [29] and therefore, most of the JIA patients used DMARDS. There is some evidence that biologics, especially etanercept, could provoke the development of IBD [30]. While three (out of five) of our patients on biologics used etanercept and had low FC values, the number of patients was too low to draw any conclusions. Recent reports suggest that patients with SpA using etanercept confer a risk of IBD [31], but we had no such patients.

All subgroups of JIA patients presented with comparable FC values, though the polyarthritis patients tended to have higher values. These higher values in polyarthritis patients were again mainly explained by NSAID use in the active joint disease. Among HLA-B27 positive JIA patients, there is a risk for evolution of IBD [32, 33], but we did not find such patients with a suspicion of IBD. Here, the proportion of HLA-B27 positive patients was quite high, though in line with earlier studies from Finland and the Nordic countries [34, 35]. In contrast, a recent study reported higher FC levels among patients with enthesitis-related arthritis (ERA, HLA-B27 positive juvenile SpA) than among other JIA patients [36]. This difference was not explained by NSAID use. However, the study reported that only one out of nine ERA patients with abdominal pain had an elevated FC value (>300 μg/g). In a recent pilot study with adult patients, elevated FC levels (cut-off value >50 μg/g) were found in 41% (of 39) patients with ankylosing spondylitis [37]. In a more recent study, the optimal cut-off value for FC detecting bowel inflammation in patients with ankylosing spondylitis was 85 μg/g [20]. In that study, the FC values were higher in patients with NSAID use, but the association with bowel inflammation remained after adjustment for the drug use. These results may indicate that ERA/SpA patients should be under careful observation for possible gut damage. The present results in pediatric patients do not support this suggestion because only one HLA-B27 positive patient had FC value greater than 100 μg/g. On the other hand, the total number of HLA-B27 positive JIA patients was limited, and more studies on this matter need to be conducted in children.

When the FC value is exceedingly high, endoscopies are recommended, but with lower values (150–300 μg/g) and minor abdominal symptoms modifying the medication and/or diet may be the primary options. One of our JIA patients had a very high FC value, which declined below the cut-off point after introducing medication for esophagitis confirmed in endoscopy and adjusting the dairy consumption. Endoscopies are invasive procedures requiring anesthesia in pediatric patients with indications to be discussed with pediatric gastroenterologists.

Taken together, we found that those JIA patients who needed NSAIDs for longer periods have often elevated FC levels. Notably, this might be a sign of suboptimal disease control. In adults e.g. chronic gastritis did not cause an increase in FC values [38]. Whether an uncontrolled joint disease could increase the risk of gut involvement remains to be seen in future studies. In the present study, one fifth of the JIA patients had an elevated FC value; none of them had signs of IBD, and only a few of the patients fulfilled indications for an endoscopy.

The fecal test was easy to carry out, and the patients readily agreed to bring a sample with them. Some patients had abdominal pains but a low FC value; those patients also had other non-specific aches and joint pains that could not be attributed to arthritis, representing the possibility of a dysfunctional pain disorder [39]. For patients with low FC levels, patients taking NSAIDs and patients experiencing minor pains, invasive and unnecessary endoscopies could be avoided [40]. Abdominal pains are common, and while another study found that 14–16% of 8-year-old Finnish children experience abdominal pain [41], in our study approximately 44% of the patients reported such pain. Notably, FC levels are low among patients with functional abdominal pain [42].

Conclusions

To conclude, we recommend determining the FC values of JIA patients who complain of abdominal pain or who regularly take NSAIDs for several weeks. If the FC value is high and remains high when cutting down exposure to NSAIDs, bowel examinations (endoscopies) should be considered. As the FC test is reliable in ruling out intestinal inflammation and can easily be repeated, it should be used more often because it is a simple non-invasive procedure for the patient.

Key messages

1) Fecal calprotectin, a surrogate marker of gut inflammation, should be measured in JIA patients complaining abdominal pain or using NSAIDs regularly.
2) When the fecal calprotectin value is consistently elevated, consider the need of endoscopies.
3) A fecal calprotectin test is a useful tool in screening for the need of gastrointestinal investigations.

Abbreviations

AI: Autoimmune; ANA: Antinuclear antibodies; CyA: Cyclosporine A; DMARDs: Disease modifying anti-rheumatic drugs; ERA: Enthesitis-related arthritis; ESR: Erythrocyte sedimentation rate; FC: Faecal calprotectin; GI: Gastrointestinal; IBD: Inflammatory bowel disease; ILAR: International League of Associations for Rheumatology; JADAS: JIA disease activity score; JIA: Juvenile idiopathic arthritis; JSpA: Juvenile spondylarthritis; MTX: Methotrexate; NSAIDs: Non-steroidal anti-inflammatory drugs; oJIA: Oligoarthritis; pJIA: Polyarthritis; PPI: Proton pump inhibitor; S-ANA: Serum antinuclear antibodies; SpA: Spondyloarthritis; SSZ: Sulphasalazine; VAS: Visual analogue scale

Acknowledgements

Not applicable.

Funding

There were no extra funding relating to this study.

Authors' contributions

All authors accompanied in designing the study, interpreted the patient data, collaborated in writing the manuscript, read and approved the final manuscript.

Competing interests

The authors declare that they have no competing interests.

Consent for publication

Not applicable.

References

1. Beukelman T, Patkar NM, Saag KG, Tolleson-Rinehart S, Cron RQ, DeWitt EM, et al. 2011 American College of Rheumatology recommendations for the treatment of juvenile idiopathic arthritis: initiation and safety monitoring of therapeutic agents for the treatment of arthritis and systemic features. Arthritis Care Res (Hoboken). 2011;63:465–82.
2. Ashorn M, Verronen P, Ruuska T, Huhtala H. Upper endoscopic findings in children with active juvenile chronic arthritis. Acta Paediatr. 2003;92:558–61.
3. Graham DY, Opekun AR, Willingham FF, Qureshi WA. Visible small-intestinal mucosal injury in chronic NSAID users. Clin Gastroenterol Hepatol. 2005;3:55–9.
4. Dowd JE, Cimaz R, Fink CW. Nonsteroidal antiinflammatory drug-induced gastroduodenal injury in children. Arthritis Rheum. 1995;38:1225–31.
5. Mulberg AE, Linz C, Bern E, Tucker L, Verhave M, Grand RJ. Identification of nonsteroidal antiinflammatory drug-induced gastroduodenal injury in children with juvenile rheumatoid arthritis. J Pediatr. 1993;122:647–9.
6. Turunen P, Ashorn M, Auvinen A, Iltanen S, Huhtala H, Kolho KL. Long-term health outcomes in pediatric inflammatory bowel disease: a population-based study. Inflamm Bowel Dis. 2009;15:56–62.
7. Orlando A, Renna S, Perricone G, Cottone M. Gastrointestinal lesions associated with spondyloarthropathies. World J Gastroenterol. 2009;15:2443–8.
8. Poullis A, Foster R, Mendall MA, Fagerhol MK. Emerging role of calprotectin in gastroenterology. J Gastroenterol Hepatol. 2003;18:756–62.
9. Sipponen T, Savilahti E, Kolho KL, Nuutinen H, Turunen U, Färkkilä M. Crohn's disease activity assessed by fecal calprotectin and lactoferrin: correlation with Crohn's disease activity index and endoscopic findings. Inflamm Bowel Dis. 2008;14:40–6.
10. Sipponen T, Kärkkäinen P, Savilahti E, Kolho KL, Nuutinen H, Turunen U, et al. Correlation of faecal calprotectin and lactoferrin with an endoscopic score for Crohn's disease and histological findings. Aliment Pharmacol Ther. 2008;28:1221–9.
11. Henderson P, Casey A, Lawrence SJ, Kennedy NA, Kingstone K, Rogers P, et al. The diagnostic accuracy of fecal calprotectin during the investigation of suspected pediatric inflammatory bowel disease. Am J Gastroenterol. 2012;107:941–9.
12. Van Rheenen PF, Van de Vijver E, Fidler V. Faecal calprotectin for screening of patients with suspected inflammatory bowel disease: diagnostic meta-analysis. BMJ. 2010;341:c3369.
13. Lewis JD. The utility of biomarkers in the diagnosis and therapy of inflammatory bowel disease. Gastroenterology. 2011;140:1817–26. e2.
14. Tibble JA, Sigthorsson G, Foster R, Scott D, Fagerhol MK, Roseth A, et al. High prevalence of NSAID enteropathy as shown by a simple faecal test. Gut. 1999;45:362–6.
15. Johne B, Fagerhol MK, Lyberg T, Prydz H, Brandtzaeg P, Naess-Andresen CF, et al. Functional and clinical aspects of the myelomonocyte protein calprotectin. Mol Pathol. 1997;50:113–23.
16. Frosch M, Strey A, Vogl T, Wulffraat NM, Kuis W, Sunderkötter C, et al. Myeloid-related proteins 8 and 14 are specifically secreted during interaction of phagocytes and activated endothelium and are useful markers for monitoring disease activity in pauciarticular-onset juvenile rheumatoid arthritis. Arthritis Rheum. 2000;43:628–37.
17. Olafsdottir E, Aksnes L, Fluge G, Berstad A. Faecal calprotectin levels in infants with infantile colic, healthy infants, children with inflammatory bowel disease, children with recurrent abdominal pain and healthy children. Acta Paediatr. 2002;91:45–50.
18. Van de Vijver E, Schreuder AB, Cnossen WR, Muller Kobold AC, van Rheenen PF, North Netherlands Pediatric IBD Consortium. Safely ruling out inflammatory bowel disease in children and teenagers without referral for endoscopy. Arch Dis Child. 2012;97:1014–8.
19. Fernell E, Fagerberg UL, Hellström PM. No evidence for a clear link between active intestinal inflammation and autism based on analyses of faecal calprotectin and rectal nitric oxide. Acta Paediatr. 2007;96:1076–9.
20. Petty RE, Southwood TR, Manners P, Baum J, Glass DN, Goldenberg J, et al. International League of Associations for Rheumatology classification of juvenile idiopathic arthritis: second revision, Edmonton, 2001. J Rheumatol. 2004;31:390–2.
21. Consolaro A, Ruperto N, Bazso A, Pistorio A, Magni-Manzoni S, Filocamo G, et al. Paediatric Rheumatology International Trials Organisation. Development and validation of a composite disease activity score for juvenile idiopathic arthritis. Arthritis Rheum. 2009;61:658–66.
22. Kolho KL, Turner D. Fecal calprotectin and clinical disease activity in pediatric ulcerative colitis. ISRN Gastroenterol. 2013;2013:179024.
23. Kolho K-L, Raivio T, Lindahl H, Savilahti E. Fecal calprotectin remains high during glucocorticoid therapy in children with inflammatory bowel disease. Scand J Gastroenterol. 2006;41:720–5.
24. Sipponen T, Kolho KL. Faecal calprotectin in children with clinically quiescent inflammatory bowel disease. Scand J Gastroenterol. 2010;45:872–7.
25. Cypers H, Varkas G, Beeckman S, Debusschere K, Vogl T, Roth J, et al.

Elevated calprotectin levels reveal bowel inflammation in spondyloarthritis. Ann Rheum Dis. 2016;75:1357–62.
26. Tibble JA, Sigthorsson G, Foster R, Forgacs I, Bjarnason I. Use of surrogate markers of inflammation and Rome criteria to distinguish organic from nonorganic intestinal disease. Gastroenterology. 2002;123:450–60.
27. Tachecí I, Bradna P, Douda T, Baštecká D, Kopáčová M, Rejchrt S, et al. Small intestinal injury in NSAID users suffering from rheumatoid arthritis or osteoarthritis. Rheumatol Int. 2016;36:1557–61.
28. Fagerberg UL, Lööf L, Merzoug RD, Hansson LO, Finkel Y. Fecal calprotectin levels in healthy children studied with an improved assay. J Pediatr Gastroenterol Nutr. 2003;37:468–72.
29. Tynjälä P, Vähäsalo P, Tarkiainen M, Kröger L, Aalto K, Malin M, et al. Aggressive combination drug therapy in very early polyarticular juvenile idiopathic arthritis (ACUTE-JIA): a multicentre randomised open-label clinical trial. Ann Rheum Dis. 2011;70:1605–12.
30. Van Dijken TD, Vastert SJ, Gerloni VM, Pontikaki I, Linnemann K, Girschick H, et al. Development of inflammatory bowel disease in patients with juvenile idiopathic arthritis treated with etanercept. J Rheumatol. 2011;38:1441–6.
31. Toussirot É, Houvenagel É, Goëb V, Fouache D, Martin A, Le Dantec P, et al. Development of inflammatory bowel disease during anti-TNF-α therapy for inflammatory rheumatic disease: a nationwide series. Joint Bone Spine. 2012;79:457–63.
32. Lionetti P, Pupi A, Veltroni M, Fonda C, Cavicchi MC, Azzari C, et al. Evidence of subclinical intestinal inflammation by 99m technetium leukocyte scintigraphy in patients with HLA-B27 positive juvenile onset active spondyloarthropathy. J Rheumatol. 2000;27:1538–41.
33. Van Praet L, Van den Bosch F, Mielants H, Elewaut D. Mucosal inflammation in spondylarthritides: past, present, and future. Curr Rheumatol Rep. 2011;13: 409–15.
34. Ylijoki H. Re-evaluation of the factors determining the long term clinical outcome of juvenile rheumatoid arthritis. Turku: PhD thesis, University of Turku; 1998.
35. Berntson L, Andersson Gäre B, Fasth A, Herlin T, Kristinsson J, Lahdenne P, et al. Nordic Study Group. Incidence of juvenile idiopathic arthritis in the Nordic countries. A population based study with special reference to the validity of the ILAR and EULAR criteria. J Rheumatol. 2003;30(10):2275–82.
36. Stoll ML, Punaro M, Patel AS. Fecal calprotectin in children with the enthesitis-related arthritis subtype of juvenile idiopathic arthritis. J Rheumatol. 2011;38:2274–5.
37. Matzkies FG, Targan SR, Berel D, Landers CJ, Reveille JD, McGovern DP, et al. Markers of intestinal inflammation in patients with ankylosing spondylitis: a pilot study. Arthritis Res Ther. 2012;14:R261.
38. Montalto M, Gallo A, Ianiro G, Santoro L, D'Onofrio F, Ricci R, et al. Can chronic gastritis cause an increase in fecal calprotectin concentrations? World J Gastroenterol. 2010;16:3406–10.
39. Walker LS, Dengler-Crish CM, Rippel S, Bruehl S. Functional abdominal pain in childhood and adolescence increases risk for chronic pain in adulthood. Pain. 2010;150:568–72.
40. Heida A, Holtman GA, Lisman-van Leeuwen Y, Berger MY, van Rheenen PF. Avoid Endoscopy in Children With Suspected Inflammatory Bowel Disease Who Have Normal Calprotectin Levels. J Pediatr Gastroenterol Nutr. 2016;62:47–9.
41. Luntamo T, Sourander A, Santalahti P, Aromaa M, Helenius H. Prevalence Changes of Pain, Sleep Problems and Fatigue Among 8-Year-Old Children: Years 1989, 1999, and 2005. J Pediatr Psychol. 2012;37:307–18.
42. Manz M, Burri E, Rothen C, Tchanguizi N, Niederberger C, Rossi L, et al. Value of fecal calprotectin in the evaluation of patients with abdominal discomfort: an observational study. BMC Gastroenterol. 2012;12:5.

28

A systematic review of psychosocial therapies for children with rheumatic diseases

Ezra M. Cohen[1,5*], Alessio Morley-Fletcher[2], Darshan H. Mehta[3] and Yvonne C. Lee[4]

Abstract

Background: To assess the quality of evidence for the effects of psychosocial therapies on pain and function in children with rheumatic diseases.

Methods: We conducted a literature search of MEDLINE and PsycINFO for randomized clinical trials of psychosocial interventions for pain and disability in children with rheumatic diseases from January 1969 to September 2015. Studies with a sample size less than 10 subjects were excluded. Study quality was assessed using the Jadad score.

Results: Five articles met inclusion criteria, for a total of 229 patients, aged 5 to 18 years. Two studies included children with fibromyalgia. Three studies included children with juvenile arthritis. Neither study in fibromyalgia reported the statistical significance of immediate between-group pre-post changes in functioning or pain. One study examining the effects of an internet-based psychosocial intervention in children with juvenile arthritis reported significant differences in post-intervention pain scores ($p = 0.03$). However, 2 studies did not show improvements in pain scores among children with juvenile arthritis treated with psychosocial interventions vs. a wait-list control or vs. an active control (massage). No studies reported significant between-group differences for functional outcomes in children with juvenile arthritis.

Conclusions: The available data were limited by the scarcity of randomized trials. Definite conclusions about the immediate effect of psychosocial interventions on pain and function in children with fibromyalgia could not be made because between-group comparisons of post-treatment change scores were not reported. For children with juvenile inflammatory arthritis, results of between-group comparisons for pain differed across studies, and analyses examining disability revealed no significant differences between groups.

Keywords: Juvenile arthritis, Juvenile fibromyalgia, Psychological therapies, Mind-body therapies, Meditation

Background

Children with rheumatic conditions often experience pain and disability [1, 2], leading to significant impairment in quality of life [3]. Pain and disability are frequently associated with mood disorders. One study noted that 67% of children with fibromyalgia have a current DSM-IV diagnosis [4]. Stress and mood problems may be associated with pain and disability [5, 6].

* Correspondence: ezra.cohen@childrens.harvard.edu
[1]Division of Immunology, Boston Children's Hospital, 300 Longwood Ave, Boston, MA 02115, USA
[5]Department of Rheumatology, Boston Children's Hospital, 300 Longwood Ave, Boston, MA 02115, USA
Full list of author information is available at the end of the article

Given the association between pain, disability and psychosocial factors, psychosocial therapies have been hypothesized to have benefit for individuals with persistent pain and disability.

Psychosocial therapies may be defined as any therapies that influence the psychosocial processes which underpin or maintain pain, disability or other symptoms [7]. Among these, mind-body therapies and cognitive-behavioral therapies are the most widely used. Mind-body therapies are defined by the National Center for Complementary and Integrative Health as "a large and diverse group of techniques that are administered or taught to others by a trained practitioner or teacher [8]." Mind-body comprises the most commonly used complementary and alternative therapies, such as acupuncture, biofeedback, hypnosis, progressive muscle relaxation, guided imagery, mindfulness, meditation, yoga, tai chi and qi gong [9].

In the last few decades, cognitive-behavioral therapy (CBT) has been a dominant approach for treating psychological disorders in children, and though it shares many similarities with mind-body therapies, it is regarded by most as distinct [10]. CBT developed as a hybrid of cognitive and behavioral therapy [11]. Cognitive therapy focuses on identifying cognitive distortions and substituting them with more rational assessments. Behavioral therapy encourages behaviors that bring pleasure and self-efficacy, while discouraging maladaptive behaviors. Over time, CBT has absorbed techniques from a wide variety of interventions, including hypnosis, imagery, biofeedback, mindfulness techniques and meditation [12]. In fact, the term "cognitive-behavioral intervention" has become so broad that it may encompass its traditional meaning in addition to any or all of these techniques [7]. For this reason, it is difficult to estimate the effects of CBT in the literature as its own separate entity.

Psychosocial therapies have shown promise for treating rheumatic diseases in adults, though results are mixed. A large systematic review of psychological treatments in adults with rheumatoid arthritis found pooled effect sizes of $d = 0.22$ for pain and $d = 0.27$ for functional disability [13]. A systematic review of mind-body therapies for fibromyalgia found that individuals treated with mind-body therapies had greater improvements in pain and global assessment than wait-list controls, but poorer outcomes than individuals who participated in moderate/high intensity exercise [14]. In addition, a more recent randomized control trial (RCT) of tai chi vs. education and stretching in fibromyalgia concluded a modest benefit in symptoms [15].

Given studies reporting that psychosocial interventions improve pain and disability in adults with rheumatic conditions, we wanted to examine the evidence for psychosocial treatments to manage pain and disability in children with rheumatic disorders.

Methods

Inclusion and exclusion criteria

We included articles in this study only if they were published in English in a peer-reviewed journal. Unpublished abstracts and posters were excluded. We included articles which examined psychosocial therapies for children with rheumatic diseases with pain or disability as an outcome. Psychosocial therapies included CBT, coping skills, meditation, mindfulness, guided imagery, hypnosis, biofeedback, breathing techniques, progressive muscle relaxation, relaxation therapy, yoga and tai chi. Only prospective studies with a randomized design and total sample size > 10 were included in this review. We focused on prospective studies with a randomized design because we were interested in examining the impact of psychosocial therapies as an intervention. The study population included children who were 0 to 18 years at the beginning of the study. Articles which reported pain and functional disability as an outcome were included. Studies of children with any rheumatic disease (as below) were included.

Two investigators (EMC and AMF) independently conducted systematic searches for articles on psychosocial interventions in children through September 2015 on MEDLINE and PsycINFO using the following terms: (cognitive behavioral therapy, hypnosis, mindfulness, meditation, relaxation, progressive muscle relaxation, breathing, guided imagery, tai chi, or yoga) AND children AND rheumatic diseases (including fibromyalgia, systemic lupus erythematosus, juvenile arthritis, dermatomyositis, polymyositis, Sjogren's, sarcoidosis, relapsing polychondritis, microscopic polyangiitis, granulomatosis with polyangiitis, eosinophilic granulomatosis with polyangiitis, polyarteritis nodosa, Takayasu arteritis, Behcet's disease, and scleroderma). The two investigators compared search results, and discrepant results were reviewed and discussed until consensus was achieved.

The following data were extracted from articles for examination: population, country of origin, gender proportion, sample size, study design (randomized), type of control used if any, primary and secondary outcome measures, results, and duration of follow-up. When possible, we contacted the authors for information that was not provided in the manuscript. We calculated percentage change in pain and disability based upon pre and immediate post-treatment measures. "Post-treatment" refers to scoring just after the intervention finishes, and is a more proximate measure of the intervention's effect, whereas end-of-study scores (i.e. after intervention-free follow-up) measure the durability of an intervention's effects after it has been withdrawn. We assessed study quality using the Jadad score (0–5), a system that evaluates blinding, randomization and accounting for all subjects [16]. The Jadad score refers primarily to RCTs, as many of its components (blinding, randomization) are unique to RCTs.

Results

Our search yielded 255 manuscripts, of which 64 were excluded based on title because they did not involve children, rheumatic disease and/or psychosocial therapies. Of the remaining 191 manuscripts, 176 were excluded after reading the abstract because these studies included the wrong population, did not represent a prospective trial, and/or did not pertain to a childhood rheumatic disease. Fifteen manuscripts were read in full. Of those, 10 were excluded for $N < 10$, lacking randomization, analysis of previously reported results or lacking pain or function as an outcome [17]. This yielded 5 RCTs (Fig. 1). We divided these into trials of juvenile fibromyalgia and trials of juvenile arthritis because the pathophysiology of these conditions differs, with fibromyalgia being a non-inflammatory condition and juvenile arthritis being a systemic inflammatory condition. Tables 1 and 2 provide a summary of our results [18–22].

We found a total of 2 studies for fibromyalgia, both from the same first author [21, 22]. These studies comprised a total sample size of 144 children. For mind-body interventions, 1 study used CBT and 1 used coping skills training. For controls, 1 study used education controls and 1 used self-monitoring, which involved symptom diaries. Treatment duration was 8 weeks for both studies. Follow-up ranged from 8 weeks to 6 months. Although there was significant drop-out (16 out of 114 subjects) in one study, there were no significant imbalances in the arms [22]. Both trials were RCTs, with a mean Jadad score 3. Both trials fully accounted for their participants and were single-blind. Neither were double-blind, underscoring the difficulty of double-blinding with psychosocial interventions. Both studies had weekly treatment sessions. Home practice was encouraged, but duration of home practice was not reported.

We found 3 studies in juvenile arthritis. These were from 3 different lead authors from 3 different countries, with a total sample size of 85 children. One study used progressive muscle relaxation as the primary intervention, while one used CBT, and one used computer-based CBT. For controls, one used an attention control (similar to self-monitoring), one used a wait-list control, and one used daily massage. 2 of the trials were RCTs, while the study by Lomholt et al. employed group randomization after stratifying by age and geographic region. These studies had a mean Jadad score of 1.6, and none were blinded. The median number of subjects in each trial was 20 with a range of 19 to 46. One had 9 subjects drop-out, with equal distribution of drop-outs between the intervention and control groups [20]. 1 of 19 subjects dropped out in the study by Lomholt et al., and drop-out was not reported in the study by Field et al. In all 3 studies, participants were followed for the duration of the interventions (4–12 weeks, median of 8 weeks), without additional follow-up beyond the intervention period. Home practice was a part of all studies' treatment conditions, though mean duration of home practice was not reported.

The choice of pain and function outcomes were the same for the fibromyalgia studies, which all had the same first author, but varied across the studies of

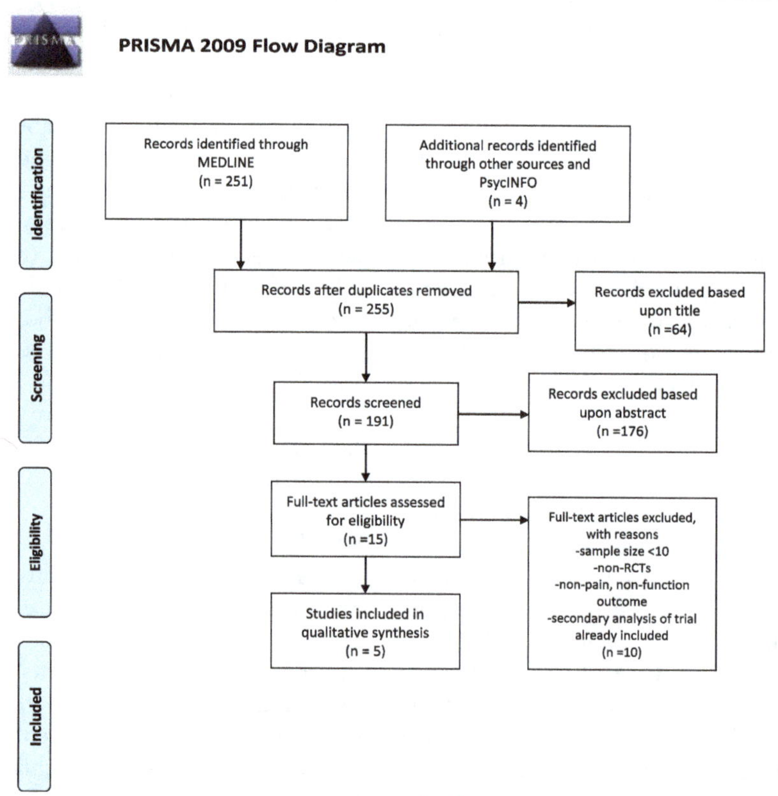

Fig. 1 The process of study selection. "Other sources" include the references or text of reviewed articles

Table 1 RCTs in juvenile fibromyalgia

Citation	N	Age (years)	Gender (%F)	Study Design	Intervention	Comparison Group	Duration of Treatment	Additional Follow-up	Pain Measure	Pain results (post-treatment)	Disability Measure	Disability results (post-treatment)	Jadad Score
Kashikar-Zuck, S. et al. (2012) [22]	114	11–18	92	RCT	Weekly CBT sessions	Education group	8 weeks	4 months	Visual Analogue Scale (0–10). Higher score implies greater pain.	Pre-post difference in CBT group: 5.7 to 5.3 (−7%; *p*-value not provided) Pre-post difference in education group: 5.8 to 6.0 (+3%; *p*-value not provided) Between groups difference of change scores: 0.6 (favoring CBT group; *p*-value not provided)	Functional Disability Inventory (0–60)	Pre-post difference in CBT group: 21.4 to 16.7 (−22%; *p*-value not provided) Pre-post difference in education group: 19.2 to 19.8 (+3%; *p*-value not provided) Between groups difference of change scores: 5.3 (favoring CBT group; *p*-value not provided)	3
Kashikar-Zuck, S. et al. (2005) [21]	30	13–17	100	RCT (Crossover)	Weekly coping skills training	Self-monitoring (8 weeks of recording VAS scores)	8 weeks	8 weeks (to finish crossover intervention)	Visual Analogue Scale (0–10)	Pre-post difference in Group A (coping skills): 5.7 to 4.4 (−23%; *p*-value not provided) Pre-post difference in Group B (self-monitoring): 5.3 to 5.9 (+11%; *p*-value not provided) Between group difference of change scores: 1.9 (favoring coping skills; *p*-value not provided)	Functional Disability Inventory (0–60)	Pre-post difference in Group A (coping skills): 21.0 to 15.1 (−28%) (*p*-values not provided) Pre-post difference in Group B (self-monitoring): 21.9 to 16.6 (−24%) (*p*-values not provided) Between group difference of change scores: mean 0.6 (favoring coping skills; *p*-value NS)	3

The crossover design assigned patients to coping skills first then self-monitoring or vice versa

Table 2 RCTs in juvenile arthritis

Citation	N	Age (years)	Gender (%F)	Study Design	Intervention	Comparison Group	Duration of Treatment	Additional Follow-up	Pain Measure	Pain Results	Disability Measure	Disability Results	Jadad Score
Field T. et al. (1997) [18]	20	5–15	70	RCT	Relaxation therapy (nightly, parent-guided)	Daily massage	30 days	None	Visual Analogue Scale (0–10) (pain in the last week)	Pre-post difference in relaxation group: 3.5 to 4.2 (+20%; *p*-value NS) Pre-post difference in massage group: 4.8 to 1.6 (−67%; $p < 0.05$) Between group difference of change scores: 3.9 (massage group with greater improvement; *p*-value not provided)			1
Lomholt J. et al. (2015) [19]	19	9–14	79	RCT with group randomization	Weekly CBT sessions	Wait-list control	8 weeks	None	Revised Faces Pain Scale (0–10). Higher score implies greater pain.	Pre-post difference in CBT group: 3.1 to 4.1 (+32%; *p*-value NS) Pre-post difference in control group: 2.7 to 2.7 (0%; *p*-value NS) Post-scores between groups adjusted for pre-scores: *p*-value NS	Functional Disability Inventory (0–60)	Pre-post difference in CBT group: 11.4 to 11.7 (+2.6%; *p*-value NS) Pre-post difference in control group: 9.8 to 9.2 (−6.1%; *p*-value NS) Between group differences in change scores: 0.9 (control group with greater improvement *p*-value NS)	2
Stinson J. et al. (2010) [20]	46	12–18	67	RCT	Internet-based education, relaxation and distraction	Attention control	12 weeks	None	Recalled Pain Inventory (0–10) in past week. Higher score implies greater pain. [24]	Pre-post difference in intervention group; 2.7 to 2.2 (−19%; *p*-value not provided) Pre-post difference in attention control 3.0 to 3.5 (+17%; *p*-value not provided) Post-score difference adjusted for pre-score significant (favoring intervention group; $p = 0.03$)	Juvenile Arthritis Quality of Life Questionnaire (JAQQ) activity (0–7; higher score implies greater dysfunction)	Pre-post difference in intervention group; 2.4 to 2.0 (−17%; *p*-value not provided) Pre-post difference in attention control 2.7 to 2.3 (−15%; *p*-value not provided) Post-score difference adjusted for pre-score: *p*-value NS	2

children with juvenile arthritis. The studies in fibromyalgia consistently used the Visual Analogue Scale (VAS; for pain) and Functional Disability Inventory (FDI; for disability). For the studies in arthritis, 1 study used the FDI while another used the Juvenile Arthritis Quality of Life Questionnaire (JAQQ), which is specifically designed to assess disability and dysfunction in children with arthritis [23]. The JAQQ assesses psychosocial, gross motor and fine motor functioning, as well as general symptoms. For pain, each of these studies used a different measure (e.g., VAS pain scale, Revised Faces Pain Scale and Recalled Pain Inventory) [24, 25].

In children with fibromyalgia, psychosocial therapies appeared to decrease disability, but documentation of statistically significant changes was frequently unavailable, particularly for immediate post-intervention scores. Percent improvement in FDI for the intervention groups ranged between 22 and 28%. In the comparison arms, improvement ranged from a worsening of 3% to an improvement of 24%. *P*-values for pre-post changes in FDI were not available for immediate post-intervention measures. Between group differences in the change in FDI score were non-significant in one study (comparing weekly coping skills training vs. self-monitoring) and not reported in the other.

For the outcome of pain among children with fibromyalgia, both studies reported VAS pain as an outcome and neither reported post-intervention significance levels. Between-group comparisons were not provided.

In children with juvenile arthritis, only two studies reported disability as an outcome measure. In these studies, between-group post-treatment disability scores did not significantly differ from each other. Pre-post significance levels were only provided in 1 of 2 studies, and this was not significant [19]. Stinson et al. reported a non-significant post-score difference (adjusted for pre-treatment baseline). This study used attention control with JAQQ as the outcome, while Lomholt et al. used wait-list control with FDI as the outcome.

For the outcome of pain in children with juvenile arthritis, no studies reported significant pre-post test results for the psychosocial intervention group. Between group comparisons of post-intervention pain scores revealed a statistically significant difference ($p = 0.03$), favoring the psychosocial intervention (internet-based education, relaxation and distraction) in one study [20], revealed no significant difference in one study [19] and were not reported in one study [18]. The latter study included an active control group (massage). Effect sizes could not be calculated because intra-class and inter-class correlations are required for these calculations, and these values were not reported in any of the studies. No adverse outcomes were reported in any of the studies.

Discussion

To our knowledge, this is the first summary of the literature for psychosocial interventions for pediatric rheumatic disease. In children with fibromyalgia, within-group comparisons suggest that CBT/coping skills training may decrease pain and disability, but definite conclusions cannot be made because these studies did not report p-values for tests directly comparing pre-post-treatment change scores between groups. In studies of children with inflammatory arthritis, between-group comparisons did not reveal any significant differences in functional outcomes, and results of between-group comparisons for pain were not consistent across studies.

In children, psychosocial interventions have been studied most in behavioral and psychiatric conditions. One meta-analysis of mindfulness interventions in children found effect sizes in the small-to-moderate range, with larger effect sizes noted for improvements in psychosocial symptoms and for children treated in clinical settings rather than schools [26]. Yoga has been studied as an aid to physical therapy in rehabilitation, and other mind-body therapies have shown benefit for headache in children [27, 28]. Biofeedback also has a history of use in the pediatric population, treating conditions ranging from fecal and urinary incontinence to ADHD and headaches [29, 30]. CBT has been used most extensively in psychiatric conditions, notably anxiety and trauma [31, 32].

A prior systematic review and meta-analysis of psychosocial therapies in children with chronic pain suggests a large effect size, although only a subset of articles could be compared directly because they used a common pain measure [7]. Another Cochrane review evaluated psychosocial therapies for needle-associated procedural pain in children, finding large effect sizes for CBT, hypnosis and distraction [33]. However, many of the component studies in these reviews suffered from small sample size and heterogeneity of methods. In this review, the analyses examining pain as an outcome were less conclusive than those of Eccleston's meta-analysis, which focused mainly on children with headaches [7]. Our study represents two smaller subpopulations (children with fibromyalgia and children with juvenile arthritis) which may respond differently to psychosocial therapies, as arthritis is thought to be primarily inflammatory in etiology, whereas fibromyalgia is driven primarily by central sensitization. One complicating feature of this distinction is that fibromyalgia can co-exist in children diagnosed with juvenile arthritis.

Our review was limited by the small number of appropriate studies, as well as the small sample size of the included studies. In addition, not all studies included both pain and disability as outcomes, limiting conclusions that could be made about both outcomes. Study quality was good in the fibromyalgia group (Jadad score of 3), though, due to the nature of the interventions, no studies were blinded. In the inflammatory arthritis group, study quality was poor (Jadad score of 1.6). Similar to the studies of children with fibromyalgia, these studies were not blinded, and many lacked adequate description of randomization methods. It should be noted that the applicability of the Jadad score has been questioned, given its emphasis on the reporting of methods rather than an evaluation of the methods themselves [16]. While there may be more consistency across the studies in the fibromyalgia, owed to their having a common first author, conclusions about their external validity are more difficult to draw. No studies in these groups reported adverse outcomes, which are likely rare with these therapies, but still essential to understand in order to assess risk-benefit ratios.

Other factors limit our ability to draw broad conclusions from these studies. In these studies, the duration of treatment ranged from 30 days to 12 weeks. It is unclear whether an intervention of this duration is long enough to have a measurable impact. We chose to assess the measurement of change in outcome immediately at the end of the intervention period because the greatest likelihood for improvement would be at this time point before the effects of the intervention fade. In future studies, it will be important to assess adherence to home therapies over time, as well as family and societal factors that may impact the effectiveness of psychosocial therapies.

In addition, there was significant heterogeneity in the length of treatment, making comparisons difficult. Though the studies were randomized, sample sizes were small and residual confounders, such as disease activity, may still be present. The generalizability of these results may also be limited because the study populations were mostly female adolescents. Since fibromyalgia and juvenile inflammatory arthritis affect females more them males, the female predominance in these studies is expected. Larger studies, however, with a larger number of males, are needed before the implications of these studies can be expanded to include boys and young men.

In addition, both studies of juvenile fibromyalgia and 1 study of juvenile arthritis excluded children less than 11 years of age [20–22]. This may reflect the perception that psychosocial therapies are easier to administer in older children, though CBT is used with regularity in children as young as 7 years old [34]. Whereas juvenile fibromyalgia disproportionately affects adolescents, juvenile arthritis generally peaks in the younger years [35, 36]. Additional studies are needed to understand whether the effectiveness of these interventions vary by age.

One of the greatest difficulties we encountered was the inconsistent reporting of outcomes and analyses. We chose to use the between-group difference in pre-post change scores as our primary outcome measure. These analyses directly compare changes in the outcome between the two groups, taking into account baseline values of the outcome. It is particularly important to consider baseline values of the outcome measure in small studies, where randomization may not yield groups with similar baseline characteristics. Although some studies reported a significant improvement in outcome measures in the treatment arm, adjustment for pre-post differences was frequently not reported.

Finally, while many studies used an education control, others used wait-list, self-monitoring and massage as comparison groups. To prove efficacy, it is important to know *over what*. This is an easier question to answer in drug trials, where placebo control groups have helped isolate drug effects from more nebulous causes. In research involving psychosocial interventions, which is the relevant comparison group– standard medical care, wait-list controls, placebo interventions or other psychosocial interventions? In fact, all of these have been studied, with differing results. Interestingly, a large meta-analysis of mindfulness studies in adults by Grossman et al. showed similar mean effect sizes whether using active or wait-list controls [37]. Another large meta-analysis of CBT for adults with chronic pain by Morley et al. found considerable variability between wait-list and active controls, with wait-list controlled trials reporting larger differences in outcomes between the intervention and control groups [38].

Conclusion

Nevertheless, many children with rheumatic conditions have pain that is incompletely treated, and there is a great demand for psychosocial and non-pharmacologic treatments. Based on this review, we conclude that the existing studies are too heterogeneous, and the reporting too inconsistent to draw convincing conclusions. In addition, although Eccleston's earlier review suggested that adverse events, when reported, tend to be evenly distributed between control and intervention arms, there is a great need for consistent documentation of adverse effects in these studies, as these treatments are often thought of as being 'risk-free' when, in actuality, this area may just be 'data-free' [7]. The emergence and consolidation of research networks and registries in the pediatric rheumatology community such as the Childhood Arthritis and Rheumatology Research Alliance represent a major opportunity for studying these therapies in a uniform and broad-based manner, and these efforts will hopefully clarify the role of these therapies in the future [39].

Abbreviations

CBT: Cognitive-behavioral therapy; FDI: Functional Disability Inventory; JAQQ: Juvenile Arthritis Quality of Life Questionnaire; RCT: Randomized controlled trial; VAS: Visual Analogue Scale.

Acknowledgements

Not applicable.

Funding
No funding was used in the production of this study. Dr. Lee's work was supported by the NIH grant AR064850.

Authors' contributions
EC wrote and edited the manuscript, and conducted the primary search. AM-F conducted a confirmatory search. YL edited the manuscript and helped to arbitrate discrepancies between the two independent searchers. DM edited the manuscript and helped to design the study. All authors read and approved the final manuscript.

Competing interests
Dr. Lee reports a research grant from Pfizer and stock in Express Scripts. No other authors report conflicts of interests. Neither company played any role in the study or in the writing of the manuscript.

Author details
[1]Division of Immunology, Boston Children's Hospital, 300 Longwood Ave, Boston, MA 02115, USA. [2]Department of Pediatrics, Massachusetts General Hospital, 55 Fruit Street, Boston, MA 02114, USA. [3]Benson-Henry Institute for Mind-Body Medicine, Massachusetts General Hospital, 151 Merrimac St., Boston, MA 02114, USA. [4]Division of Rheumatology, Immunology and Allergy, Brigham and Women's Hospital, 60 Fenwood Road, Boston, MA 02115, USA. [5]Department of Rheumatology, Boston Children's Hospital, 300 Longwood Ave, Boston, MA 02115, USA.

References

1. Gäre BA, Fasth A. The natural history of juvenile chronic arthritis: a population based cohort study. II. Outcome. J Rheumatol. 1995;22:308–19.
2. Reid GJ, Lang BA, McGrath PJ. Primary juvenile fibromyalgia. Psychological adjustment, family functioning, coping, and functional disability. Arthritis Rheum. 1997;40:752–60.
3. Ruperto N, Buratti S, Duarte-Salazar C, Pistorio A, Reiff A, Bernstein B, Maldonado-Velázquez MR, Beristain-Manterola R, Maeno N, Takei S, Falcini F, Lepore L, Spencer CH, Pratsidou-Gertsi P, Martini A, Ravelli A. Health-related quality of life in juvenile-onset systemic lupus erythematosus and its relationship to disease activity and damage. Arthritis Rheum. 2004;51:458–64.
4. Kashikar-Zuck S, Parkins IS, Graham TB, Lynch AM, Passo M, Johnston M, Schikler KN, Hashkes PJ, Banez G, Richards MM. Anxiety, mood, and behavioral disorders among pediatric patients with juvenile fibromyalgia syndrome. Clin J Pain. 2008;24:620–6.
5. Fifield J, Mcquillan J, Armeli S, Tennen H, Reisine S, Affleck G. Chronic strain, daily work stress and pain among workers with rheumatoid arthritis: Does job stress make a bad day worse? Work Stress. 2004;18:275–91.
6. Lenze EJ, Rogers JC, Martire LM, Mulsant BH, Rollman BL, Dew MA, Schulz R, Reynolds CF. The Association of Late-Life Depression and Anxiety With Physical Disability: A Review of the Literature and Prospectus for Future Research. Am J Geriatr Psychiatry. 2001;9:113–35.
7. Eccleston C, Palermo TM, Williams AC, Lewandowski Holley A, Morley S, Fisher E, Law E. Psychological therapies for the management of chronic and recurrent pain in children and adolescents. Cochrane Database Syst Rev. 2014;5:CD003968.
8. Mind and Body Practices. https://nccih.nih.gov/health/mindbody. Accessed 5 Oct 2016.
9. Astin JA, Shapiro SL, Eisenberg DM, Forys KL. Mind-Body Medicine: State of the Science, Implications for Practice. J Am Board Fam Med. 2003;16:131–47.
10. Reinecke MA, Ryan NE, DuBois DL. Cognitive-behavioral therapy of depression and depressive symptoms during adolescence: a review and meta-analysis. J Am Acad Child Adolesc Psychiatry. 1998;37:26–34.
11. Beck J, Beck JS. Cognitive Behavior Therapy: Basics and Beyond. 2nd ed. New York: Guilford Press; 2011.
12. Teasdale JD, Segal ZV, Williams JM, Ridgeway VA, Soulsby JM, Lau MA. Prevention of relapse/recurrence in major depression by mindfulness-based cognitive therapy. J Consult Clinical Psychol. 2000;68:615–23.
13. Astin JA, Beckner W, Soeken K, Hochberg MC, Berman B. Psychological interventions for rheumatoid arthritis: a meta-analysis of randomized controlled trials. Arthritis Rheum. 2002;47:291–302.
14. Hadhazy VA, Ezzo J, Creamer P, Berman BM. Mind-body therapies for the treatment of fibromyalgia. A systematic review. J Rheumatol. 2000;27:2911–8.
15. Wang C, Schmid CH, Rones R, Kalish R, Yinh J, Goldenberg DL, Lee Y, McAlindon T. A Randomized Trial of Tai Chi for Fibromyalgia. N Engl J Med. 2010;363:743–54.
16. Berger V. Is the Jadad score the proper evaluation of trials? J Rheumatol. 2006;33:1710–1.
17. Kashikar-Zuck S, Sil S, Lynch-Jordan AM, Ting TV, Peugh J, Schikler KN, Hashkes PJ, Arnold LM, Passo M, Richards-Mauze MM, Powers SW, Lovell DJ. Changes in pain coping, catastrophizing, and coping efficacy after cognitive-behavioral therapy in children and adolescents with juvenile fibromyalgia. J Pain. 2013;14:492–501.
18. Field T, Hernandez-Reif M, Seligman S, Krasnegor J, Sunshine W, Rivas-Chacon R, Schanberg S, Kuhn C. Juvenile rheumatoid arthritis: benefits from massage therapy. J Pediatr Psychol. 1997;22:607–17.
19. Lomholt JJ, Thastum M, Christensen AE, Leegaard A, Herlin T. Cognitive behavioral group intervention for pain and well-being in children with juvenile idiopathic arthritis: a study of feasibility and preliminary efficacy. Pediatr Rheumatol Online J. 2015;13:35.
20. Stinson JN, McGrath PJ, Hodnett ED, Feldman BM, Duffy CM, Huber AM, Tucker LB, Hetherington CR, Tse SML, Spiegel LR, Campillo S, Gill NK, White ME. An internet-based self-management program with telephone support for adolescents with arthritis: A pilot randomized controlled trial. J Rheumatol. 2010;37:1944–52.
21. Kashikar-Zuck S, Swain NF, Jones BA, Graham TB. Efficacy of cognitive-behavioral intervention for juvenile primary fibromyalgia syndrome. J Rheumatol. 2005;32:1594–602.
22. Kashikar-Zuck S, Ting TV, Arnold LM, Bean J, Powers SW, Graham TB, Passo MH, Schikler KN, Hashkes PJ, Spalding S, Lynch-Jordan AM, Banez G, Richards MM, Lovell DJ. Cognitive behavioral therapy for the treatment of juvenile fibromyalgia: a multisite, single-blind, randomized, controlled clinical trial. Arthritis Rheum. 2012;64:297–305.
23. Degotardi P. Pediatric measures of quality of life: The Juvenile Arthritis Quality of Life Questionnaire (JAQQ) and the Pediatric Quality of Life (PedsQL). Arthritis Rheum. 2003;49:S105–12.
24. Stinson J, Stevens BJ, Feldman BM, Streiner D, McGrath PJ, Dupuis A, Gill N, Petroz GC. Construct validity of a multidimensional electronic pain diary for adolescents with arthritis. Pain. 2008;136:281–92.
25. Hicks C, von Baeyer C, Spafford P. The Faces Pain Scale–Revised: toward a common metric in pediatric pain measurement. Pain. 2001;93:173–83.
26. Zoogman S, Goldberg S, Hoyt W, Miller L. Mindfulness interventions with youth: A meta-analysis. Mindfulness (N Y). 2015;6:290–302.
27. Galantino M, Galbavy R, Quinn L. Therapeutic effects of yoga for children: a systematic review of the literature. Pediatr Phys Ther. 2008;20:66–80.
28. Eccleston C, Morley S, Williams A, Yorke L, Mastroyannopoulou K. Systematic review of randomised controlled trials of psychological therapy for chronic pain in children and adolescents, with a subset meta-analysis of pain relief. Pain. 2002;99:157–65.
29. Amon KL, Campbell A. Can Children with AD/HD Learn Relaxation and Breathing Techniques through Biofeedback Video Games? Aust J Educ Dev Psychol. 2008;8:72–84.
30. Glazier D, Ankem M, Ferlise V, Gazi M, Barone J. Utility of biofeedback for the daytime syndrome of urinary frequency and urgency of childhood. Urology. 2001;57:791–3.
31. Kendall PC, Hudson JL, Gosch E, Flannery-Schroeder E, Suveg C. Cognitive-behavioral therapy for anxiety disordered youth: A randomized clinical trial evaluating child and family modalities. J Consult Clin Psychol. 2008;76:282–97.
32. COHEN JA, MANNARINO AP, BERLINER L, DEBLINGER E. Trauma-Focused Cognitive Behavioral Therapy for Children and Adolescents: An Empirical Update. J Interpers Violence. 2000;15:1202–23.
33. Uman LS, Birnie KA, Noel M, Parker JA, Chambers CT, McGrath PJ, Kisely SR. Psychological interventions for needle-related procedural pain and distress

in children and adolescents. In: Chambers CT, editor. Cochrane Database of Systematic Reviews. Chichester: John Wiley & Sons, Ltd; 2013.
34. Mendlowitz SL, Manassis K, Bradley S, Scapillato D, Miezitis S, Shaw BE. Cognitive-Behavioral Group Treatments in Childhood Anxiety Disorders: The Role of Parental Involvement. J Am Acad Child Adolesc Psychiatry. 1999;38:1223–9.
35. Siegel D, Janeway D, Baum J. Fibromyalgia syndrome in children and adolescents: clinical features at presentation and status at follow-up. Pediatrics. 1998;101:377–82.
36. Sullivan D, Cassidy J, Petty R. Pathogenic implications of age of onset in juvenile rheumatoid arthritis. Arthritis Rheum. 1975;18:251–5.
37. Grossman P, Niemann L, Schmidt S, Walach H. Mindfulness-based stress reduction and health benefits. A meta-analysis. J Psychosom Res. 2004;57:35–43.
38. Morley S, Eccleston C, Williams A. Systematic review and meta-analysis of randomized controlled trials of cognitive behaviour therapy and behaviour therapy for chronic pain in adults, excluding headache. Pain. 1999;80:1–13.
39. Oliveira S, Ravelli A, Pistorio A, Castell E, Malattia C, Prieur AM, Saad-Magalhães C, Murray KJ, Bae S-C, Joos R, Foeldvari I, Duarte-Salazar C, Wulffraat N, Lahdenne P, Dolezalova P, de Inocencio J, Kanakoudi-Tsakalidou F, Hofer M, Nikishina I, Ozdogan H, Hashkes PJ, Landgraf JM, Martini A, Ruperto N. Proxy-reported health-related quality of life of patients with juvenile idiopathic arthritis: the Pediatric Rheumatology International Trials Organization multinational quality of life cohort study. Arthritis Rheum. 2007;57:35–43.

29

TLR4 rs41426344 increases susceptibility of rheumatoid arthritis (RA) and juvenile idiopathic arthritis (JIA) in a central south Chinese Han population

Yan Wang[1,2,3], Lianghui Chen[1,2,3], Fang Li[1,2], Meihua Bao[1,2], Jie Zeng[1,2], Ju Xiang[1,2], Huaiqing Luo[1,2,3], Jianming Li[1,4*] and Liang Tang[1,2*]

Abstract

Background: The aim of the study was to determine whether polymorphisms in toll-like receptor 4 (*TLR4*) confer susceptibility to rheumatoid arthritis (RA) and juvenile idiopathic arthritis (JIA) in a central south Chinese Han population.

Methods: Genotyping for six well studied polymorphisms (rs4986790, rs4986791, rs10759932, rs41426344, rs11536889 and rs7873784) in *TLR4* gene were conducted in 1074 unrelated patients with RA and 1692 healthy control subjects, as well as in 217 unrelated patients with JIA and 378 healthy control subjects using direct sequencing technique. Comparisons between cases and controls in alleles, genotypes and haplotypes were carried out using Fisher's exact test.

Results: Significant genetic associations were detected between the 3'UTR rs41426344C and RA ($p < 0.001$, $p_{adj} < 0.001$, OR = 2.24) and JIA ($p < 0.001$, $p_{adj} < 0.001$, OR = 2.05). In addition, rs4986790G was found to be significantly associated with the susceptibility for RA ($p = 0.005$, $p_{adj} = 0.03$, OR = 3.43), but not for JIA ($p = 0.06$, $p_{adj} = 0.36$, OR = 2.65). Furthermore, significant increasing in the distributions of haplotypes H4 and H10 in RA (H4: $p = 0.001$, OR = 1.13; H10: $p = 0.001$, OR = 1.15) and JIA (H4: $p = 0.04$, OR = 2.06; H10: $p = 0.02$, OR = 2.47) were also found. Moreover, the frequency of rs41426344C significantly increased in RF-positive and anti-CCP positive subjects both in RA (RF^+: $p < 0.0001$, OR = 2.33; anti-CCP^+: $p = 0.008$, OR = 2.79) and JIA (RF^+: $p = 0.02$, OR = 2.91; anti-CCP^+: $p = 0.02$, OR = 2.78).

Conclusions: Our study suggested that rs41426344 and rs4986790 of *TLR4* might contribute to RA, and rs41426344 might contribute to JIA pathogenesis in central south Chinese Han population.

Keywords: Genetic association, Toll like receptors 4 (*TLR4*), Rheumatoid arthritis (RA), Juvenile idiopathic arthritis (JIA), Chinese Han population

Background

Rheumatoid arthritis (RA) is an autoimmune disease characterized by progressive particular damage caused by inflammatory cells and synoviocytes and was thought to be caused by complex interaction of multiple susceptibility genes and environmental factors [1]. It affects approximately 0.32% Chinese Han population and 1% Caucasian respectively. Juvenile idiopathic arthritis (JIA) refers to a group of chronic childhood arthropathies of unknown aetiology [2]. Chronic arthritis is a common feature of RA and JIA. Familiar and twins studies have provided robust evidence for the role of genetic factors in these diseases [3, 4].

Toll-like receptors (TLRs) play important roles in the recognition of inflammatory diseases caused by invading microorganisms. They have been also increasingly suggested to have important roles in RA and JIA [5, 6].

* Correspondence: tlcool318@163.com
[1]Department of Human Anatomy, Histology and Embryology, Institute of Neuroscience, Changsha Medical University, No. 1501 Lei Feng Road,, Wangcheng District, Changsha City, Hunan Province 410219, People's Republic of China
Full list of author information is available at the end of the article

There are 13 structurally unique members identified in TLRs family. Toll-like receptor 4 (TLR4), one of the important member of TLRs, plays a key role in the process of the innate immune response, and activates the nuclear factor-κB (NF-κB) signaling pathway by binding to lipopolysaccharide (LPS), which was identified to be an important mechanism in the development of rheumatic diseases [7–11].

The *TLR4* gene consisting of three exons is located on chromosome 9q32–33 [12]. Previous studies have reported that some polymorphisms in the *TLR4* coding/non-coding region, in particular Asp299Gly polymorphism, are associated with a blunted receptor activity and a subsequently diminished inflammatory response in humans [13–16]. Furthermore, variants in the *TLR4* were also reported to be associated with lymphoid tissue lymphoma [17], Hodgkin lymphoma [17], cancer [18] and ischemic cerebrovascular disease [19]. Surprisingly, relatively few genetic studies reported significant associations of polymorphisms in *TLR4* with RA and JIA susceptibility. Most studies have focused on the correlation between two well known *TLR4* polymorphisms (Asp299Gly and Thr399Ile) and RA and JIA, while inconclusive or contradictory results were observed [20, 21]. To our knowledge, only three studies with relatively small sample size have investigated the association between variants in the *TLR4* and RA in Chinese Han population [22–24], and negative result was also reported [23, 24]. In addition, no research conducted on the association between *TLR4* polymorphisms and JIA in central Chinese Han population was found. Thus, the role of *TLR4* in RA and JIA in central Chinese Han population remains unclear.

In present study, we aimed to examine the possible associations of *TLR4* polymorphisms with auto-antibody levels in RA and JIA susceptibility in a central south Chinese Han population.

Methods

Sample collection

The study was approved by the Ethical Committee at Changsha Medical University (EC/14/013, 06/11/2014). Written, informed consents for genetic analysis were obtained from all subjects or their guardians. A total of 1074 unrelated patients (Female/Male: 842/232; age: 41.7 ± 11.6 years) who met the American College of Rheumatology (The American Rheumatism Association) 1987 revised criteria for RA [25] and 217 unrelated patients (boy/girl: 178/39; age: 6.3 ± 3.1 years) who fulfilled the EULAR JIA criteria were recruited from the first affiliated hospital, Changsha Medical University. Rheumatoid factor (RF) and anti-cyclic citrullinated peptide (anti-CCP) status were determined for all the patients. The erythrocyte sedimentation rate (ESR) was tested by Westergren method. The auto-antibody levels were detected by Enzyme-linked immunosorbent assay (ELISA). In addition, 1692 unrelated control subjects without the history of RA and 378 unrelated control subjects without the history of JIA (matched for ethnicity, gender and age) for this study were also enrolled. The control subjects were healthy individuals who took the health examination in the first affiliated hospital, Changsha Medical University. All participants were Chinese Han population in origin.

Genotyping

A combination of 6 well-studied informative *TLR4* SNPs (Two functional variants [rs4986790 (Asp299Gly) and rs4986791 (Thr399Ile) in exon 3, one variant (rs10759932) in 5'UTR and three variants (rs41426344, rs11536889 and rs7873784) in 3'UTR were genotyped in RA, JIA and healthy controls. Genomic DNA was extracted from peripheral leukocytes using the standard phenol–chloroform method [26]. The multiplex PCR was carried out on the ABI Veriti Thermal Cycler (Applied Biosystems, Foster City, CA). Genotyping was conducted using direct sequencing by the ABI 3730XL DNA Sequencer (Applied Biosystems, Foster City, CA). The PCR primers and sequencing probes were shown in Additional file 1: Table S1.

Statistical analysis

Hardy-Weinberg equilibrium (HWE) was tested in the cases and controls using a classic chi-square test with 1° of freedom. The statistical analysis was performed using SHESIS (http://analysis.bio-x.cn/SHEsisMain.htm). Individual analyses of associations between *TLR4* polymorphisms and RA and JIA, as well as clinical features were performed by comparing alleles and genotypes in cases and controls using Fisher's exact test. The corresponding ORs and 95% confidence intervals (CI) were assessed using a standard logistic regression analysis. Bonferroni correction was applied to adjust the p value (P_{adj}) in multiple comparisons. Analysis of haplotype diversity was performed using the expectation-maximization algorithm (EM). Specific P values and ORs and 95% confidence intervals (CI) were obtained by comparing each haplotype with the more common haplotype in the population using Fisher's exact test. Statistical significance was set at $p < 0.05$.

Results

Clinical features such as erythrocyte sedimentation rate (ESR), C-reactive protein (CRP), IgA, IgG, IgM were shown in Table 1. For JIA, the patients can be classified into five subtypes (systemic JIA, polyarticular (RF^+ and RF^-) JIA, pauciarticular JIA, psoriatic JIA and other JIA). There were 21 (9.6%), 52 (23.7%) (RF^+: 15 (6.9%); RF^-: 37 (16.8%)), 111 (51.2%), 28 (12.9%) and 5 (2.3%) separately for each subtype.

Table 1 Clinical characteristics of RA and JIA patients and heathy controls

Clinical characteristics	RA (Mean ± SD)	Control (Mean ± SD)	p	JIA (Mean ± SD)	Control (Mean ± SD)	p
Sex ratio (Female/Male)	3.63 (842/232)	3.47 (1314/378)	0.17	4.56 (178/39)	4.72 (312/66)	0.89
Age (years)	41.7 ± 11.6	39.6 ± 13.2	0.75	6.3 ± 3.1	6.7 ± 2.5	0.75
Onset age, years	49.5 ± 7.9	–	–	7.5 ± 4.9	–	–
Bone erosions n (%)	421 (39.1%)	–	–	46 (21.3%)	–	–
Shared epitope	467 (43.5%)	–	–	79 (36.4%)	–	–
DAS28	4.7 ± 1.3	–	–	3.4 ± 1.1	–	–
ESR (mm/h) (0–10 mm/h)	33.2 ± 12.5	4.5 ± 2.2	<0.001	34.5 ± 19.3	4.3 ± 2.4	<0.001
CRP (mg/l) (0.8–8 mg/l)	25.8 ± 12.2	4.9 ± 1.3	<0.001	19.3 ± 37.5	3.77 ± 1.4	<0.001
IgA mg/mL (0.71–3.35 mg/mL)	12.2 ± 2.7	2.88 ± 1.4	<0.001	10.2 ± 2.4	2.59 ± 1.7	<0.001
IgG mg/mL (7.6–16.6 mg/mL)	45.7 ± 5.4	10.3 ± 4.1	<0.001	29.6 ± 5.1	9.7 ± 1.3	<0.001
IgM mg/mL (0.48–2.12 mg/mL)	6.6 ± 1.3	1.78 ± 2.1	<0.001	5.4 ± 1.7	1.88 ± 1.02	<0.001
RF^+, %	826 (76.9%)	0 (0%)		37 (16.9%)	0 (0%)	
CCP^+, %	766 (71.3%)	0 (0%)		33 (15.4%)	0 (0%)	

Abbreviation: *SD* Standard Deviation, *ESR* erythrocyte sedimentation rate, *CRP* C-reactive protein, *RF* rheumatoid factor, *JIA* juvenile idiopathic arthritis, *RA* Rheumatoid arthritis
Disease activity score 28(DAS28): a score for evaluation of RA activity by assessing the state of 28 joints; anti-CCP: anti-cyclic citrullinated peptide

Single-locus association

All variants in cases and controls were in Hardy-Weinberg equilibrium (HWE) ($p > 0.05$). Genotype data for the 6 *TLR4* SNPs successfully typed in the central south Chinese Han population cases and controls were examined by single-marker analysis (Tables 2 and 3). Genotype analysis showed that the distribution of rs41426344 CC was significantly higher in RA and JIA patients compared with controls, even after the Bonferroni's correction (RA: $p < 0.001$, $p_{adj} < 0.001$, OR [CI95%]: 3.75 [2.51–5.6]; JIA: $p = 0.0002$, $p_{adj} = 0.0006$, OR [CI95%]: 4.79 [1.97–11.67]). The frequencies of rs41426344C in RA and JIA were 0.21 and 0.25 separately. Significant associations between rs41426344C and RA and JIA were observed in further allelic analysis (RA: $p < 0.001$, $p_{adj} < 0.001$, OR [CI95%]: 2.24 [1.76–2.85]; JIA: $p < 0.001$, $p_{adj} < 0.001$, OR [CI95%]: 2.05 [1.52–2.77]).

The distribution of the rs4986790GA in RA cases was significantly higher than that in controls ($p < 0.001$, $p_{adj} < 0.001$, OR [CI95%]: 3.47 [2.06–5.87]). And allelic analysis of the RA cohort revealed that the frequency of the rs4986790G was significantly higher in patients (2%) compared with controls (0.06%) with an OR equal to 3.43 ($p = 0.005$, $p_{adj} = 0.03$, OR [CI95%]: 3.43 [1.39–8.45]), which indicated that G allele in rs4986790 might reveal a strong risk factor for RA in central south Chinese Han population.

No association was detected between other SNPs in the 3'UTR (rs11536889 and rs7873784) and 5'UTR (rs10759932) of the *TLR4* gene and RA and JIA ($p > 0.05$).

Table 2 Allele distributions of *TLR4* gene polymorphisms in RA, JIA and healthy controls

SNPs (MAF)	Region	Position	RA Case (freq.)	RA Control (freq.)	P	P^a_{adj}	OR [95%CI][b]	JIA Case (freq.)	JIA Control (freq.)	P	P^a_{adj}	OR [95%CI][b]
rs10759932(C)	5'UTR	27786349	0.32	0.29	0.37	–	1.10 [0.89–1.34]	0.26	0.26	0.86	–	1.03 [0.78–1.34]
rs4986790 (G)	Exon 3	27796507	0.02	0.006	**0.005**	**0.03**	**3.43 [1.39–8.45]**	0.02	0.008	0.06	–	2.65 [0.93–7.49]
rs4986791 (T)	Exon 3	27796807	0.05	0.04	0.03	0.18	1.75 [1.09–2.82]	0.07	0.05	0.12	–	1.46 [0.90–2.37]
rs41426344 (C)	3'UTR	27799138	0.21	0.13	**<0.001**	**<0.001**	**2.24 [1.76–2.85]**	0.25	0.14	**<0.001**	**<0.001**	**2.05 [1.52–2.77]**
rs11536889 (C)	3'UTR	27799336	0.22	0.19	0.07	–	1.24 [0.98–1.56]	0.23	0.19	0.19	–	1.21 [0.91–1.61]
rs7873784 (C)	3'UTR	27800141	0.15	0.12	0.03	0.18	1.35 [1.03–1.77]	0.13	0.14	0.68	–	0.93 [0.66–1.31]

Abbreviation: *SNP*, single nucleotide polymorphism, *MAF* minor allele frequency, *OR* odds ratio, *95% CI* 95% confidence intervals, not calculated, *RA* Rheumatoid arthritis, *JIA* juvenile idiopathic arthritis, *Freq* frequency; p_{adj}, $p_{adjusted}$
[a]The Bonferroni's correction was carried out to adjust the *p* value
[b]OR and 95% CI are calculated for the minor allele of each SNP

Table 3 Distribution of the genotypes of *TLR4* gene polymorphisms in RA and JIA cases and controls

SNPs	Genotype	Control no.	RA no.	OR [95%CI]	p^a	p^b_{adj}	Control no.	JIA no.	OR [95%CI]	p^a	p^b_{adj}
rs10759932 (C)	TT	844	498	0.87 [0.74–1.01]	0.07	–	204	125	1.16 [0.83–1.62]	0.39	–
	CT	696	466	1.09 [0.94–1.28]	0.24	–	151	73	0.76 [0.54–1.08]	0.13	–
	CC	143	108	1.21 [0.93–1.57]	0.15	–	23	19	1.48 [0.79–2.79]	0.22	–
rs4986790 (G)	AA	1671	1029	**0.28 [0.17–0.49]**	**<0.001**	**<0.001**	372	208	0.37 [0.13–1.06]	0.06	–
	GA	21	45	**3.47 [2.06–5.87]**	**<0.001**	**<0.001**	6	9	2.68 [0.94–7.64]	0.06	–
	GG	0	0	–	–	–	0	0	–	–	–
rs4986791 (T)	CC	1590	986	0.72 [0.53–0.96]	0. 03	0.09	399	186	0.58 [0.35–0.97]	0.04	0.12
	CT	100	85	1.37 [1.01–1.84]	0.04	0.12	39	30	1.65 [0.99–2.73]	0.05	–
	TT	2	3	–	–	–	0	1	–	–	–
rs41426344 (C)	GG	1287	615	**0.42 [0.36–0.49]**	**<0.001**	**<0.001**	280	127	**0.49 [0.35–0.70]**	**<0.001**	**<0.001**
	GC	369	378	**1.94 [1.64–2.31]**	**<0.001**	**<0.001**	91	72	1.57 [1.08–2.26]	0.02	0.06
	CC	36	81	**3.75 [2.51–5.6]**	**<0.001**	**<0.001**	7	18	**4.79 [1.97–11.67]**	**0.0002**	**0.0006**
rs11536889 (C)	GG	1113	647	**0.79 [0.67–0.92]**	**0.003**	**0.009**	242	133	0.89 [0.63–1.26]	0.51	–
	GC	518	372	1.20 [1.02–1.41]	0.03	0.09	125	70	0.96 [0.67–1.37]	0.84	–
	CC	60	54	1.44 [0.99–2.09]	0.06	–	11	14	2.3 [1.02–5.16]	0.04	0.12
rs7873784 (C)	GG	1308	790	0.81 [0.68–0.97]	0.02	0.06	278	165	1.14 [0.78–1.68]	0.50	–
	GC	358	268	1.24 [1.03–1.48]	0.02	0.06	96	48	0.83 [0.56–1.23]	0.37	–
	CC	25	16	1.01 [0.54–1.89]	1.00	–	4	4	1.76 [0.43–7.09]	–	–

Abbreviation: *SNP* single nucleotide polymorphism, *OR* odds ratio, *95% CI* 95% confidence intervals; –, not calculated, *RA* Rheumatoid arthritis, *JIA* juvenile idiopathic arthritis

[a] *P* value were calculated using Fisher's exact test

[b] The Bonferroni's correction was carried out to adjust the *P* value

And no notable association was detected between both genotypes and alleles in rs4986790 and JIA ($p > 0.05$).

Haplotype analysis

Haplotypes were predicted for 6 SNPs using PLINK 1.09 (http://pngu.mgh.harvard.edu/~purcell/plink/). Ten haplotypes in RA and JIA separately with a frequency > 1% were predicted in both cases and controls accounting for > 90% of all the haplotypes. The haplotype 1(H1) (TACGGG) containing rs10759932T, rs4986790A, rs4986791C, rs41426344G, rs11536889G, rs7873784G was the most common haplotype with a frequency of approximately 43% in RA and 42% in JIA. However, no association was found between H1 and RA and JIA ($p > 0.05$). Additionally, we observed a marginally significant increase in the distribution of H4 (TGTCCG) and H10 (CGTCCG) in RA compared with that in the controls (H4: $p = 0.001$, OR [95%CI] = 1.13 [0.77–1.26]; H10: $p = 0.001$, OR [95%CI] = 1.15 [1.02–1.56]) (Table 4). Similar results were found in H4 and H10 in JIA and controls (TGTCCG: $p = 0.04$, OR [95%CI] = 2.06[1.01–4.21]; H10: $p = 0.02$, OR [95%CI] = 2.47[1.11–5.49]) (Table 4).

Allelic/Genotypic distribution of RF and anti-CCP in RA and JIA

Data were available on autoantibody levels including information on circulating RF and anti-CCP. Carriage of rs41426344C significantly increased in RF-positive (RF^+ vs. RF^- : 0.17 vs. 0.08) and anti-CCP positive (anti-CCP^+ vs. anti-CCP^- : 0.15 vs. 0.06) subjects in RA (RF^+: p <0.0001, OR [95%CI] = 2.33 [1.65–3.01]; anti-CCP^+: p =0.008, OR [95%CI] = 2.79[1.28–6.11]) and JIA (RF^+ vs. RF^- : 0.19 vs. 0.08; anti-CCP^+ vs. anti-CCP^- : 0.16 vs. 0.05) (RF^+: p =0.02, OR [95%CI] = 2.91 [1.11–7.56]; anti-CCP^+: p =0.02, OR [95%CI] = 2.78 [1.21–6.74]) (Table 5). Allele and genotype frequencies were not different after stratification by anti-CCP status for rs4986790 that was shown to be associated with RA and JIA in our study (Table 5).

Discussion

In the current study, 1074 RA, 217 JIA and 2070 healthy controls were genotyped for six polymorphisms in the *TLR4* gene that was previously reported to be associated with autoimmune diseases. The data showed that the frequencies of *TLR4* rs4986790G in RA cases, as well as rs41426344C in JIA cases significantly increased than that in the controls, which was, to our knowledge, the first study to demonstrate associations between the two common polymorphisms and RA and JIA in central Chinese Han population using case-control design.

TLRs play important roles in both innate and adaptive immune responses that invading by microorganisms [27]. The chronic inflammation and the well-recognized interactions of TLRs with numerous endogenous ligands

Table 4 Haplotype analysis of RA and JIA cases and the healthy controls in the *TLR4* genes

NO.	haplotype[a]	RA		OR [95CI%], P^b	JIA		OR [95CI%], P^b
		Control (freq.)	Case (freq.)		Control (freq.)	Case (freq.)	
H1	TACGGG	0.47	0.43	1.03 [0.99–1.17],0.29	0.45	0.42	0.72 [0.52–1.01],0.06
H2	TACGGC	0.06	0.12	1.07 [0.83–1.33],0.07	0.06	0.10	1.74 [0.95–3.21],0.07
H3	TACGCG	0.11	0.09	0.54 [0.22–1.11],0.13	0.10	0.07	0.66 [0.36–1.23],0.19
H4	TGTCCG	0.02	0.08	**1.13 [0.77–1.26],0.001**	0.04	0.08	**2.06 [1.01–4.21] 0.04**
H5	TACCCC	0.003	0.01	1.09 [0.76–1.45],0.06	0.003	0.006	1.75 [0.11–2.86],0.39
H6	CACGGG	0.06	0.06	1.01 [0.99–1.03],0.89	0.04	0.06	1.54 [0.72–3.31],0.26
H7	CACGCG	0.01	0.02	1.10 [0.98–1.24],0.57	0.02	0.02	0.87 [0.26–2.93],0.78
H8	CACGCC	0.003	0.001	0.86 [0.63–1.05],0.69	0.002	0.003	1.74 [0.11–2.04],0.54
H9	CACCGG	0.14	0.11	0.98 [0.97–0.99],0.07	0.15	0.11	0.70 [0.42–1.16],0.17
H10	CGTCCG	0.03	0.13	**1.15 [1.02–1.56],0.001**	0.03	0.07	**2.47 [1.11–5.49],0.02**

Abbreviation: *SNP* single nucleotide polymorphism, *OR* odds ratio, *95% CI* 95% confidence intervals; –, not calculated, *RA* Rheumatoid arthritis, *JIA* juvenile idiopathic arthritis, *Freq* frequency

[a]Haplotype structure of *TLR4* for RA and JIA were rs4986790, rs4986791, rs10759932,rs41426344, rs11536889, rs7873784

[b]*P* value were calculated using Fisher's exact test

have implicated this pathway in a number of disease states including RA and JIA [27, 28]. As a member of TLRs, TLR4 has been considered to recognize not only the LPS component of gram-negative bacteria but also the mouse mammary tumor virus [29, 30]. In particular, TLR4 has been identified as an important part of investigation in understanding arthritides pathogenesis. It has been also demonstrated that TLR4 is over-expressed in RA synovium [31]. Investigations using animal models of inflammatory arthritis also implicate TLR4 in RA. Mice with non-functional TLR4 or mice deficient of MyD88 are protected from inflammatory arthritis [32]. As for JIA, Donn R et al. indicated that the macrophage migration inhibitory factor (MIF) have been reported to be associated with JIA [33]. And a relationship between MIF and TLR4 was found in a study of MIF-deficient mice [34], which supported the hypothesis that TLR4 is a risk factor for investigation in JIA.

The *TLR4* Asp299Gly (rs4986790) is a functional allele located in the exon 3 region of *TLR4* gene and was known to cause an aspartic acid to glycine replacement, which alter its extracellular domain and potentially modify its binding affinity. The strong association between *TLR4* Asp299Gly polymorphism and RA disease susceptibility has been reported in a Dutch cohort [35], but not in Irish, British and Spanish populations [35–37]. And no positive results was found between *TLR4* Asp299Gly and JIA in UK Caucasian and Indian [5, 38]. In our study, the frequency of Asp299Gly polymorphism in central south Chinese Han population was higher than that in other Chinese Han population populations [23, 39, 40], but was similar with that in Caucasian populations [41–44]. And a significant association was detected between *TLR4* Asp299Gly and RA in central south Chinese Han population compared to healthy controls. To our knowledge, this is the first study that a significant association between *TLR4* Asp299Gly and RA in Chinese Han population was reported. Interestingly, negative result was shown by Zheng [23] and Yuan [24]. The complex genetic ethnic specificity in Chinese Han populations might contribute to the difference.

Notable, the rs41426344 appeared to be significantly associated with both RA and JIA in central south Chinese Han population. Both rs41426344C allele and CC genotype are increased in RA cases, which was similar with the result reported by Zheng [22]. There were already evidences suggesting that the rs41426344 may act as susceptibility loci with diseases [44]. Cheng et al. suggested that rs41426344 may be a functional site, which could attenuate the LPS-induced transmembrane signaling through the alteration of post-transcriptional regulation of 3'UTR and target gene expression [41]. In addition, no significant association was found between other two 3'UTR SNPs (rs11536889 and rs7873784) and RA and JIA. Though the absence of association in these two loci was detected in our present study, we cannot exclude the possible effect of these two SNPs on RA and JIA development in other populations for genetic polymorphisms often vary between ethnic groups. Thus, replication in other populations is needed before these results can be generalized.

Conclusions

We observed significant associations between RA and JIA disease susceptibility and a *TLR4* variant (rs41426344) in a set of RA and JIA patients, as well as rs4986790 in RA patients and healthy individuals in central south Chinese Han population. Our finding needs to

Table 5 Rs4986790 and rs41426344 allele/genotype frequencies and autoantibody levels in patients with RA and JIA

SNPs	Allele/ Genotypes	RA		P^a,OR [95%CI]	JIA		P^a,OR [95%CI]	RA		P^a,OR [95%CI]	JIA		P^a,OR [95%CI]
		RF$^+$ (freq.)	RF$^-$ (freq.)		RF$^+$ (freq.)	RF$^-$ (freq.)		Anti-CCP$^+$ (freq.)	Anti-CCP$^-$ (freq.)		Anti-CCP$^+$ (freq.)	Anti-CCP$^-$ (freq.)	
rs4986790	G	0.11	0.13		0.15	0.14		0.25	0.21		0.13	0.11	
	A	0.89	0.87	0.74,0.94 [0.65–1.36]	0.85	0.86	0.82,1.07 [0.59–1.97]	0.75	0.79	0.55,1.19 [0.66–2.15]	0.87	0.89	0.84,1.26 [0.97–1.93]
	GG	0.0	0.0	–	–	–	–	0.0	0.0	–	0.0	0.0	–
	GA	0.33	0.29	0.51,1.17 [0.73–1.86]	0.31	0.30	0.84,1.06 [0.57–1.99]	0.34	0.32	0.75,0.88 [0.42–1.86]	0.29	0.27	0.64,1.22 [0.79–1.88]
	AA	0.67	0.71	0.92,0.98 [0.63–1.52]	0.69	0.70	0.84,0.94 [0.50–1.76]	0.66	0.68	0.84,0.93 [0.45–1.90]	0.71	0.73	0.79,0.46 [0.22–0.97]
rs41426344	C	0.17	0.08		0.19	0.08		0.15	0.06		0.16	0.05	
	G	0.83	0.92	**<.0001,2.33 [1.65–3..01]**	0.82	0.92	**0.02,2.91 [1.11–7.56]**	0.85	0.94	**0.008,2.79 [1.28–6.11]**	0.84	0.95	**0.02,2.78 [1.21–6.74]**
	CC	0.04	0.01	**0.01,1.45 [0.48–4.26]**	0.04	0.015	**0.001,3.23 [0.39–26.79]**	0.03	0.01	–,2.34 [0.27–20.45]	0.02	0.01	–,2.45 [0.36–18.75]
	CG	0.30	0.13	**<.0001,2.82 [1.90–4.19]**	0.30	0.13	**0.009,2.76 [1.26–6.05]**	0.23	0.09	**0.003,3.37 [1.48–9.43]**	0.22	0.10	**0.002,2.94 [1.39–8.25]**
	GG	0.66	0.86	**<.0001,0.37 [0.25–0.53]**	0.65	0.85	**0.002,0.32 [0.15–0.69]**	0.74	0.90	**<.0001,0.21 [0.09–0.48]**	0.76	0.89	**<.0001,0.34 [0.11–0.85]**

Abbreviation: *SNP* single nucleotide polymorphism, *OR* odds ratio, *95% CI* 95% confidence intervals; –, not calculated, *RF* rheumatoid factor, *anti-CCP* anti-cyclic citrullinated peptide

[a]*P* value were calculated using Fisher's exact test

be confirmed in other larger numbers of Chinese Han population cohorts. And to identify the potential mechanisms by which variant in rs41426344 and rs4986790 affects *TLR4* and RA and JIA is necessary.

Acknowledgements

We are grateful to the patients and control individuals for participating in this study. In addition, we should thanks Dr. Bifeng Chen from Chinese University of Hongkong and Peter R. Patrylo, Ph. D from Departments of Physiology and Anatomy Southern Illinois University School of Medicine for Language polishing.

Funding

This study was supported in part by the Foundation of the Education Department of Hunan (11C0141, 15C0513, 16C0162), the key Foundation of the Education Department of Hunan (15A023,16A027), National Science Foundation of Hunan province (2015JJ6010), Foundation of the health department of Hunan (B2016096) and the construct program of the key discipline in Hunan province.

Authors' contributions

LT and JML designed the experiments and drafted the manuscript. YW, LHC, FL and JZ collected the samples and carried out the genotyping. MHB and JX contributed to the statistical analysis. JML and HQ L are project leader and planned the study. All authors read and approved the final manuscript.

Competing interests

The authors declare that they have no competing interests.

Consent for publication

Consents to publish have obtained from all subjects or their guardians.

Author details

[1]Department of Human Anatomy, Histology and Embryology, Institute of Neuroscience, Changsha Medical University, No. 1501 Lei Feng Road,, Wangcheng District, Changsha City, Hunan Province 410219, People's Republic of China. [2]School of Basic Medical Science, Changsha Medical University, Changsha, People's Republic of China. [3]Experiment center for Function, Changsha Medical University, Changsha, People's Republic of China. [4]Department of Neurology, Xiang-ya Hospital, Central South University, Changsha City, Hunan Province, China.

References

1. Davidson A, Diamond B. Autoimmune diseases. N Engl J Med. 2001;345:340–50.
2. Goulielmos GN, Chiaroni-Clarke RC, Dimopoulou DG, Zervou MI, Trachana M, Pratsidou-Gertsi P, Garyfallos A, Ellis JA. Association of juvenile idiopathic arthritis with PTPN22 rs2476601 is specific to females in a Greek population. Pediatr Rheumatol. 2016;14:25.
3. Kirchner M, Sonnenschein A, Schoofs S, Schmidtke P, Umlauf VN, Mannhardt-Laakmann W. Surface expression and genotypes of Toll-like receptors 2 and 4 in patients with juvenile idiopathic arthritis and systemic lupus erythematosus. Pediatr Rheumatol. 2013;11:9.
4. Malievsky VA, Viktorova TV, Danilko KV, Nazarova LS. PReS-FINAL-2113: The association of the NFKB1 gene polymorphism with systemic onset juvenile idiopathic arthritis in Russia. Pediatr Rheumatol. 2013;11 Suppl 2:125.
5. Lamb R, Zeggini E, Thomson W, Donn R. Toll-like receptor 4 gene polymorphisms and susceptibility to juvenile idiopathic arthritis. Ann Rheum Dis. 2005;64:767–9.
6. Kuuliala K, Orpana A, Leirisalo-Repo M, Kautiainen H, Hurme M, Hannonen P, Korpela M, Mo¨tto¨nen T, Paimela L, Puolakka K, Karjalainen A, Repo H. Polymorphism at position +896 of the toll-like receptor 4 gene interferes with rapid response to treatment in rheumatoid arthritis. Ann Rheum Dis. 2006;65:1241–3.
7. Ospelt C, Brentano F, Rengel Y, Stanczyk J, Kolling C, Tak PP, Gay RE, Gay S, Kyburz D. Overexpression of Toll-like receptors 3 and 4 in synovial tissue from patients with early rheumatoid arthritis. Toll-like receptor expression in early and longstanding arthritis. Arthritis Rheum. 2008;58:3684–92.
8. Akira S, Takeda K, Kaisho T. Toll-like receptors: critical proteins linking innate and acquired immunity. Nat Immunol. 2001;2:675–80.
9. Schröder NW, Schumann RR. Single nucleotide polymorphisms of toll-like receptors and susceptibility to infectious disease. Lancet Infect Dis. 2005;5: 156–64.
10. Candore G, Colonna-Romano G, Balistreri CR, Di CD, Grimaldi MP. Biology of longevity: role of the innate immune system. Rejuvenation Res. 2006;9:143–8.
11. Turner MW, Hamvas RM. Mannose-binding lectin: structure, function, genetics and disease associations. Rev Immunogenet. 2000;2:305–22.
12. Buraczynska M, Baranowicz-Gaszczyk I, Ksiazek A. Toll-like receptor 4 gene polymorphism and early onset of diabetic retinopathy in patients with type 2 diabetes. Hum Immunol. 2009;70:121–4.
13. Arbour NC, Lorenz E, Schutte BC, Zabner J, Kline JN. TLR4 mutations are associated with endotoxin hyporesponsiveness in humans. Nat Genet. 2000;25:187–91.
14. Hemming NV, Blanco JCG, Segal DM, Medvedev SA, Lorenz E, Arditi M, Rallabhandi VGP, Bell J, Boukhvalova MS. Analysis of TLR4 polymorphic variants: new insights into TLR4/MD-2/CD14 stoichiometry, structure, and signaling. J Immunol. 2006;177:322–32.
15. Kinane DF, Shiba H, Stathopoulou PG, Zhao H, Lappin DF, Singh A, Eskan MA, Beckers S, Waigel S, Alpert B, Knudsen TB. Gingival epithelial cells heterozygous for toll-like receptor 4 polymorphisms Asp299Gly and Thr399ile are hypo-responsive to Porphyromonas gingivalis. Genes Immun. 2006;7:190–200.
16. Montes AH, Asensi V, Alvarez V, Valle E, Ocaña MG, Meana A, Carton JA, Paz J, Fierer J, Celada A. The toll-like receptor (Asp299Gly) polymorphism is a risk factor for gram-negative and haematogenous osteomyelitis. Clin Exp Immunol. 2006;143:404–13.
17. Nuolivirta K, Hurme M, Halkosalo A, Koponen P, Korpp M. Gene polymorphism of IFNG+ 874 T/A and TLR4 + 896A/G and recurrent infections and wheezing in toddlers with history of bronchiolitis. Pediatr Infect Dis J. 2009;28:1121–3.
18. Zhang K, Zhou B, Wang Y, Rao L, Zhang L. The TLR4 gene polymorphisms and susceptibility to cancer: a systematic review and meta-analysis. Eur J Cancer. 2013;49:946–54.
19. Yin YW, Li JC, Li BH. Toll-like receptor 4 gene Asp299Gly polymorphism in ischemic cerebrovascular disease: a meta-analysis. Int J Neurosci. 2014;124:252–60.
20. Xu WD, Liu SS, Pan HF, Ye DQ. Lack of association of TLR4 polymorphisms with susceptibility to rheumatoid arthritis and ankylosing spondylitis: A meta-analysis. Joint Bone Spine. 2012;79:566–9.
21. Tizaoui K, Naouali A, Kaabachi W, Hamzaoui A, Hamzaoui K. Association of Toll like receptor Asp299Gly with rheumatoid arthritis risk: A systematic review of case–control studies and meta-analysis. Pathol Res Pract. 2015;211:219–25.
22. Yang HJ, Wei CY, Li Q, Shou T, Yang Y, Xiao CJ, Yu M, Li M, Yang ZL, Zhang JY, Zheng BR. Association of TLR4 gene non-missense single nucleotide polymorphisms with rheumatoid arthritis in Chinese Han population. Rheumatol Int. 2013;33:1283–8.
23. Zheng BR, Li Q, Wei CY, Qin J, Shou T, Zhou R, Shao J, Yang Y, Xiao C. Lack of association of TLR4 gene Asp299Gly and Thr399Ile polymorphisms with rheumatoid arthritis in Chinese Han population of Yunnan Province. Rheumatol Int. 2010;30:1249–52.
24. Yuan M, Xia J, Ma L, Xiao B, Yang Q. Lack of the toll-like receptor 4 gene polymorphisms Asp299Gly and Thr399ile in a Chinese population. Int J Neurosci. 2010;120(6):415–20.

25. Arnett FC: The American Rheumatism Association. revised criteria for the classification of rheumatoid arthritis. Arthritis Rheum. 1987;1988(31):315–24.
26. Di PF, Ortenzi F, Tilio M, Concetti F, Napolioni V. Genomic dna extraction from whole blood stored from 15- to 30-years at −20 °c by rapid phenol-chloroform protocol: a useful tool for genetic epidemiology studies. Mol Cell Probes. 2010;25:44–8.
27. Beutler B. Inferences, questions and possibilities in Toll-like receptor signalling. Nature. 2004;430:257–63.
28. Foell D, Wittkowski H, Roth J. Mechanisms of disease: a "DAMP" view of inflammatory arthritis. Nat Clin Pract Rheumatol. 2007;3:382–90.
29. Erridge C. Endogenous ligands of TLR2 and TLR4: agonists or assistants? J Leukoc Biol. 2010;87:989–99.
30. Dhaouadi T, Sfar I, Haouami Y, Abdelmoula L, Turki S, Hassine LB. Polymorphisms of toll-like receptor-4 and cd14 in systemic lupus erythematosus and rheumatoid arthritis. Biomarker Res. 2013;1:20.
31. Sanchez-Pernaute O, Filkova M, Gabucio A. Citrullination enhances the pro-inflammatory response to fibrin in rheumatoid arthritis synovial fibroblasts. Ann Rheum Dis. 2013;72:1400–6.
32. van den Berg WB, van Lent PL, Joosten LA, Abdollahi-Roodsaz S, Koenders MI. Amplifying elements of arthritis and joint destruction. Ann Rheum Dis. 2007;66 Suppl 3:iii45–8.
33. Donn R, Alourfi Z, Zeggini E, Lamb R, Jury F, Lunt M, the British Paediatric Rheumatology Study Group, Meazza C, De Benedetti F, Thomson W, Ray D. A functional promoter haplotype of macrophage migration inhibitory factor (MIF) is linked and associated with juvenile idiopathic arthritis. Arthritis Rheum. 2004;50:1604–10.
34. Roger T, David J, Glauser MP, Calandra T. MIF regulates innate immune responses through modulation of Toll-like receptor 4. Nature. 2001;414:920–4.
35. Kilding R, Akil M, Till S, Amos R, Winfield J, Iles MM, Wilson AG. A biologically important single nucleotide polymorphism within the toll-like receptor-4 gene is not associated with rheumatoid arthritis. Clin Exp Rheumatol. 2003;21:340–2.
36. Sánchez E, Orozco G, López-Nevot MÁ, Jiménez-Alonso J, Martín J. Polymorphisms of toll-like receptor 2 and 4 genes in rheumatoid arthritis and systemic lupus erythematosus. Tissue Antigens. 2004;63:54–7.
37. Sheedy F, Marinou IL, Wilson A. The Mal/TIRAP S180L and TLR4 G299D polymorphisms are not associated with susceptibility to or severity of rheumatoid arthritis. Ann Rheum Dis. 2008;67:1328–31.
38. Myles A, Aggarwal A. Lack of association of single nucleotide polymorphisms in toll-like receptors 2 and 4 with enthesitis-related arthritis category of juvenile idiopathic arthritis in Indian population. Rheumatol Int. 2013;33:417–21.
39. Guo QS, Xia B, Jiang Y, Morre SA, Cheng L, Li J, Crusius JBA, Pen˜a AS. Polymorphisms of CD14 gene and TLR4 gene are not associated with ulcerative colitis in Chinese patients. Postgrad Med J. 2005;81:526–9.
40. Cheng L, Eng HL, Chou MH, You, Lin TM. Genetic polymorphisms of viral infection associated Toll-like receptors in Chinese population. Transl Res. 2007;150:311–8.
41. Radstake TRDJ, Franke B, Hanssen S, Netea MG, Welsing P, Barrera P, Joosten LAB, van Riel PLCM, van den Berg WB. The Toll-like receptor 4 Asp299Gly functional variant is associated with decreased rheumatoid arthritis disease susceptibility but does not influence disease severity and/or outcome. Arthritis Rheum. 2004;50:999–1001.
42. Adam R, Sturrock RD, Gracie JA. TLR4 mutations (Asp299Gly and Thr399Ile) are not associated with ankylosing spondylitis. Ann Rheum Dis. 2006;65:1099–101.
43. Paulus SC, Hirschfeld AF, Victor RE, Brunstein J, Thomas E, Turvey SE. Common human toll-like receptor 4 polymorphisms-role in susceptibility to respiratory syncytial virus infection and functional immunological relevance. Clin Immunol. 2007;123:252–7.
44. Hishida A, Matsuo K, Goto Y, Mitsuda Y, Hiraki A. Toll-like receptor 4 + 3725 G/C polymorphism, Helicobacter pylori seropositivity, and the risk of gastric atrophy and gastric cancer in Japanese. Helicobacter. 2009;14:47–53.

The spectrum of rheumatic in-patient diagnoses at a pediatric hospital in Kenya

Angela Migowa[1], Inés Colmegna[2], Carol Hitchon[3], Eugene Were[4], Evelyn Ng'ang'a[5], Thomas Ngwiri[4], John Wachira[4], Sasha Bernatsky[6] and Rosie Scuccimarri[1*]

Abstract

Background: Pediatric rheumatic diseases are chronic illnesses that can cause considerable disease burden to children and their families. There is limited epidemiologic data on these diseases in East Africa. The aim of this study was to assess the spectrum of pediatric rheumatic diagnoses in an in-patient setting and determine the accuracy of ICD-10 codes in identifying these conditions.

Methods: Medical records from Gertrude's Children's Hospital in Kenya were reviewed for patients diagnosed with "diseases of the musculoskeletal system and connective tissue" as per ICD-10 diagnostic codes assigned at discharge between January and December 2011. Cases were classified as "rheumatic" or "non-rheumatic". Accuracy of the assigned ICD-10 code was ascertained. Death records were reviewed. Longitudinal follow-up of "rheumatic" cases was done by chart review up to March 2014.

Results: Twenty six patients were classified as having a "rheumatic" condition accounting for 0.32% of patients admitted. Of these, 11 (42.3%) had an acute inflammatory arthropathy, 6 (23.1%) had septic arthritis, 4 (15.4%) had Kawasaki disease, 2 (7.7%) had pyomyositis, and there was one case each of septic bursitis, rheumatic fever, and a non-specific soft tissue disorder. No cases of juvenile idiopathic arthritis (JIA) were identified. One case of systemic lupus erythematosus was documented by death records. The agreement between the treating physician's discharge diagnosis and medical records ICD-10 code assignment was good (Kappa: 0.769). On follow-up, one child had recurrent knee swelling that was suspicious for JIA.

Conclusions: Pediatric rheumatic conditions represented 0.32% of admissions at a pediatric hospital in Kenya. Acute inflammatory arthropathies, septic arthritis and Kawasaki disease were the most frequent in-patient rheumatic diagnoses. Chronic pediatric rheumatic diseases were rare amongst this in-patient population. Despite limitations associated with the use of administrative diagnostic codes, they can be a first step in evaluating the spectrum of pediatric rheumatic conditions in Kenya and other countries in East Africa.

Keywords: Pediatric rheumatology, Global health, Kenya, Juvenile arthritis, Lupus, Kawasaki disease, ICD-10, Diagnostic codes

Background

Pediatric rheumatic diseases are chronic illnesses that can cause considerable disease burden to children and their families. They are associated with the potential for physical disability, diminished quality of life and significant direct and indirect costs [1–3]. This underscores the importance of early diagnosis and treatment.

One of the aims of the "Bone and Joint Decade" (2000–2010) was to increase the recognition and understanding of the impact of musculoskeletal conditions throughout the world and to improve health-related quality of life for patients living with these conditions [4, 5]. Understanding the burden of pediatric rheumatic diseases is a critical first step in developing and implementing policies to improve patient outcomes. Multiple studies suggest that pediatric rheumatic conditions are not rare in Africa [6–11] yet there are limited data available from epidemiological studies. Although children

* Correspondence: rosie.scuccimarri@muhc.mcgill.ca
[1]Division of Pediatric Rheumatology, Department of Pediatrics, McGill University Health Centre, 1001 Decarie Boulevard, Room A04.6306, Montreal, QC, CanadaH4A 3J1
Full list of author information is available at the end of the article

represent 53% of the Kenyan population (38.5 million in 2010) [12], the spectrum and frequency of pediatric rheumatic disorders remains to be defined.

We undertook this study to assess the spectrum of pediatric rheumatic diagnoses among children hospitalized in 2011 at Gertrude's Children's Hospital (GCH) in Kenya and to determine the accuracy of the use of musculoskeletal ICD-10 diagnostic codes in identifying these conditions.

Methods

Setting

GCH is a private, not-for-profit hospital located in Nairobi, the capital of Kenya. The hospital serves the population of Nairobi and its environs with a combined population of approximately 4 million people [12]. It is a tertiary level hospital with a bed capacity of 103, an emergency department and 24 subspecialty clinics ranging from cardiology, neurology, pulmonology, dermatology, orthopedics etc. At the time this study was conducted, there were no pediatric rheumatologists in Kenya. GCH was selected because it is one of the largest pediatric centers in East Africa, it is the only dedicated pediatric hospital in Nairobi and it has an electronic medical record system that was implemented at the end of 2010.

At GCH, the primary physician makes a final diagnosis at discharge. Trained medical records' clerks assign an International Classification of Disease 10th edition (ICD-10) code based on the physician's discharge diagnosis.

Study procedures

Following ethical approval from the Institutional Review Boards of McGill University (Montreal, Canada) and Gertrude's Children's Hospital (Nairobi, Kenya), a retrospective cross-sectional study was undertaken. Medical records of patients diagnosed with "diseases of the musculoskeletal system and connective tissue" as per ICD-10 diagnostic codes (M00 to M99, "M-codes") at discharge between January 1st and December 31st 2011 were identified by the electronic medical records system and selected for review. For in-patients, only the discharge diagnosis is recorded electronically. Data from the patient's history, clinical examination, laboratory and microbiology investigations were extracted (AM) from paper charts using a structured case report form. After assessing the clinical information of each case, two rheumatologists (RS-pediatric rheumatologist and IC) classified cases as having a "rheumatic" condition if they had a chronic rheumatic disease; or if they had an acute inflammatory or infectious condition involving the joints, bursae, muscles, or ligaments. All other cases were considered "non-rheumatic". Any discrepancies between the two rheumatologists were resolved by consensus.

For the "rheumatic" cases, we assessed the agreement between the ICD-10 code at discharge assigned by the medical records' clerks with the discharge diagnosis given to the patient by the treating physician. In addition, we report the agreement between the diagnosis assigned by the treating physician at discharge and that considered by the rheumatologists upon chart review.

In addition, the medical records of all in-patients who died at GCH between January and December 2011were reviewed to ascertain if there were any fatal "musculoskeletal system and connective tissue" cases, which may not have been identified by the electronic medical record system. As well, to assess whether any of the patients diagnosed with a "rheumatic" condition in 2011 progressed to develop a chronic inflammatory disease, longitudinal follow-up of "rheumatic" cases was done by chart review up to March 2014 by a pediatric rheumatologist (RS).

Statistics

Descriptive statistics were used. Kappa coefficients were reported to quantify the degree of agreement between the diagnoses given by the GCH treating physician, medical records' clerks and rheumatologists.

Results

In 2011, there were a total of 8011 admissions at GCH of which 45 were assigned an "M-code" at discharge (Fig. 1). The medical records of 44 cases were reviewed (1 chart could not be retrieved). From the information documented in the medical records, 3 were misassigned as an "M-code", 15 were classified as "non-rheumatic" and 26 were classified as having a "rheumatic" condition. The chart that could not be retrieved had a discharge diagnosis of scoliosis and would have likely been considered "non-rheumatic".

Of the charts reviewed, surgical cases accounted for 7 of the "non-rheumatic" conditions. Examples of these included ganglion and dermoid cyst excisions. From the non-surgical "non-rheumatic" conditions, examples included musculoskeletal pain from sickle cell crises, neck pain from suspected meningitis, and torticollis from a viral infection. Only one patient was identified as being HIV positive; the patient with neck pain from suspected meningitis.

"Rheumatic" conditions accounted for 0.32% of the in-patient admissions at GCH in 2011. The median age of the "rheumatic" patients was 3 years (range: 3 months – 15 years); 58% (15/26) were male. "Rheumatic" diagnoses included: acute inflammatory arthropathies ($n = 11$, 42.3%), septic arthritis ($n = 6$, 23.1%), Kawasaki disease (KD) ($n = 4$, 15.4%), pyomyositis ($n = 2$, 7.7%), septic bursitis ($n = 1$, 3.8%), rheumatic fever ($n = 1$, 3.8%) and non-specific soft tissue disorder ($n = 1$, 3.8%). In the patients with an

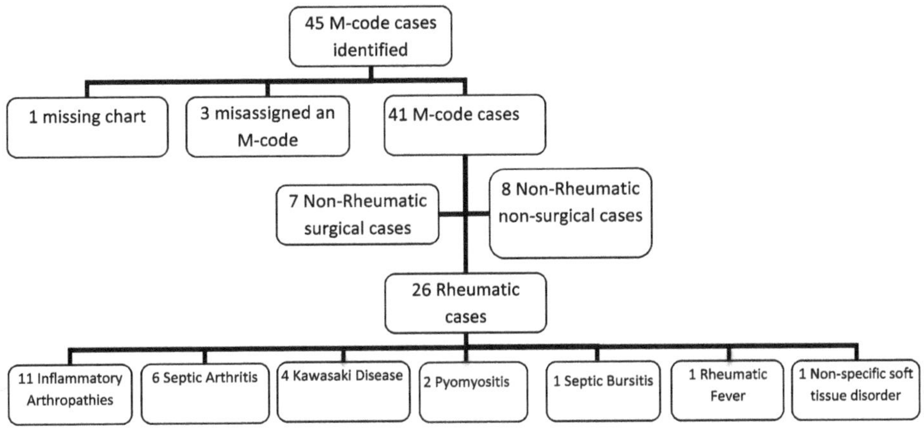

Fig. 1 Spectrum of Pediatric Rheumatic Conditions

inflammatory arthropathy, HIV or TB arthritis was not suspected by the treating physicians.

The agreement between the ICD-10 code assigned by the medical records' clerk and that of the treating physician for "rheumatic" conditions was 76.9% (20/26; Kappa: 0.769). The agreement between the ICD-10 code assigned by the treating physician and that given by the rheumatologist upon the medical record's review for the "rheumatic" conditions was 84.6% (22/26; Kappa: 0.846). Perfect agreement was found between the clerk, treating physician and rheumatologist in cases of KD, rheumatic fever and pyomyositis (Table 1).

The charts of the 26 patients deemed to have a "rheumatic" condition were reviewed again in March 2014 to assess if any had progressed to develop a chronic inflammatory disease on follow-up. Only one patient had a recurrent episode of knee swelling suspicious for the diagnosis of juvenile idiopathic arthritis (JIA). No other patients had a chronic disease course. The discharge diagnosis of the child with suspected JIA was "reactive arthritis versus septic arthritis". Upon initial chart review, and before the longitudinal follow-up, the patient had been categorized as an "acute inflammatory arthropathy" for this study.

From the 46 in-patient deaths from 2011, 45 charts were available and each was reviewed in detail. From this review, only 1 patient with a "rheumatic" condition was identified. This patient had systemic lupus erythematosus (SLE) and had died from sepsis. This patient had two admissions in 2011 and the discharge diagnosis assigned by the treating physician was "SLE". However the medical records' clerk had not assigned an "M-code" for either admissions and thus the electronic medical record system had not identified these admissions in the 2011 search.

Table 1 Agreement between Rheumatic Diagnoses assigned by the Rheumatologist, Treating Physician and Records Clerk

Diagnosis by Rheumatologist	Agreement between Records Clerk and Treating Physician	Agreement between Treating Physician and Rheumatologist
	n (%) = 20/26 (76.9%)	*n* (%) = 22/26 (84.6%)
Inflammatory Arthropathies (11)	8 (72.73)	9 (81.82)
Septic Arthritis (6)	4 (66.67)	5 (83.33)
Kawasaki Disease (4)	4 (100)	4 (100)
Pyomyositis (2)	2 (100)	2 (100)
Septic Bursitis (1)	0 (0)	0 (0)
Rheumatic Fever (1)	1 (100)	1 (100)
Non-Specific Soft Tissue Disorder (1)	1 (100)	1 (100)

Discussion

Rheumatic conditions accounted for 0.32% of all admissions at GCH in 2011. Acute inflammatory arthropathies were the most common in-patient "rheumatic" diagnoses accounting for 42.3% of all "rheumatic" cases. These patients had a short duration of symptoms, suggesting a post-infectious etiology. No cases of JIA requiring admission were identified during the study period. Septic arthropathies and pyomyositis combined were as common as the inflammatory arthropathies. KD was the only vasculitis diagnosed and accounted for 15.4% of the "rheumatic" cases. One case of SLE was identified, but only when the death records were reviewed. This suggests the possibility that other patients with "rheumatic" conditions may have been missed due to administrative errors in diagnostic code assignment.

The follow-up chart review, performed in 2014 to assess the evolution of the 26 "rheumatic" cases identified in 2011, confirmed that only one patient had a chronic disease course with recurrent episodes of knee swelling suspicious for the diagnosis of JIA. However, this does not exclude the possibility that some of these patients were followed elsewhere. This is a limitation of a retrospective study.

The male predominance of the "rheumatic" cases (58%) reflects the disease entities seen in this study. Chronic rheumatic diseases such as JIA and SLE are more common among females however, these diseases were not found in this in-patient population and therefore a female predominance should not be expected. All 3 cases of pyomyositis and septic bursitis were male. These entities are more commonly seen post-trauma which would be expected to be more frequent in males. As well, KD is slightly more common in males and in this study, 3 of the 4 patients with KD were male.

In our study, there were no children admitted for JIA and only one for SLE. This could reflect the low prevalence of these conditions as a cause for hospital admission, the lack of awareness / expertise of pediatricians in diagnosing these conditions, the limited use of specific M codes, the underestimation of the real frequency of these diagnoses based on their ascertainment through ICD-10 codes (i.e. coding errors) or the limitation of M-codes in identifying multisystem diseases such as SLE. Furthermore, an in-patient population may not be the ideal target population to assess conditions like JIA, which may be more likely assessed in out-patient clinics.

In this study, we chose to use M-codes to identify cases. However it is possible, that other cases could have been captured by the use of other specific codes (i.e. renal or hematologic impairments for SLE) and that M-codes underestimate the frequency of multisystem diagnoses. In the case of SLE, despite having a specific diagnostic M-code, discharge diagnosis may reflect the patient's reason for admission (i.e. renal failure) rather than the patient's diagnosis, which is another limitation of the use of administrative diagnostic codes to identify cases. As well, it is important to note that misdiagnoses are difficult to capture no matter what tool is used to identify cases. For example, if the treating physician could not identify that the child being treated for fever, rash and pericarditis was a child with systemic JIA and the discharge diagnosis was pericarditis or viral illness, this case would not have been captured. The absence of these diseases may reflect the limitations associated with the use of administrative diagnostic codes to capture cases in addition to the lack of expertise of pediatricians to diagnose specific rheumatic diseases rather than the true absence of disease.

JIA and pediatric SLE cases have been identified in various countries across the African continent such as in Nigeria, South Africa and Zambia [6–11]. In the Nigerian studies, they identified 11 children with SLE who were admitted to a hospital over a 5 year period [9, 10]. The rates reported for SLE in our study appear lower than those reported in Nigeria. With regard to JIA, all previous reported cases reflected out-patient data and thus are not comparable.

The first pediatric case of KD was described in Africa in 1979 [13]. In our study, four cases of KD were identified over a one year period, which is comparable, or a bit higher, than a few of the larger African case series in the literature [14–16]. Rheumatic fever is still the most common cause of acquired cardiac disease in children in developing countries [17] yet in this study, only one case of rheumatic fever was admitted. It is possible that most cases were managed as out-patients.

In Kenya, there is both a private and public medical system with several private hospitals and one main public national referral hospital that provide pediatric care in Nairobi. In 2008, the Government of Kenya provided resources for 48% of the country's health care facilities, while 49% was provided by the private sector (both for-profit and not-for-profit) [18]. Although private, GCH is the only dedicated pediatric hospital providing care exclusively to children; whereas the other hospitals have pediatric units. GCH has fewer but comparable in-patient admissions as compared to the main national public referral hospital (GCH: 8011 in 2011; public hospital: 9656 in 2007) [19]. We chose to undertake this study at GCH because it had the infrastructure to support this study particularly with the electronic medical records system. However, given that GCH only sees pediatric patients, it does not have access to adult rheumatology services. It is possible that if this study was conducted at the main public national referral hospital that has both adult and pediatric units, with access to adult rheumatology, more defined "rheumatic" cases could have been identified. In addition, given that GCH is a private hospital, the population that accesses it is different socioeconomically than those who can only access the public system.

It is important to highlight that at the time this study was conducted, there were no pediatric rheumatologists in Kenya. Global variability in the prevalence rates of pediatric musculoskeletal diseases has been attributed to varying levels of awareness of rheumatic diseases, combined with the lack of personnel and infrastructure to diagnose and manage these conditions [20]. This is particularly relevant in a setting where diverse and frequent entities such as infections, rickets and hemoglobinopathies [21] can lead to misdiagnosis and delays in the treatment of more rare rheumatic disorders. Olowu suggested that the paucity of pediatric rheumatologists, low level of lupus awareness, malaria endemicity (since malaria shares certain clinical features with lupus) contributed to misdiagnosis of lupus in the Nigerian pediatric population [10]. In his series, all SLE cases were misdiagnosed prior to referral (36.4% as malaria) suggesting a low level of awareness [10]. Prospective studies assessing rheumatic diagnoses made by pediatric rheumatologists now working in Kenya will be relevant to estimate the real burden of rheumatic conditions in this setting. We suspect that disease awareness and the presence of pediatric rheumatologists locally will improve case ascertainment and provide more accurate estimates of the frequency and spectrum of disease.

The agreement in the use of ICD-10 diagnostic codes by the records clerks and the diagnosis of the treating physician was good (Kappa 0.769). However there are challenges and limitations in using administrative databases in estimating disease prevalence. As expected, the more specific the treating physician's discharge diagnosis, the more accurate was the assigned code as reflected by the 100% agreement for the diagnosis of KD. In contrast, the missed SLE coding likely occurred due to the use of an acronym ("SLE") that was not interpreted by the medical record's clerk. This highlights the importance of promoting a clear and precise record of discharge diagnoses by physicians as a way to increase the accuracy of administrative data in estimating frequencies of diagnostic categories.

The aim of pediatric global health priorities has been to reduce infant and childhood mortality. Infectious diseases and injuries account for 75% of cause-specific mortality among children 5–14 years of age [22]. Musculoskeletal disease only comprises 0.1% of all-cause mortality in the same age group [22]. Therefore musculoskeletal disease has not been considered a health priority for most African countries. Most medical efforts have been directed towards preventable diseases such as acute respiratory infections, malaria, measles, diarrhea, HIV, malnutrition and trauma [22]. However, as preventable diseases are better controlled and treated, there is an expected health priority shift towards chronic conditions including rheumatic diseases [20, 22]. Therefore the importance of rheumatic disease awareness and building medical expertise capacity cannot be overstated.

Conclusions

To our knowledge, this is the first report of the spectrum of pediatric rheumatic conditions amongst in-patients in Kenya. Pediatric rheumatic conditions represented 0.32% of admissions at a pediatric hospital in Nairobi. Acute inflammatory arthropathies, septic arthritis and Kawasaki disease were the most frequent in-patient rheumatic diagnoses. Chronic pediatric rheumatic diseases were rare amongst this in-patient population. This may reflect the limitations associated with the use of administrative diagnostic codes and lack of expertise of pediatricians to diagnose specific rheumatic diseases rather than the true absence of disease. Increasing awareness of pediatric rheumatic diseases amongst health care professionals as well as the recruitment of pediatric rheumatologists to the region will allow for better identification of cases and estimation of the burden of these diseases among Kenyan children. Despite the limitations associated with the use of administrative diagnostic codes, they can be a first step in evaluating the spectrum and frequency of pediatric rheumatic conditions in Kenya and other countries in East Africa.

Abbreviations

GCH: Gertrude's Children's Hospital; HIV: Human immunodeficiency virus; ICD-10: International classification of disease 10th edition; JIA: Juvenile idiopathic arthritis; KD: Kawasaki disease; M-codes: Diagnostic codes for "diseases of the musculoskeletal system and connective tissue" as per ICD-10 (M00 to M99); SLE: Systemic lupus erythematosus

Acknowledgements

The authors would like to thank the medical records department of Gertrude's Children's Hospital for their assistance with this study.

Funding

This work was supported by a Canada-Africa Research Exchange Grant (CAREG) from Universities Canada.

Authors' contributions

AM, RS, IM conceived the study, participated in its design and coordination, were involved in the collection of the data, in the statistical analysis and drafting of the manuscript. CH conceived the study, participated in its design and contributed to the drafting of the manuscript. SB participated in the design of the study. EN, EW participated in the collection of data. EW, TN, JW participated in the coordination of the study. All authors read, revised and approved the final manuscript.

Competing interests

The authors declare that they have no competing interests.

Consent for publication

Not applicable.

Author details

[1]Division of Pediatric Rheumatology, Department of Pediatrics, McGill University Health Centre, 1001 Decarie Boulevard, Room A04.6306, Montreal, QC, CanadaH4A 3J1. [2]Division of Rheumatology, Department of Medicine, McGill University Health Centre, Montreal, QC, Canada. [3]Division of Rheumatology, Department of Internal Medicine, University of Manitoba, Winnipeg, MB, Canada. [4]Department of Pediatrics, Gertrude's Children's Hospital, Nairobi, Kenya. [5]Department of Pediatrics, The Nairobi Hospital, Nairobi, Kenya. [6]Division of Rheumatology & Division of Clinical Epidemiology, Department of Medicine & Department of Epidemiology, Biostatistics and Occupational Health, McGill University Health Centre, McGill University, Montreal, QC, Canada.

References

1. Moorthy LN, Peterson MG, Hassett AL, Lehman TJ. Burden of childhood-onset arthritis. Pediatr Rheumatol Online J. 2010;8:20.

2. Minden K, Niewerth M, Listing J, et al. The economic burden of juvenile idiopathic arthritis-results from the German paediatric rheumatologic database. Clin Exp Rheumatol. 2009;27(5):863–9.
3. Bernatsky S, Duffy C, Malleson P, Feldman DE, St Pierre Y, Clarke AE. Economic impact of juvenile idiopathic arthritis. Arthritis Rheum. 2007;57(1):44–8.
4. WHO Scientific Group on the Burden of Musculoskeletal Conditions at the Start of the New Millenium. The burden of musculoskeletal conditions at the start of the new millenium. World Health Organ Tech Rep Ser. 2003; 919(i-x):1–218.
5. Woolf AD. The bone and joint decade 2000–2010. Ann Rheum Dis. 2000; 59(2):81–2.
6. Chipeta J, Njobvu P, Wa-Somwe S, Chintu C, McGill PE, Bucala R. Clinical patterns of juvenile idiopathic arthritis in Zambia. Pediatr Rheumatol Online J. 2013;11(1):33.
7. Adelwoo OO, Umar A. Juvenile idiopathic arthritis among Nigerians: a case study. Clin Rheumatol. 2010;29(7):757–61.
8. Weakley K, Esser M, Scott C. Juvenile idiopathic arthritis in two tertiary centres in the Western Cape, South Africa. Pediatr Rheumatol Online J. 2012;10(1):35.
9. Olowu WA, Adelusola KA, Senbanjo IO. Clinicopathology of childhood-onset renal systemic lupus erythematosus. Nephrology (Carlton). 2007;12(4):364–70.
10. Olowu W. Childhood-onset systemic lupus erythematosus. J Natl Med Assoc. 2007;99(7):777–84.
11. Kanyerezi BR, Mbidde E. Juvenile chronic polyarthritis in Ugandan African children. East Afr Med J. 1980;57(7):484–9.
12. Kenya. Kenya National Bureau of Statistics. Kenya facts and figures, 2014. Nairobi: Director General Kenya National Bureau of Statistics; 2014. p. 83.
13. Elamin AM. Kawasaki disease in two African siblings. Trop Doct. 1979;9(4): 153–4.
14. Kibel MA, Jaffe IP, Ryder C. Kawasaki disease. S Afr Med J. 1980;58(1):6.
15. Badoe EV, Neequaye J, Oliver-Commey JO, et al. Kawasaki disease in Ghana: case reports from Korle Bu teaching hospital. Ghana Med J. 2011;45(1):38–42.
16. Mabiala Babela JR, Ollandzobo Ikobo LC, Nika RE, Moyen G. Study of 11 new cases of Kawasaki disease Congolese. Bull Soc Pathol Exot. 2015;108(4):250–4.
17. Watson G, Jallow B, Le Doare K, Pushparajah K, Anderson ST. Acute rheumatic fever and rheumatic heart disease in resource-limited settings. Arch Dis Child. 2015;100(4):370–5.
18. Turin, D. R. "Health Care Utilization in the Kenyan Health System: Challenges and Opportunities." Inquiries Journal/Student Pulse. 2010;2(09). Retrieved from http://www.inquiriesjournal.com/a?id=284. Accessed 2 Dec 2016.
19. Gichobi D, Wanzala P, Mutai J, Kamweya A. Factors associated with disease outcome in children at Kenyatta National Hospital (KNH). J Public Health Epidemiol. 2010;2(9):262–6.
20. Scott C, Webb K. Pediatric rheumatology in sub-Saharan Africa. Rheumatology (Oxford). 2014;53(8):1357–8.
21. McGill PE, Oyoo GO. Rheumatic disorders in Sub-saharan Africa. East Afr Med J. 2002;79(4):214–6.
22. Henrickson M. Policy challenges for the pediatric rheumatology workforce: Part III. the international situation. Pediatr Rheumatol Online J. 2011;9:26.

Permissions

All chapters in this book were first published in PR, by BioMed Central; hereby published with permission under the Creative Commons Attribution License or equivalent. Every chapter published in this book has been scrutinized by our experts. Their significance has been extensively debated. The topics covered herein carry significant findings which will fuel the growth of the discipline. They may even be implemented as practical applications or may be referred to as a beginning point for another development.

The contributors of this book come from diverse backgrounds, making this book a truly international effort. This book will bring forth new frontiers with its revolutionizing research information and detailed analysis of the nascent developments around the world.

We would like to thank all the contributing authors for lending their expertise to make the book truly unique. They have played a crucial role in the development of this book. Without their invaluable contributions this book wouldn't have been possible. They have made vital efforts to compile up to date information on the varied aspects of this subject to make this book a valuable addition to the collection of many professionals and students.

This book was conceptualized with the vision of imparting up-to-date information and advanced data in this field. To ensure the same, a matchless editorial board was set up. Every individual on the board went through rigorous rounds of assessment to prove their worth. After which they invested a large part of their time researching and compiling the most relevant data for our readers.

The editorial board has been involved in producing this book since its inception. They have spent rigorous hours researching and exploring the diverse topics which have resulted in the successful publishing of this book. They have passed on their knowledge of decades through this book. To expedite this challenging task, the publisher supported the team at every step. A small team of assistant editors was also appointed to further simplify the editing procedure and attain best results for the readers.

Apart from the editorial board, the designing team has also invested a significant amount of their time in understanding the subject and creating the most relevant covers. They scrutinized every image to scout for the most suitable representation of the subject and create an appropriate cover for the book.

The publishing team has been an ardent support to the editorial, designing and production team. Their endless efforts to recruit the best for this project, has resulted in the accomplishment of this book. They are a veteran in the field of academics and their pool of knowledge is as vast as their experience in printing. Their expertise and guidance has proved useful at every step. Their uncompromising quality standards have made this book an exceptional effort. Their encouragement from time to time has been an inspiration for everyone.

The publisher and the editorial board hope that this book will prove to be a valuable piece of knowledge for researchers, students, practitioners and scholars across the globe.

List of Contributors

Claudia Bracaglia, Giusi Prencipe and Fabrizio De Benedetti
Division of Rheumatology, Ospedale Pediatrico Bambino Gesù IRCCS, Piazza S. Onofrio 4, 00165 Rome, Italy

Babatunde Hakeem Olaosebikan and Olufemi Oladipo Adelowo
Department of Medicine, Lagos State University Teaching Hospital, Ikeja, Lagos State, Nigeria

Barakat Adeola Animashaun
Department of Paediatrics, Lagos State University Teaching Hospital, Ikeja, Lagos State, Nigeria

Richard Oluyinka Akintayo
Department of Medicine, University of Ilorin Teaching Hospital, Ilorin, Kwara State, Nigeria

Maria Ekelund
Department of Pediatrics, Ryhov County Hospital, Jönköping, Sweden
Department of Women's and Children's Health, Uppsala University, Uppsala, Sweden

Lillemor Berntson
Department of Women's and Children's Health, Uppsala University, Uppsala, Sweden

Kristiina Aalto and Suvi Peltoniemi
Department of Pediatrics, Children's Hospital, Helsinki University Hospital, Helsinki, Finland

Anders Fasth
Department of Pediatrics, Institute of Clinical Sciences, Sahlgrenska Academy, University of Gothenburg, Gothenburg, Sweden

Troels Herlin
Department of Pediatrics, Århus University Hospital, Århus, Denmark

Susan Nielsen and Marek Zak
Pediatric Rheumatology Department, Pediatric Clinic II, Copenhagen University Hospital, Rigshospitalet, Copenhagen, Denmark

Ellen Nordal
Department of Pediatrics, University Hospital of North Norway, Tromsø, Norway
Department of Clinical Medicine, UIT The Arctic University of Norway, Tromsø, Norway

Marite Rygg
Department of Laboratory Medicine, Children's and Women's Health, Norwegian University of Science and Technology, Trondheim, Norway
Department of Pediatrics, St. Olav's Hospital, Trondheim, Norway

Lily Siok Hoon Lim
Children's Hospital Research Institute of Manitoba, University of Manitoba, Winnipeg, Canada
Department of Pediatrics, University of Manitoba, Winnipeg, Canada
Institute of Health Policy Management and Evaluation, University of Toronto, Toronto, Canada

Eleanor Pullenayegum
The Child Health Evaluative Sciences Program, SickKids Research Institute, Toronto, Canada

Rahim Moineddin
Department of Family and Community Medicine, University of Toronto, Toronto, Canada

Dafna D Gladman
Department of Medicine, Toronto Western Research Institute, University of Toronto, Toronto, Canada
Centre for Prognosis Studies, University Health Network, Toronto Western Hospital, Toronto, Canada

Earl D Silverman
Division of Rheumatology, SickKids, Toronto, Canada
Physiology and Experimental Medicine Program, SickKids Research Institute, Toronto, Canada
Department of Pediatrics and Immunology, University of Toronto, Toronto, Canada

Brian M Feldman
Institute of Health Policy Management and Evaluation, University of Toronto, Toronto, Canada
The Child Health Evaluative Sciences Program, SickKids Research Institute, Toronto, Canada
Division of Rheumatology, SickKids, Toronto, Canada
Department of Pediatrics and Immunology, University of Toronto, Toronto, Canada
The Dalla Lana School of Public Health, University of Toronto, Toronto, Canada

Veronica Lundberg and Catharina Eriksson
Department of Clinical Sciences, Pediatrics, Umeå University, SE 901 85 Umeå, Sweden

Chack-Yung Yu, Brent Adler, Sharon Bout-Tabaku, Katherine E. Lintner, Melissa Moore-Clingenpeel and Charles H. Spencer
Nationwide Children's Hospital, 700 Children's Dr, Columbus, OH 43205, USA

Rabheh Abdul-Aziz
Nationwide Children's Hospital, 700 Children's Dr, Columbus, OH 43205, USA
Women & Children's Hospital of Buffalo, 219 Bryant Street, Buffalo, NY 14222, USA

Shannon E. Peters
School of Medicine and Medical Sciences, University College Dublin, Dublin, Ireland

Ronald M. Laxer
Division of Rheumatology, Department of Pediatrics and Medicine, The Hospital for Sick Children and University of Toronto, Toronto, ON, Canada

Bairbre L. Connolly and Dimitri A. Parra
Image Guided Therapy, Department of Diagnostic Imaging, The Hospital for Sick Children and University of Toronto, Toronto, ON, Canada

Yukiko Kimura and Jennifer E. Weiss
Pediatric rheumatology, Joseph M. Sanzari Children's Hospital, Hackensack University Medical Center, 30 Prospect Ave, Hackensack, NJ 07601, USA

Sriharsha Grevich and Sarah Ringold
Pediatric rheumatology, Seattle Children's Hospital, Seattle, USA

Timothy Beukelman
Pediatric rheumatology, University of Alabama at Birmingham, Birmingham, USA

Esi Morgan
Rheumatology, Cincinnati Children's Hospital Medical Center, Cincinnati, USA

Peter A. Nigrovic
Rheumatology, Immunology and Allergy, Brigham and Women's Hospital, Boston, USA

Kelly Mieszkalski
Childhood Arthritis & Rheumatology Research Alliance, Milwaukee, USA

T Brent Graham
Pediatric rheumatology, Vanderbilt University, Nashville, USA

Maria Ibarra
Pediatric rheumatology, Children's Mercy Hospital, Kansas City, USA

Norman Ilowite
Pediatric rheumatology, Children's Hospital at Montefiore, Bronx, NY, USA

Marisa Klein-Gitelman
Pediatric rheumatology, Ann & Robert H. Lurie Children's Hospital of Chicago, Chicago, USA

Karen Onel
Pediatric rheumatology, University of Chicago, Chicago, USA

Sampath Prahalad
Pediatric rheumatology, Emory University School of Medicine, Atlanta, USA

Marilynn Punaro
Pediatric rheumatology, Texas Scottish Rite Hospital, Dallas, USA

Dana Toib
Pediatric rheumatology, St. Christopher's Hospital, Philadelphia, USA

Heather Van Mater and Laura E. Schanberg
Pediatric rheumatology, Duke University, Durham, NC, USA

Pamela F. Weiss
Pediatric rheumatology, Children's Hospital of Philadelphia, Philadelphia, USA

Nele Herregods, Koenraad Verstraete and Lennart Jans
Department of Radiology and Medical Imaging, Ghent University Hospital, De Pintelaan 185, 9000 Ghent, Belgium

Joke Dehoorne, Joke Van Vlaenderen and Rik Joos
Department of Pediatric Rheumatology, Ghent University Hospital, De Pintelaan 185, 9000 Ghent, Belgium

Filip Van den Bosch, Gaëlle Varkas and Dirk Elewaut
Department of Rheumatology and VIB Inflammation Research Center, Unit for Molecular Immunology and Inflammation, Ghent University Hospital, De Pintelaan 185, 9000 Ghent, Belgium

Jacob Lester Jaremko
Department of Radiology & Diagnostic Imaging, University of Alberta Hospital, 8440-112 Street, Edmonton T6G 2B7, AB, Canada

Xenofon Baraliakos
Rheumazentrum Ruhrgebiet, Ruhr-University Bochum, Claudiusstr. 45, 44649 Herne, Germany

Timothy Beukelman
Division of Pediatric Rheumatology, The University of Alabama at Birmingham, 1600 7th Avenue South, CPP 210, Birmingham, AL 35233-1711, USA

Yukiko Kimura
Hackensack University Medical Center, Hackensack, USA

Norman T. Ilowite
Children's Hospital at Montefiore, Bronx, USA

Kelly Mieszkalski, Grendel Burrell, Brian Best and Jason Jones
Childhood Arthritis and Rheumatology Research Alliance, Durham, USA

Marc D. Natter
Children's Hospital Boston, Boston, USA

Laura E. Schanberg
Duke University, Durham, USA

Timothy Beukelman
University of Alabama at Birmingham, Birmingham, USA
Division of Pediatric Rheumatology, The University of Alabama at Birmingham, 1600 7th Avenue South, CPP 210, Birmingham, AL 35233-1711, USA

Janneke Anink and Lisette van Suijlekom-Smit
Erasmus Medical Center, Rotterdam, The Netherlands

Lillemor Berntson
Uppsala University Hospital, Uppsala, Sweden

Ciaran Duffy
Children's Hospital of Eastern Ontario, Ottawa, Canada

Justine A. Ellis
Murdoch Children's Research Institute, Genes, Environment & Complex Disease, Parkville, Australia

Maria Jose Santos
Hospital Garcia de Orta, Almada, Portugal

Laura E. Schanberg
Duke University, Durham, USA

Nico Wulffraat
University Medical Center Utrecht, Utrecht, The Netherlands

Kimme Hyrich
University of Manchester and Central Manchester Foundation Trust, Manchester, UK

Krzysztof Orczyk, Joanna Świdrowska-Jaros and Elżbieta Smolewska
Department of Pediatric Rheumatology, Medical University of Lodz, Sporna
36/50, 91-738 Lodz, Poland

Parveen Bhatti and Beth A. Mueller
Department of Epidemiology, School of Public Health, University of Washington, Seattle, WA, USA
Public Health Sciences Division, Fred Hutchison Cancer Research Center, Seattle, WA, USA

Susan Shenoi
Department of Pediatrics, Division of Rheumatology, Seattle Children's Hospital, University of Washington School of Medicine, Seattle, WA, USA

J. Lee Nelson
Public Health Sciences Division, Fred Hutchison Cancer Research Center, Seattle, WA, USA

Samantha W. Bell
Department of Epidemiology, School of Public Health, University of Washington, Seattle, WA, USA
School of Medicine, University of California, San Francisco, San Francisco, CA, USA
University of California, San Francisco, 513 Parnassus Ave., Room S245, San Francisco, CA 94143, USA

Andrea Coda
School of Health Sciences, Faculty of Health and Medicine, The University of Newcastle, Ourimbah, Australia

Dean Sculley
School of Biomedical Sciences and Pharmacy, Faculty of Health and Medicine, The University of Newcastle, Ourimbah, Australia

Derek Santos
School of Health Sciences, Queen Margaret University, Edinburgh, UK

Xavier Girones
Faculty of Health Sciences at Manresa, University of Vic-Central University of Catalonia, Manresa, Barcelona, Spain

Lucie Brosseau
School of Rehabilitation, Ottawa University, Ottawa, Canada

Derek R. Smith
James Cook University, Townsville, Australia

Joshua Burns
The Children's Hospital at Westmead & the University of Sydney, Hawkesbury Rd & Hainsworth St, Sydney, NSW 2000, Australia

Keith Rome
AUT University, Auckland, New Zealand

Jane Munro
Department of General Medicine, Royal Children's Hospital, Parkville, VIC, Australia

Davinder Singh-Grewal
The Children's Hospital at Westmead & the University of Sydney, Hawkesbury Rd & Hainsworth St, Sydney, NSW 2000, Australia
Sydney Children Hospitals Network & Clinical A/Prof- The University of Sydney, Sydney, Australia

Khulood Khawaja and Mustafa Al-Maini
Department of Rheumatology, Allergy and Immunology, Al-Mafraq Hospital, Abu Dhabi, United Arab Emirates

Serdar Cantez
Department of Pediatrics, Istanbul University, Istanbul Faculty of Medicine, Istanbul, Turkey

Gil J. Gross
Department of Pediatrics, University of Toronto, Division of Cardiology, The Hospital for Sick Children, Toronto, Canada

Ian MacLusky
Department of Pediatrics, University of Ottawa; Division of Respirology, the Childrens' Hospital of Eastern Ontario, Ottawa, Canada

Brian M. Feldman
Department of Pediatrics, Faculty of Medicine and the Institute of Health Policy, Management & Evaluation, the Dalla Lana School of Public Health, University of Toronto, Division of Rheumatology, The Hospital for Sick Children, Toronto, Canada

Danielle R. Bullock, Richard K. Vehe and Colleen K. Correll
Division of Pediatric Rheumatology, Department of Pediatrics, University of Minnesota, East Bldg Rm M668, 2450 Riverside Ave, Minneapolis, MN 55454, USA

Lei Zhang
Clinical and Translational Sciences Institute, University of Minnesota, 717 Delaware Street SE, Minneapolis, MN 55414, USA

A. B. Orandi and K. W. Baszis
Department of Pediatrics, Division of Rheumatology, Washington University School of Medicine, 660 S. Euclid Ave, Campus Bo 8116, St. Louis, Missouri 63110, USA

V. R. Dharnidharka
Department of Pediatrics, Division of Nephrology, Washington University School of Medicine, St. Louis, Missouri, USA

A. M. Huber
Department of Pediatrics, Division of Rheumatology, IWK Health Centre and Dalhousie University, Halifax, Nova Scotia, Canada

M. F. Hoeltzel
Department of Pediatrics, Division of Rheumatology, University of Michigan Medical School, Ann Arbor, Michigan, USA

Mohsen Karami, Mehryar Soleimani and Reza Shiari
Mofid Children Hospital, Shahid Beheshti University of Medical Sciences, Shariati Ave., Tehran 15514-15468, Iran

Yonatan Butbul-Aviel
Department of Pediatrics B, Ruth Rappaport Children's Hospital, Rambam Medical Center, Haifa, Israel
Pediatric Rheumatology Service, Ruth Rappaport Children's Hospital, Rambam Medical Center, Haifa, Israel
The Ruth and Bruce Rappaport Faculty of Medicine, The Technion - Israel Institute of Technology, Haifa, Israel

Riva Brik
Department of Pediatrics B, Ruth Rappaport Children's Hospital, Rambam Medical Center, Haifa, Israel
Pediatric Rheumatology Service, Ruth Rappaport Children's Hospital, Rambam Medical Center, Haifa, Israel
The Ruth and Bruce Rappaport Faculty of Medicine, The Technion - Israel Institute of Technology, Haifa, Israel
Sackler Faculty of Medicine, Tel Aviv University, Ramat Aviv, Israel

Nofar Hezkelo
Sackler Faculty of Medicine, Tel Aviv University, Ramat Aviv, Israel

Yosef Uziel
Sackler Faculty of Medicine, Tel Aviv University, Ramat Aviv, Israel
Pediatric Rheumatology Unit, Department of Pediatrics, Meir Medical Center, Kfar Saba, Israel

Gil Amarilyo
Sackler Faculty of Medicine, Tel Aviv University, Ramat Aviv, Israel
Pediatric Rheumatology Unit, Schneider Children's Medical Center of Israel, 14 Kaplan St., 4920235 Petach Tikva, Israel

Claas H. Hinze and Dirk Foell
Department of Pediatric Rheumatology and Immunology, University Hospital Münster, Albert-Schweitzer-Campus 1, Building D3, 48149 Münster, Germany

Prasad T. Oommen
Department of Pediatric Oncology, Hematology and Clinical Immunology, University Hospital Düsseldorf, Düsseldorf, Germany

Frank Dressler
Department of Pediatric Pulmonology, Allergy and Neonatology, Hanover Medical School, Hanover, Germany

Andreas Urban
Department of Pediatrics, St. Mary's Hospital, Amberg, Germany

Frank Weller-Heinemann
Division of Pediatric Rheumatology, Prof. Hess Children's Hospital, Bremen, Germany

Fabian Speth
Division of Pediatric Rheumatology, University Medicine, Rostock, Germany
Division of Immunology, Bone Marrow Transplantation and Rheumatology, University Hospital Ulm, Ulm, Germany

Elke Lainka and Ulrich Neudorf
Department of Pediatrics, University Hospital Essen, Essen, Germany

Jürgen Brunner
Department of Pediatrics, Medical University Innsbruck, Innsbruck, Austria

Heike Fesq and Johannes-Peter Haas
German Center for Pediatric and Adolescent Rheumatology, Garmisch-Partenkirchen Department of Dermatology, Oberammergau Center for Rheumatic Diseases, Oberammergau, Germany

Wolfgang Müller-Felber
Department of Pediatric Neurology, University Hospital Munich, Munich, Germany

Christoph Rietschel
Department of Pediatrics, Clementine Children's Hospital, Frankfurt, Germany

Tobias Schwarz
Department of Pediatric Rheumatology, St. Josef Hospital, Sendenhorst, Germany

Ulrike Schara
Department of Pediatric Neurology, University Hospital Essen, Essen, Germany

Hermine I. Brunner, Edward H. Giannini and Daniel J. Lovell
Division of Rheumatology, Cincinnati Children's Hospital Medical Center & Cincinnati Children's Research Foundation, MLC 4010, Cincinnati, OH 45229, USA

Lisa G. Rider
Environmental Autoimmunity Group, Clinical Research Branch, National Institute of Environmental Health Sciences, National Institutes of Health, Bethesda, MD, USA

Daniel J. Kingsbury
Randall Children's Hospital at Legacy Emanuel, Portland, OR, USA

Dominic Co
University of Wisconsin School of Medicine and Public Health, Madison, WI, USA

Rayfel Schneider
The Hospital for Sick Children, University of Toronto, Toronto, Canada

Ellen Goldmuntz
Division of Allergy, Immunology and Transplantation, Rheumatologic Autoimmune Diseases Section, National Institutes of Health, Bethesda, MD, USA

Karen B. Onel
Hospital for Special Surgery, Weill Cornell Medicine, New York, NY, USA

Ausra Snipaitiene, Rima Sileikiene, Edita Jasinskiene, Rimantas Uktveris and Lina Jankauskaite
The Lithuanian University of Health Sciences, A. Mickevičiaus g. 9, Kaunas, Lithuania
The Hospital of Lithuanian University of Health Sciences Kauno Klinikos, Eiveniu g. 2, Kaunas, Lithuania

Justina Klimaite
The Hospital of Lithuanian University of Health Sciences Kauno Klinikos, Eiveniu g. 2, Kaunas, Lithuania

Margot Walter, Philomine van Pelt, Annemarie de Vroed and Johanna M. W. Hazes
Department of Rheumatology, Erasmus University Medical Centre, Postal 3000, CA, Rotterdam, the Netherlands

Sylvia Kamphuis
Department of Pediatric Rheumatology, Sophia Children's Hospital - Erasmus University Medical Centre, Rotterdam, the Netherlands

Amir B. Orandi
Division of Pediatric Rheumatology, Department of Pediatric and Adolescent Medicine, Mayo Clinic, 200 First Street SW, Rochester, MN 55902, USA
Division of Pediatric Rheumatology, Department of Pediatrics, St. Louis, MO, USA

Kevin W. Baszis
Division of Pediatric Rheumatology, Department of Pediatrics, St. Louis, MO, USA

Vikas R. Dharnidharka
Division of Pediatric Nephrology, Department of Pediatrics, St. Louis, MO, USA

Noor Al-Hammadi
Division of Biostatistics, Washington University School of Medicine, St. Louis, MO, USA

Clara Westwell-Roper, Kelly L. Brown, Kimberly A. Morishita, Cherry Mammen and David A. Cabral
Clinical Professor, Division of Rheumatology, Department of Pediatrics, University of British Columbia, BC Children's Hospital, Room K4-119 4480 Oak Street Vancouver, Vancouver, BC V6H 3V4, Canada

Joanna M. Lubieniecka
Simon Fraser University, Burnaby, BC, Canada

Linda Wagner-Weiner
University of Chicago Comer Children's Hospital, Chicago, USA

Eric Yen
University of California - Los Angeles, Los Angeles, CA, USA

Suzanne C. Li
Joseph M. Sanzari Children's Hospital, Hackensack, NJ, USA

Kathleen M. O'Neil
Riley Hospital for Children at IU Health, Indianapolis, IN, USA

Sivia K. Lapidus
Morristown Medical Center, Morristown, NJ, USA

Paul Brogan
Great Ormond Street Hospital NHS Foundation Trust, London, UK

Rolando Cimaz
Ospedale Pediatrico Meyer Firenze, Florence, Italy

Kristiina Aalto, Pekka Lahdenne and Kaija-Leena Kolho
Helsinki University Central Hospital, Children's Hospital, University of Helsinki, Helsinki 00029 HUCH, Finland

Ezra M. Cohen
Division of Immunology, Boston Children's Hospital, 300 Longwood Ave, Boston, MA 02115, USA
Department of Rheumatology, Boston Children's Hospital, 300 Longwood Ave, Boston, MA 02115, USA

Alessio Morley-Fletcher
Department of Pediatrics, Massachusetts General Hospital, 55 Fruit Street, Boston, MA 02114, USA

Darshan H. Mehta
Benson-Henry Institute for Mind-Body Medicine, Massachusetts General Hospital, 151 Merrimac St., Boston, MA 02114, USA

Yvonne C. Lee
Division of Rheumatology, Immunology and Allergy, Brigham and Women's Hospital, 60 Fenwood Road, Boston, MA 02115, USA

Fang Li, Meihua Bao, Jie Zeng, Ju Xiang and Liang Tang
Department of Human Anatomy, Histology and Embryology, Institute of Neuroscience, Changsha Medical University, No. 1501 Lei Feng Road, Wangcheng District, Changsha City, Hunan Province 410219, People's Republic of China
School of Basic Medical Science, Changsha Medical University, Changsha, People's Republic of China

Yan Wang, Lianghui Chen and Huaiqing Luo
Department of Human Anatomy, Histology and Embryology, Institute of Neuroscience, Changsha Medical University, No. 1501 Lei Feng Road, Wangcheng District, Changsha City, Hunan Province 410219, People's Republic of China
School of Basic Medical Science, Changsha Medical University, Changsha, People's Republic of China
Experiment center for Function, Changsha Medical University, Changsha, People's Republic of China

Jianming Li
Department of Human Anatomy, Histology and Embryology, Institute of Neuroscience, Changsha Medical University, No. 1501 Lei Feng Road, Wangcheng District, Changsha City, Hunan Province 410219, People's Republic of China
Department of Neurology, Xiang-ya Hospital, Central South University, Changsha City, Hunan Province, China

Angela Migowa and Rosie Scuccimarri
Division of Pediatric Rheumatology, Department of Pediatrics, McGill University Health Centre, 1001 Decarie Boulevard, Room A04.6306, Montreal, QC, CanadaH4A 3J1

Inés Colmegna
Division of Rheumatology, Department of Medicine, McGill University Health Centre, Montreal, QC, Canada

Carol Hitchon
Division of Rheumatology, Department of Internal Medicine, University of Manitoba, Winnipeg, MB, Canada

Eugene Were, Thomas Ngwiri and John Wachira
Department of Pediatrics, Gertrude's Children's Hospital, Nairobi, Kenya

Evelyn Ng'ang'a
Department of Pediatrics, The Nairobi Hospital, Nairobi, Kenya

Sasha Bernatsky
Division of Rheumatology & Division of Clinical Epidemiology, Department of Medicine & Department of Epidemiology, Biostatistics and Occupational Health, McGill University Health Centre, McGill University, Montreal, QC, Canada

Index

www.ingramcontent.com/pod-product-compliance
Lightning Source LLC
LaVergne TN
LVHW080912210926
848485LV00004B/637